# Central Neural Mechanisms in Cardiovascular Regulation

George Kunos    John Ciriello

Editors

# Central Neural Mechanisms in Cardiovascular Regulation

With 80 Illustrations in 167 Parts

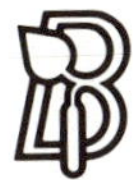

Birkhäuser
Boston   Basel   Berlin

George Kunos
Chief, LPPS,
National Institute on Alcohol Abuse
  and Alcoholism
12501 Washington Avenue
Rockville, Maryland 20852
USA

John Ciriello
Department of Physiology
University of Western Ontario
Health Science Centre
London, Ontario, N6A 5Cl
Canada

Library of Congress Cataloging-in-Publication Data
Central neural mechanisms in cardiovascular regulation / George Kunos,
  John Ciriello, editors.
        p.  cm.
     Includes bibliographical references and index.
     ISBN 0-8176-3545-9 (alk. paper).—ISBN 3-7643-3545-9 (alk.
paper)
     1. Blood—Circulation—Regulation.   2. Heart—Innervation.
3. Nervous system, Vasomotor.   4. Medulla oblongata.   I. Kunos,
George.   II. Ciriello, John.
     [DNLM:   1. Cardiovascular System—physiology.   2. Medulla
Oblongata—physiology.   3. Neuroregulators—pharmacology.
4. Sympathetic Nervous System—physiology.   WL 310 C3966]
QP109.C48   1991
612.1—dc20
DNLM/DLC
for Library of Congress                                      90-14566

Printed on acid-free paper.



Typeset by Asco Trade Typesetting Ltd., Hong Kong.
Printed and bound by Edwards Brothers, Inc., Ann Arbor, Michigan.
Printed in the United States of America.

9  8  7  6  5  4  3  2  1

ISBN 0-8176-3545-9
ISBN 3-7643-3545-9

# Preface

With the help of recent technological advances in the study of central nervous system function, important strides have been made in our knowledge regarding the pathophysiology of high blood pressure. The understanding of neural mechanisms involved in the regulation of the cardiovascular system is of critical importance to the development of rational approaches to both the treatment and prevention of this disease. It was in this spirit that a satellite symposium of the 13th Scientific Meeting of the International Society of Hypertension was held in June 1990, in Bethesda, Maryland. The chapters, in this first of two volumes on the same general theme, are based on lectures presented at the symposium and it is hoped that these summaries of recent research findings from prominent laboratories around the world will provide a stimulus for future research. The symposium would not have been possible without generous support from the National Institute on Alcohol Abuse and Alcoholism, Merck Frosst Canada, G.D. Searle Co., Squibb Institute of Medical Research, Smith, Kline & Beecham Co., Pfizer Co., E.I. Dupont de Nemours Co., Merck, Sharp & Dohme Co., The UpJohn Co., and Wyeth-Ayerst Co.

While this volume was being prepared for publication, one of its contributors, Dr. Michael J. Brody, died suddenly. It is with deep sorrow and sympathy that we mourn the loss of our colleague. Dr. Brody was a worldwide leader in cardiovascular research whose work had a major impact on our current knowledge of neural mechanisms controlling the circulation, as his chapter in this volume attests to this fact. We dedicate this book to the memory of Dr. Michael J. Brody. Although his unexpected and untimely death has deeply saddened his many friends around the world, his presence in the scientific community as an eminent scientist and warm human being will never be forgotten.

George Kunos
John Ciriello

v

# Contents

# List of Contributors

Alföldi, Alexander, M.D., Department of Medicine, Elizabeth Teaching Hospital, Budapest, Hungary

Allen, Andrew M., Ph.D., Department of Research (Neuroscience), Loeb Research Institute, Ottawa Civic Hospital, Ottawa, Ontario, Canada

Aston-Jones, Gary, Ph.D., Department of Mental Health Science, Hahnemann University, Philadelphia, Pennsylvania

Averill, David B., Ph.D., Department of Brain and Vascular Research, The Cleveland Clinic Foundation, Cleveland, Ohio

Badoer, Emilio, Ph.D., Department of Medicine, Flinders Medical Center, Bedford Park, S.A., Australia

Baradziej, Stanislaw, M.D., Department of Physiology, Medical Academy of Warsaw, Warsaw, Poland

Barman, Susan M., Ph.D., Department of Pharmacology, Michigan State University, East Lansing, Michigan

Beck, Carol, Pharm.D., Division of Clinical Pharmacology, Vanderbilt University Medical Center, Nashville, Tennessee

Blessing, William W., M.D., Ph.D., Department of Medicine, Flinders Medical Center, Bedford Park, S.A., Australia

Bogdanov, Michael B., M.D., USSR Cardiology Research Center, Institute of Experimental Cardiology, Moscow, USSR

*Brody, Michael J., Ph.D., Department of Pharmacology and Cardiovascular Center, University of Iowa College of Medicine, Iowa City, Iowa

*Deceased.

Chalmers, John P., Ph.D., Department of Medicine, Flinders Medical Center, Bedford Park, S.A., Australia

Ciriello, John, Ph.D., Department of Physiology, University of Western Ontario, London, Ontario, Canada

Cox-van Put, Joke, Mrs., Rudolf Magnus Institute for Pharmacology, University of Utrecht, Utrecht, The Netherlands

Dampney, Roger A.L., Ph.D., Department of Physiology, University of Sydney, Sydney, Australia

de Jong, Wybren, M.D., Ph.D., Marion Merrell Dow Research Institute, Strasbourg, France

de Kloet, E. Ronald, Ph.D., Division of Neuroendocrine Pharmacology, University of Leiden, Leiden, The Netherlands

Drolet, Guy, Ph.D., Department of Medicine, Flinders Medical Center, Bedford Park, S.A., Australia

Eijgelshoven, Marcel H.J., M.Sc., Rudolf Magnus Institute for Pharmacology, University of Utrecht, Utrecht, The Netherlands

Ernsberger, Paul R., Ph.D., Division of Hypertension, Case Western Reserve University School of Medicine, Cleveland, Ohio

Farsang, Csaba, M.D., D. Sc., Department of Medicine, Elisabeth Teaching Hospital, Budapest, Hungary

Ferrario, Carlos M., M.D., Department of Brain and Vascular Research, The Cleveland Clinic Foundation, Cleveland, Ohio

Gebber, Gerard L., Ph.D., Departments of Pharmacology and Physiology, Michigan State University, East Lansing, Michigan

Gjulumjan, Ararat D., M.D., USSR Cardiology Research Center, Institute of Experimental Cardiology, Moscow, USSR

Grosskreutz, Cynthia L., Ph.D., Department of Medicine, Carney Hospital, Boston, Massachusetts

Hoque, Azizul M., M.D., USSR Cardiology Research Center, Institute of Experimental Cardiology, Moscow, USSR

Irigoyen, Maria C., Ph.D., Heart Institute, University of Sao Paolo, Sao Paulo, Brazil

Kapoor, Vimal, Ph.D., Department of Medicine, Flinders Medical Center, Bedford Park, S.A., Australia

Kenney, Michael J., Ph.D., Department of Biology, Rhodes College, Memphis, Tennessee

Kocsis, Bernat, M.D., Department of Pharmacology, Michigan State University, East Lansing, Michigan

Krieger, Eduardo M., M.D., Heart Institute, University of Sao Paolo, Sao Paulo, Brazil

Kunos, George, M.D., Ph.D., National Institute on Alcohol Abuse and Alcoholism, NIH, Bethesda, Maryland

Kuzmin, Alexander I., M.D., USSR Cardiology Research Center, Institute of Experimental Cardiology, Moscow, USSR

Lewis, Stephen J., Ph.D., Departments of Pharmacology and Cardiovascular Center, University of Iowa College of Medicine, Iowa City, Iowa

Llewellyn-Smith, Ida J., Ph.D., Department of Medicine, Flinders University, Bedford Park, S.A., Australia

Machado, Benedito H., Ph.D., Department of Physiology, School of Medicine of Ribeirao Preto, University of Sao Paulo, Brazil

Madalin, Karla J., M.D., Departments of Neurology and Brain and Vascular Research, The Cleveland Clinic Foundation, Cleveland, Ohio

Mastrianni, James A., Ph.D., M.D., National Institute on Alcohol Abuse and Alcoholism, NIH, Bethesda, Maryland

McCormick, Michael, Ph.D., Department of Pharmacology, Vanderbilt University School of Medicine, Nashville, Tennessee

Medvedev, Oleg S., M.D., USSR Cardiology Research Center, Institute of Experimental Cardiology, Moscow, USSR

Meeley, Mary P., Ph.D., Department of Neurology, Laboratory of Neurobiology, Cornell University Medical College, New York, New York

Mendelsohn, Frederick A.O., M.D., Ph.D., Department of Medicine, University of Melbourne, Austin Hospital, Heidelberg, Victoria, Australia

Minson, Jane B., Ph.D., Department of Medicine, Flinders Medical Center, Bedford Park, S.A., Australia

Moreira, Edson D., Ph.D., Heart Institute, University of Sao Paolo, Sao Paulo, Brazil

Moreira, Robinson D., Ph.D., Heart Institute, University of Sao Paolo, Sao Paulo, Brazil

Morilak, David, Ph.D., Department of Medicine, Flinders Medical Center, Bedford Park, S.A., Australia

Mosqueda-Garcia, Rogelio, M.D., Ph.D., Division of Clinical Pharmacology, Vanderbilt University School of Medicine, Nashville, Tennessee

Muratani, Hiromi, M.D., Department of Brain and Vascular Research, The Cleveland Clinic Foundation, Cleveland, Ohio

Nishi, Syogoro, M.D., Ph.D., Department of Physiology, Kurume University School of Medicine, Kurume, Japan

Palkovits, Miklós, M.D., D. Sc., First Department of Anatomy, Semmelweis University Medical School, Budapest, Hungary and National Institute of Mental Health, Bethesda, Maryland

Pilowsky, Paul M., Ph.D., Department of Medicine, Flinders University, Bedford Park, S.A., Australia

Polosa, Canio, M.D., Ph.D., Department of Physiology, McGill University, Montreal, Quebec, Canada

Qadri, Fatimunnisa, Ph.D., Department of Pharmacology and German Institute for High Blood Pressure Research, University of Heidelberg, Heidelberg, Germany

Reis, Donald J., M.D., Departments of Neurology and Neuroscience, Cornell University Medical College, New York, New York

Robertson, David, M.D., Clinical Research Center, Vanderbilt University, Nashville, Tennessee

Sapru, Hreday, Ph.D., Departments of Neurosurgery and Pharmacology, New Jersey Medical School, Newark, New Jersey

Sasaki, Shuichi, Ph.D., Department of Physiology, University of Sydney, Sydney, Australia

Selivanov, Vladimir N., M.D., USSR Cardiology Research Center, Institute of Experimental Cardiology, Moscow, USSR

Simon, Jason J., Ph.D., Department of Pharmacology and Cardiovascular Center, University of Iowa, Iowa City, Iowa

Somogyi, Peter, M.D., MRC Unit, Department of Pharmacology, Oxford, U.K.

Stadler, Thilo, Ph.D., Department of Pharmacology and German Institute for High Blood Pressure Research, University Heidelberg, Heidelberg, Germany

Tjurmina, Olga A., M.D., USSR Cardiology Research Center, Institute of Experimental Cardiology, Moscow, USSR

Trzebski, Andrzej, M.D., Medical Academy of Warsaw, Institute of Physiological Sciences, Warsaw, Poland

Tseng, Ching-Jiunn, M.D., Department of Pharmacology, National Defense Medical Center, Taipei, Taiwan

Unger, Thomas, M.D., Department of Pharmacology and German Institute for High Blood Pressure Research, University of Heidelberg, Heidelberg, Germany

Van Bockstaele, Elisabeth J., Ph.D., Division of Behavioral Neurobiology, Department of Mental Health Science, Hahneman University, Philadelphia, Pennsylvania and Department of Biology, New York University, New York, New York

van den Berg, Desirée TWM, M.Sc., Rudolf Magnus Institute for Pharmacology, University of Utrecht, Utrecht, The Netherlands

van den Berg, Maria H., M.Sc., Rudolf Magnus Institute for Pharmacology, University of Utrecht, Utrecht, The Netherlands

van Giersbergen, Paul LM, Ph.D., Marion Merrell Dow Research Institute, Cincinnati, Ohio

Varga, Karoly, M.D., Ph.D., National Institute of Alcohol Abuse and Alcoholism, NIH, Bethesda, Maryland

Varner, Kurt J., Ph.D., Department of Pharmacology and Cardiovascular Center, University of Iowa College of Medicine, Iowa City, Iowa

Vasquez, Elisardo C., Ph.D., Department of Physiology, School of Medicine of Ribeirao Preto, University of Sao Paulo, Brazil

Veltmar, Annette, Ph.D., Department of Pharmacology and German Institute for High Blood Pressure Research, University of Heidelberg, Heidelberg, Germany

Yoshimura, Megumu, M.D., Ph.D., Department of Physiology, Kurume University School of Medicine, Kurume, Japan

Zhang, Ting-Xin, M.D., Department of Physiology, The University of Western Ontario, London, Ontario, Canada

# Section I
## Ventral Medullary Mechanisms

# 1
# Afferent Inputs to Ventrolateral Medulla

JOHN P. CHALMERS, EMILIO BADOER, DAVID MORILAK, GUY DROLET, JANE B. MINSON, IDA J. LLEWELLYN-SMITH, PETER SOMOGYI, VIMAL KAPOOR, AND PAUL PILOWSKY

Recent studies from our laboratory have reported the existence of two pathways arising in the nucleus tractus solitarius in the dorsomedial medulla and terminating in the ventrolateral medulla. One of these pathways contains excitatory amino acids (Somogyi et al., 1989) and the other contains enkephalin (Morilak et al., 1989; Fig. 1.1). This chapter describes these projections and their possible contribution to the regulation of blood pressure. First, however, the importance of the ventrolateral medulla in the regulation of blood pressure is summarized briefly and the major bulbospinal projections descending from this region to innervate the sympathetic outflow from the intermediolateral cell column in the thoracic spinal cord are described.

## The Pressor and Depressor Areas of the Ventrolateral Medulla

The pressor function of the ventral surface of the medulla was first demonstrated by Feldberg and Guertzenstein (1972), who produced striking reductions in arterial pressure by the bilateral application of pentobarbital sodium. Subsequent experiments using the application of glycine localized the pressor region to the rostral aspect of the surface of the ventrolateral medulla (Guertzenstein and Silver, 1974). In much the same way, clues to the existence of vasodepressor neurons in the ventral medulla also come from Feldberg (1976) and Feldberg and Guertzenstein (1976), who demonstrated large falls in blood pressure following the application of nicotine to the ventral surface of the medulla.

Further interest in the pressor areas arose from the study of the possible role of the C1 adrenaline-containing neurons (Dampney and Moon, 1980; Ross et al., 1983, 1984) and of the B3 group of serotonin-containing neurons (Howe et al., 1983) in the rostral ventral medulla. Renewed interest in the caudal depressor region was kindled by the evidence that the

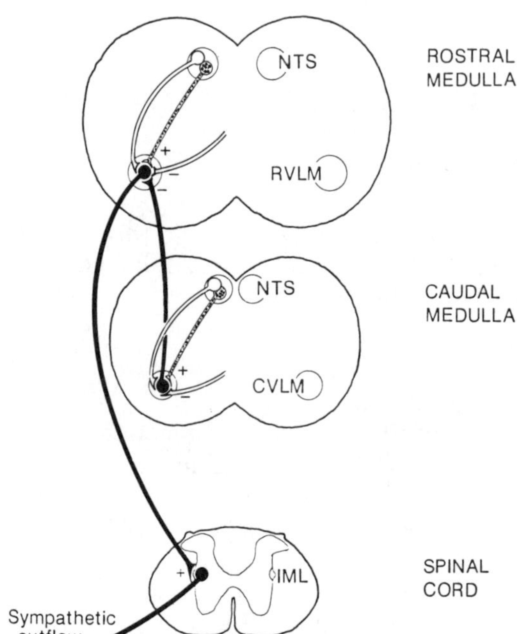


FIGURE 1.1. A schematic representation of some of the pathways in the medulla and spinal cord that regulate the sympathetic outflow. Excitatory amino acid-containing neurons (stippled) and inhibitory enkephalin-containing neurons (white) project from the nucleus tractus solitarius (NTS) to both the caudal (CVLM) and rostral (RVLM) ventrolateral medulla. In addition, enkephalin-containing neurons with local or distant cell bodies also provide an inhibitory input to the CVLM and RVLM. Sympathoexcitatory bulbospinal neurons in the RVLM (black) receive an inhibitory input from neurons in the CVLM (black). Stimulation of the RVLM increases sympathetic activity, whereas stimulation of the CVLM inhibits the bulbospinal neurons and decreases sympathetic activity.

A1 noradrenaline-containing neurons might be responsible (Blessing et al., 1981; West et al., 1981). While it is now clear that the pressor and depressor functions of these areas are not simply expressions of the individual activities of the C1 adrenaline, B3 serotonin, or A1 noradrenaline cell groups, it is well established that the ventrolateral medulla is a critically important integrative area in the regulation of blood pressure and of circulation.

The sympathoexcitatory bulbospinal neurons arise in the rostral ventrolateral medulla extending from the obex to the nucleus of the facial nerve. Bulbospinal neurons are found in the area of the C1 adrenaline-containing neurons first described by Hökfelt et al. (1974). Neurons containing other putative transmitters such as neuropeptide Y (NPY), enkephalin, and amino acids, which are colocalized in a variety of combinations, are also found in the area. Bulbospinal neurons are also found more medially in the areas of the serotonin-containing neurons that make up the lateral elements of the B3 cell group (Howe et al., 1983; Pilowsky et al., 1986b; Minson et al., 1987). Some of these neurons contain substance P and other putative neurotransmitters (Johansson et al., 1981; Sasek et al., 1990). Cox and Brody (1989 a,b) have suggested that these two regions should be termed the rostral ventrolateral medulla corresponding to the C1 region and the rostral ventromedial medulla corresponding to the B3 region. Bulbospinal neurons from both of these rostral pressor regions send axons to the inter-mediolateral cell column of the thoracic spinal cord (Fig. 1.1; Blessing et al., 1987; Johansson et al., 1981; Minson et al., 1987; Pilowsky et al., 1986a). Furthermore, synapses on identified sympathetic preganglionic neurons have been demonstrated from nerve terminals containing phenylethanolamine-N-methyltransferase (PNMT), NPY, serotonin, substance P, and glutamate (Bacon and Smith, 1988; Kohno et al., 1988; Llewellyn-Smith et al., 1990; Morrison et al., 1989; Reis et al., 1988).

The caudal ventrolateral medulla is now well established as a depressor region and it seems likely that it operates at least in part through the tonic activity of a short ascending inhibitory projection (Fig. 1.1) that acts to inhibit the pressor effects of the sympathoexcitatory bulbospinal pressor neurons descending from the rostral ventrolateral medulla (Fig. 1.1; Pilowsky et al., 1986b; Blessing and Li, 1989; Dembowsky et al., 1989). The identity of the neurotransmitter in this short ascending projection has not been clearly established but there is evidence suggesting it might be gamma-aminobutyric acid (GABA) (Blessing and Li, 1989).

## Afferent Inputs to the Ventrolateral Medulla

Although there is now a great deal of knowledge about the pressor and depressor regions in the rostral and caudal ventrolateral medulla and their descending bulbospinal projections, there has been much less work on the afferent inputs that regulate the activity of bulbospinal neurons. It has long been established that arterial baroreceptor neurons terminate in the nucleus tractus solitarius in the dorsomedial medulla. However, whereas it is clear that there is a substantial projection from the nucleus tractus solitarius to the ventrolateral medulla (Blessing and Li, 1989; Dampney et al., 1987; Loewy and Burton, 1978; Ross et al., 1985; Spyer, 1981), there is little knowledge of what neurotransmitters these afferent fibers contain.

Recent reports from our laboratory have identified two such pathways, one containing excitatory amino acids (Somogyi et al., 1989) and the other containing enkephalin (Morilak et al., 1989). These two projections are described below, together with physiological and pharmacological studies on their possible participation in the regulation of blood pressure.

## Excitatory Amino Acid Projection from Nucleus Tractus Solitarius to Ventrolateral Medulla

This study was prompted partly by the observations that baroreceptor reflexes can be blocked by excitatory amino acid antagonists injected into the ventrolateral medulla (Gordon 1987; Guyenet et al., 1987; Kubo and Kihara, 1988).

Retrograde axonal transport of tritiated-D-aspartate was used in our experiments as fully described elsewhere (Somogyi et al., 1989). This compound has been used extensively for the specific identification of central pathways using excitatory amino acids as transmitters (Cuenod and Streit, 1984). In order to trace excitatory amino acid projections to the ventrolateral medulla, tritiated-D-aspartate was injected into the pressor region of the rostral ventrolateral medulla or into the depressor region of the caudal ventrolateral medulla of rats. When injected into the rostral pressor region, tritiated-D-aspartate evoked a pressor response whereas when it was injected into the caudal depressor area it caused a fall in blood pressure.

After injections of labeled aspartate into either the rostral or caudal ventrolateral medulla, more than 90% of the neurons that selectively accumulated the marker in the medulla were in the nucleus tractus solitarius, mainly ipsilaterally, with few cells labeled in the ventrolateral medulla. None of the neurons labeled in the nucleus tractus solitarius were immunoreactive for GABA or for PNMT. Injections of the nonspecific retrograde tracers wheatgerm-gold or wheatgerm-horseradish peroxidase (HRP) into the ventrolateral medulla resulted in comparable density of labeling of the nucleus tractus solitarius, suggesting that most neurons projecting from the nucleus tractus solitarius to the ventrolateral medulla also accumulate tritiated-D-aspartate. However, in contrast to the specific amino acid marker, the nonspecific wheatgerm conjugated tracers labeled numerous neurons around the injection site as well as others in both the rostral and caudal ventrolateral medulla. These data thus confirmed previous reports of connections between the rostral and caudal ventrolateral medulla (Blessing et al., 1987; Reis et al., 1988; Ross et al., 1985). Furthermore, the sparsity of labeling with the specific amino acid marker suggested that most of these neurons do not use excitatory amino acids as transmitters (Somogyi et al., 1989).

The functional significance of this excitatory amino acid pathway was tested using injections of the selective N-methyl-D-aspartate (NMDA) receptor antagonist 2-amino-5-phosphonovalerate (2APV) (Davies et al., 1981) into physiologically identified depressor sites in the caudal ventrolateral medulla. These injections caused a rise in arterial pressure in the rat and completely abolished the depressor effects of L-glutamate injected into the ipsilateral nucleus tractus solitarius. In other experiments in anesthetized rabbits, bilateral injection of 2APV into the caudal ventrolateral medulla produced a rise in blood pressure and blocked the depressor response evoked by electrical stimulation of the aortic depressor nerve (Somogyi et al., 1989). These experiments are therefore in agreement with previous reports that the excitatory amino acid projections from the nucleus tractus solitarius participate in both tonic and reflex regulation of the circulation (Gordon, 1987; Guyenet et al., 1987; Kubo and Kihara, 1988; Urbanski and Sapru, 1988).

Since there is evidence that both the rostral pressor and the caudal depressor neurons are tonically active, it might seem somewhat paradoxical that the excitatory amino acid pathway from the nucleus tractus solitarius should project to both regions (Somogyi et al., 1989). One explanation might be that the distribution of the depressor neurons overlap with the pressor neurons more rostrally. Such depressor neurons, possibly containing GABA as an inhibitory neurotransmitter acting directly on the pressor neurons, might be targets for the excitatory amino acid projections from the nucleus tractus solitarius. It is also possible that the excitatory amino acid projection to the rostral ventrolateral medulla is a pressor pathway whose activity could account for the reversal of the effects of nucleus tractus solitarius stimulation from a depressor to a pressor response after injections of muscimol (Urbanski and Sapru, 1988) or 2APV (Somogyi et al., 1989) into the caudal ventrolateral medulla, or of bicuculline into the rostral ventrolateral medulla (Urbanski and Sapru, 1988).

It should be noted that Blessing (1989) has reported that whereas injection of 2APV into the caudal ventrolateral medulla blocks the vasodepressor response and the renal sympathoinhibitory response evoked by electrical stimulation of the aortic depressor nerve, it does not affect the baroreceptor vasomotor responses to raising or lowering arterial pressure (Blessing, 1989). Although these discrepancies are difficult to reconcile, one possibility is that the residual baroreceptor reflexes reflect activation of afferents from the carotid zones or from low pressure receptors. Another possibility is that renal sympathetic nerve activity is not representative of peripheral sympathetic activity as a whole, as has been illustrated by the experiments of Cox and Brody (1989a,b), who have shown selective activation of renal and mesenteric sympathetic nerves by stimulation of the rostral ventrolateral or the rostral ventromedial medulla, respectively.

## *Enkephalin Projection from Nucleus Tractus Solitarius to Ventrolateral Medulla*

Previous studies have demonstrated the presence of enkephalin-containing cell bodies in the nucleus tractus solitarius (Armstrong et al., 1981; Finley et al., 1981; Khachaturian et al., 1983; Yamazoe et al., 1984) and of enkephalin-containing nerve terminals in the ventrolateral medulla (Elde et al., 1976; Finley et al., 1981; Khachaturian et al., 1983; Simantov et al., 1977), but none has established the presence of an opiate pathway connecting these regions. Accordingly, we sought to determine the origin of intramedullary enkephalin-containing pathways terminating in the pressor area in the rostral ventrolateral medulla of the rabbit (Morilak et al., 1989).

A technique combining retrograde tracing of wheatgerm conjugated colloidal gold particles with immunohistochemical demonstration of enkephalin-like immunoreactivity was used for this purpose. The rostral ventrolateral medullary pressor region was first localized by injections of L-glutamate, and slow injections of wheatgerm-gold were then made at the same coordinates. A restricted injection site resulted, corresponding to the C1 pressor area, as verified by the presence of tyrosine hydroxylase and neuropeptide Y-containing neurons (Morilak et al., 1989).

After silver intensification, wheatgerm-gold particles transported retrogradely appeared as black granules in the cytoplasm of neurons. Double-labeled cells contained both the black silver granules indicative of retrograde transport and homogeneous brown immunoperoxidase reaction product, indicative of enkephalin immunoreactivity. Within the nucleus tractus solitarius, gold labeled enkephalin-containing cells were observed in the commissural nucleus and in the intermediate subnucleus at the level of the obex and rostral to the obex (Morilak et al., 1989). Cells in the nucleus tractus solitarius containing other transmitters such as substance P, galanin, neuropeptide Y, and catecholamines did not show the same degree or pattern of double labeling, suggesting that the transport was not due to nonspecific silver reduction or spread. This opiate pathway from the nucleus tractus solitarius to the rostral ventrolateral medulla could represent a major central substrate underlying opiate effects on the cardiovascular system.

## Functional Studies of Opioid Inputs to Ventrolateral Medulla

More recently we have studied the cardiovascular effects of microinjection of the nonspecific opioid antagonist naloxone as well as microinjection of selective opioid antagonists into the rostral and caudal ventrolateral medulla of the anesthetized rabbit (Morilak et al., 1990a,b; Drolet et al., unpublished observations).

Bilateral administration of naloxone directly into the pressor area of the rostral ventrolateral medulla induced a gradual and prolonged increase in mean arterial pressure (Morilak et al., 1990a). When naloxone was administered into the rostral ventrolateral medulla immediately after a moderately severe hemorrhage (20 ml of blood per kg of body weight), it improved recovery of blood pressure relative to saline controls, again inducing a gradual but long-lasting pressor response. The effects of naloxone on the baroreflex of intact animals was transient and minimal. These experiments suggest that endogenous opioids exert a tonic inhibitory influence on pressor neurons of the rostral ventrolateral medulla. This input remains active after hemorrhage and could be responsible for mediating the beneficial effects of naloxone in preventing circulatory collapse after hemorrhage (Ludbrook and Rutter, 1988).

In subsequent experiments we have examined the specific opioid receptor subtypes that could be activated by this endogenous opioid input. Specific blockade of mu receptors following bilateral injection of beta-funaltrexamine or of kappa receptors following bilateral injection of nor-binaltorphimine into the rostral ventrolateral medulla had no effects on either blood pressure or heart rate (Morilak et al., 1990b). However, specific blockade of delta receptors in the rostral ventrolateral medulla following bilateral injection of the specific antagonist ICI 174 864 caused a significant pressor response, which was rapid in onset and lasted approximately 15 min (Morilak et al., 1990b). Injection of vehicle or of the inactive analog ICI 178 173 had no effects. These experiments therefore suggest that the enkephalinergic input to the rostral ventrolateral medulla tonically inhibits the descending sympathoexcitatory pressor neurons via activation of delta opioid receptors (Morilak et al., 1990b).

The caudal ventrolateral medulla also receives inputs from enkephalin-containing nerve terminals (Elde, et al., 1976; Finley et al., 1981; Khachaturian et al., 1983; Simantov et al., 1977). Microinjection of the non-specific opioid antagonist naloxone to the caudal ventrolateral medulla produces a dose-dependent depressor response that is also seen after microinjection of selective kappa and delta antagonists but not after administration of mu antagonists (Drolet et al., unpublished observations). These experiments suggest that there are tonically active endogenous opioid inputs to the caudal ventrolateral medulla that serve to inhibit the depressor neurons situated in this area that may use either enkephalin or dynorphin as neurotransmitters.

These studies suggest the presence of distinct opioid inputs to both the rostral and the caudal ventrolateral medulla, which contribute to the control of blood pressure through inhibition of the rostral sympathoexcitatory pressor neurons and of the caudal depressor neurons. The site of origin of these inhibitory opioid inputs has not been identified, but it is clearly possible that they arise in the medulla, conceivably in the nucleus tractus solitarius because such a pathway has now been described (Morilak et al., 1989).


## Possible Interaction Between Excitatory Amino Acid and Opioid Inputs to Caudal Ventrolateral Medulla

The possible interaction between excitatory amino acid and opioid inputs to the caudal ventrolateral medulla has been studied in some preliminary experiments (Badoer and Chalmers, unpublished observation). Pretreatment by injection of 2APV into the caudal ventrolateral medulla markedly enhanced the depressor effect of naloxone injected into the same area 15 min later. On the other hand, pretreatment with naloxone injected into the caudal ventrolateral medulla significantly attenuated the pressor response to 2APV, given 15 min later into the same site (Badoer and Chalmers, unpublished observations). The specificity of these results is currently being tested using pretreatment with muscimol and bicuculline injected into the caudal ventrolateral medulla before administration of naloxone and 2APV, respectively (Badoer and Chalmers, unpublished observations).

## Conclusions

We have demonstrated that excitatory amino acid-containing neurons project from the nucleus tractus solitarius to the ventrolateral medulla and have confirmed that this pathway is involved in the tonic and reflex control of blood pressure. We have also shown an enkephalin-containing pathway connecting these two areas but do not yet know whether it has a role in cardiovascular regulation. Nevertheless, opioid pathways of unknown origin that terminate in the ventrolateral medulla have been implicated in blood pressure control by pharmacological studies in our own and other laboratories.

## References


Armstrong DM, Pickel VM, Joh TH, Reis DJ, Miller RJ (1981): Immunocytochemical localization of catecholamine synthesizing enzymes and neuropeptides in area postrema and medial nucleus tractus solitarius of rat brain. *J Comp Neurol* 196:505–517.

Bacon SJ, Smith AD (1988): Preganglionic sympathetic neurones innervating the rat adrenal medulla: Immunocytochemical evidence of synaptic input from nerve terminals containing substance P, GABA or 5-hydroxytryptamine. *J Auton Nerv Syst* 24:97–122.

Blessing WW (1989): Baroreceptor-vasomotor reflex after N-methyl-D-asparate receptor blockade in rabbit caudal ventrolateral medulla. *J Physiol* 416:67–78.

Blessing WW, Li YW (1989): Inhibitory vasomotor neurons in the caudal ventrolateral region of the medulla oblongata. *Brain Res* 81:83–97.

Blessing WW, Oliver JR, Hodgson AH, Joh TH, Willoughby JO (1987): Neuropeptide Y-like immunoreactive C1 neurons in the rostral ventrolateral medulla of the rabbit project to sympathetic preganglionic neurons in the spinal cord. *J Auton Nerv Syst* 18:121–129.

Blessing WW, West MJ, Chalmers JP (1981): Hypertension, bradycardia and pulmonary oedema in the conscious rabbit after lesions of the ventrolateral medulla oblongata coinciding with the A1 group of catecholamine neurons. *Circ Res* 49:949–958.

Cox BF, Brody MJ (1989a): Mechanisms of respiration-induced changes in vaso-motor control exerted by rostral ventrolateral medulla. *Am J Physiol* 257:R626–R634.

Cox BF, Brody MJ (1989b): Subregions of rostral ventral medulla control arterial pressure and regional hemodynamics. *Am J Physiol* 257:R635–R640.

Cuenod M, Streit P (1984): Neuronal tracing using retrograde migration of labeled transmitter-related compounds. In Handbook of Chemical Neuroanatomy. Volume 1. Methods in Chemical Neuroanatomy. Elsevier. Amsterdam, Björklund A, Hökfelt T eds. 365–397.

Dampney RAL Czachurski J, Dembowsky K, Goodchild AK, Seller HJ (1987): Afferent connections and spinal projections of the pressor region in the rostral ventrolateral medulla of the cat. *J Auton Nerv Syst* 20:73–86.

Dampney RAL, Moon EA (1980): Role of ventrolateral medulla in vasomotor response to cerebral ischemia. *Am J Physiol* 239:H349–H358.

Davies J, Francis A, Jones AW, Watkins JC (1981): 2-Amino-5-phosphonovalerate (2-APV), a potent and selective antagonist of amino acid-induced and synaptic excitation. *Neurosci Lett* 21:77–81.

Dembowsky K, Czachurski J, Seller H (1989): Some properties of the sympathoinhibition from the caudal ventrolateral medulla oblongata in the cat. *Brain Res* 81:143–157.

Elde R, Hökfelt T, Johansson O, Terenius L (1976): Immunohistochemical studies using antibodies to leucine-enkephalin: Initial observations on the nervous system of the rat. *Neuroscience* 1:349–351.

Feldberg W (1976): The ventral surface of the brainstem: A scarcely explored region of pharmacological sensitivity. *Neuroscience* 1:427–441.

Feldberg W, Guertzenstein PG (1972): A vasodepressor effect of pentobarbitone sodium. *J Physiol* 224:83–103.

Feldberg W, Guertzenstein PG (1976): Vasodepressor effects obtained by drugs acting on the ventral surface of the brainstem. *J Physiol* 258:337–355.

Finley JCW, Maderdrut JL, Petrusz P (1981): The immunocytochemical localization of enkephalins in the central nervous system of the rat. *J Comp Neurol* 198:541–565.

Gordon FJ (1987): Aortic baroreceptor reflexes are mediated by NMDA receptors in caudal ventrolateral medulla. *Am J Physiol* 252:R628–R633.

Guertzenstein PG, Silver A (1974): Fall in blood pressure produced from discrete regions of the ventral surface of the medulla by glycine and lesions. *J Physiol (Lond)* 242:489–503.

Guyenet PG, Filtz TM, Donaldson SR (1987): Role of excitatory amino acids in rat vagal and sympathetic baroreflexes. *Brain Res* 407:272–284.

Hökfelt T, Fuxe K, Goldstein M, Johansson O (1974): Immunohistochemical evidence for the existence of adrenaline neurons in the rat brain. *Brain Res* 66:235–251.

Howe PRC, Kuhn DM, Minson JB, Stead BH, Chalmers JP (1983): Evidence for a bulbospinal serotonergic pressor pathway in the rat brain. *Brain Res* 270:29–36.

Johansson O, Hökfelt T, Pernow B, et al., (1981): Immunohistochemical support for three putative transmitters in one neuron: Coexistence of 5-hydroxytryptamine, substance P and thyrotropin releasing hormone like immunoreactivity in medullary neurons projecting to the spinal cord. *Neuroscience* 6:1857–1881.

Khachaturian H, Lewis ME, Watson SJ (1983): Enkephalin systems in diencephalon and brainstem of the rat. *J Comp Neurol* 220:310–320.

Kohno J, Shinoda K, Kawai Y, Ohuchi T, Ono K, Shiotani Y (1988): Interaction between adrenergic fibers and intermediate cholinergic neurons in the rat spinal cord: A new double-immunostaining method for correlated light and electron microscopic observations. *Neuroscience* 25(1):113–121.

Kubo T, Kihara M (1988): N-Methyl-D-aspartate receptors mediate tonic vasodepressor control in the caudal ventrolateral medulla of the rat. *Brain Res* 45:366–370.

Llewellyn-Smith IS, Minson JB, Morilak DA, Oliver JR, Chalmers JP (1990): Neuropeptide Y-immunoreactive synapses in the intermediolateral cell column of rat and rabbit thoracic spinal cord. *Neurosci Lett* 108:243–248.

Loewy AD, Burton H (1978): Nuclei of the solitary tract: Efferent projections to the lower brain stem and spinal cord of the cat. *J Comp Neurol* 181:421–450.

Ludbrook J, Rutter PC (1988): Effect of naloxone on haemodynamic responses to acute blood loss in unanesthetized rabbits. *J Physiol* 400:1–15.

Milner TA, Morrison SF, Abate C, Reis DJ (1988): Phenylethanolamine N-methyltransferase-containing terminals synapse directly on sympathetic preganglionic neurons in the rat. *Brain Res* 448:205–222.

Minson JB, Chalmers JP, Caon AC, Renaud B (1987): Separate areas of rat medulla oblongata with populations of serotonin- and adrenaline-containing neurons alter blood pressure after L-glutamate stimulation. *J Auton Nerv Syst* 19:39–50.

Morilak DA, Somogyi P, McIlhinney RAJ, Chalmers J (1989): An enkephalin-containing pathway from nucleus tractus solitarii to the pressor area of the rostral ventrolateral medulla of the rabbit. *Neuroscience* 1:427–441.

Morilak DA, Drolet G, Chalmers J (1990a): Cardiovascular effects of the opioid antagonist naloxone in the rostral ventrolateral medulla of rabbits. *Am J Physiol* 258:R325–333.

Morilak DA, Drolet G, Chalmers J (1990b): Tonic opioid inhibition of the pressor region of the rostral ventrolateral medulla of rabbits is mediated by delta receptors. *J Pharmacol Exp Ther* 254:671–676.

Morrison SF, Calloway J, Milner TA, Reis DJ (1989): Glutamate in the spinal sympathetic intermediolateral nucleus: Localization by light and electron microscopy. *Brain Res* 503:5–15.

Pilowsky PM, Kapoor V, Minson JB, West MJ, Chalmers JP (1986a): Spinal cord serotonin release and raised blood pressure after brainstem kainic acid injection. *Brain Res* 366:354–357.

Pilowsky PM, Morris MJ, Minson JB, et al. (1986b): Inhibition of vasodepressor neurons in the caudal ventrolateral medulla of the rabbit increases both arterial pressure and the release of neuropeptide Y-like immunoreactivity from the spinal cord. *Brain Res* 420:380–384.

Reis DJ, Morrison S, Ruggiero DA (1988): The C1 area of the brainstem in tonic and reflex control of blood pressure. *Hypertension* II (suppl I): I8–I13.

Ross CA, Ruggiero DA, Reis DJ (1985): Projections from the nucleus tractus solitarii to the rostral ventrolateral medulla. *J Comp Neurol* 242:511–534.

Ross CA, Ruggiero DA, Joh TH, Reis DJ (1983): Adrenaline synthesizing neurons in the rostral ventrolateral medulla: A possible role in tonic vasomotor control. *Brain Res* 273:356–361.

Ross CA, Ruggiero DA, Park DH, et al. (1984): Tonic vasomotor control by the rostral ventrolateral medulla: Effect of electrical or chemical stimulation of the area containing C1 adrenaline neurons on arterial pressure, heart rate, and plasma catecholamines and vasopressin. *J Neurosci* 4:474–494.

Sasek CA, Wessendorf MW, Helke CJ (1990): Evidence for co-existence of thyrotropin-releasing hormone, substance P and serotonin in ventral medullary neurons that project to the intermediolateral cell column in the rat. *Neuroscience* 35:105–119.

Simantov R, Kuhar MJ, Uhl GR, Snyder SH (1977): Opioid peptide enkephalin: immunohistochemical mapping in rat central nervous system. *Proc Natl Acad Sci USA* 74:2167–2171.

Somogyi P, Minson JB, Morilak D, Llewellyn-Smith IS, McIlhinney JRA, Chalmers J (1989): Evidence for an excitatory amino acid pathway in the brainstem and for its involvement in cardiovascular control. *Brain Res* 496:401–407.

Spyer KM (1981): Neural organization and control of the baroreceptor reflex. *Rev Physiol Biochem Pharmacol* 88:24–124.

Urbanski RW, Sapru HN (1988): Evidence for a sympathoexcitatory pathway from the nucleus tractus solitarii to the ventrolateral medullary pressor area. *J Auton Nerv Syst* 23:161–174.

West MJ, Blessing WW, Chalmers J (1981): Arterial baroreceptor reflex function in the conscious rabbit after brain lesions coinciding with the A1 group of catecholamine neurons. *Circ Res* 49:959–970.

Yamazoe M, Shisaka S, Shibaski T, et al. (1984): Distribution of six neuropeptides in the nucleus tractus solitarii of the rat: An immunohistochemical analysis. *Neuroscience* 13:1243–1266.

# 2
# Widespread Autonomic Afferents to the Nucleus Paragigantocellularis of the Rostral Ventrolateral Medulla

ELISABETH J. VAN BOCKSTAELE AND GARY ASTON-JONES

## Introduction

The nucleus paragigantocellularis (PGi) was first described in the human brain (Olzewski and Baxter, 1954) and later in the rat (Andrezik et al., 1981) on the basis of cytoarchitectonics in Nissl-stained material. This nucleus covers a large region in the rostral ventral medulla extending rostrally from the lateral reticular nucleus to the caudal pole of the superior olivary nucleus. It is bordered medially by the inferior olivary nucleus and nucleus gigantocellularis pars ventralis in its caudal division, laterally by the spinal trigeminal nucleus and tract, and dorsally by the nucleus ambiguus. Caudally, this area has been termed the "retrofacial PGi" (Taber, 1961), corresponding to its location immediately caudal to the facial nucleus and ventral to the nucleus ambiguus. Rostrally, the PGi is bordered medially by the pyramidal tract and laterally by the facial nucleus. As the facial nucleus progresses rostrally, it extends more medially to encompass most of the ventral medulla thereby displacing the rostral pole of the PGi. The rostral medial component of PGi is designated here as juxtafacial PGi.

Anatomical and physiological studies have implicated the PGi in many autonomic processes (for review see Ciriello et al., 1986; Loewy and McKellar, 1980; McAllen et al., 1987). Specifically, in the lateral PGi these functions include 1) control of resting arterial pressure (Dampney and Moon, 1980; Guertzenstein and Silver, 1974; Ross et al., 1984), 2) cardiopulmonary reflexes, 3) respiration (Feldman, 1986; McAllen, 1986), and 4) parasympathetic function (Bieger and Hopkins, 1987; Nosaka et al., 1979). These functions are consistent with subdivisions of the lateral PGi defined by others, which include the nucleus rostroventrolateralis (Ross et al., 1984), the external formation of the nucleus ambiguus (Bieger and Hopkins, 1987), and the ventral respiratory group corresponding to the Bötzinger complex (Feldman, 1986), respectively. Neurons in the medial aspect of the ventral PGi have also been implicated in blood pressure regulation (Howe et al., 1983; Minson et al., 1987) as well as in antinociception and analgesia (Azami et al., 1982; Punnen et al., 1984; Satoh et al., 1979; Sun and Guyenet, 1986).

The PGi has also been implicated in vigilance and attention because of its prominent projection to noradrenergic neurons in the locus coeruleus (LC; Aston-Jones et al., 1986; Guyenet and Young, 1987). Activation of PGi predominantly excites LC neurons via the release of an excitatory amino acid transmitter (Ennis and Aston-Jones, 1988).

Therefore, the PGi appears to be a region in which many functionally related processes converge for integration. To understand the basis for such integration, a comprehensive knowledge of the afferent projections to the PGi is necessary. Previous studies have revealed that major afferents to PGi arise from the spinal cord, midline pontine and medullary nuclei, vestibular nuclei, nucleus of the solitary tract, nucleus of the lateral lemniscus (Andrezik et al., 1981 ), and lateral hypothalamus (Andrezik et al., 1981; Beitz et al., 1983; Fardin et al., 1984; Li and Lovick, 1985). In addition, less prominent afferents have been reported from several central structures (Andrezik et al., 1981; Carlton et al., 1983).

Studies to date, however, have not examined the possible topographic specificity of afferents terminating within PGi. Given that the PGi covers a large area of the ventral medulla, knowledge of differential connectivity from its inputs is critical in elucidating the functional correlates of substructures within this region.

In the studies reviewed here (for details, see Van Bockstaele et al., 1989), we have used the retrograde transport of wheat germ agglutinin-conjugated horseradish peroxidase (WGA-HRP), Fluoro-Gold (FG) or WGA-HRP coupled with 20-nm gold particles (WGA-apoHRP-Gold) to examine afferent projections to the PGi. To examine the topographic specificity of inputs to PGi, we extended the retrograde tracing results with the anterograde transport of WGA-HRP or of *Phaseolus vulgaris*-leucoagglutinin (PHA-L) from selected afferent areas shown to contain retrogradely labeled neurons. We find that many diverse brain areas project to the PGi and that many of these projections innervate topographically specific regions of the PGi. Most of the afferent nuclei are restricted to the brain stem but there are also projections from the diencephalon and telencephalon.

# Results

## *Retrograde Tracing Studies from Retrofacial PGi*

Discrete iontophoretic injections of either WGA-HRP, FG, or small pressure injections of WGA-apoHRP-Gold within the retrofacial division of the PGi yielded numerous retrogradely labeled neurons throughout the brain and spinal cord of the rat. The pattern of retrograde labeling for each tracer was similar. Most brain areas containing labeled neurons also contained anterograde labeling following WGA-HRP injections into PGi. All cases with WGA-HRP injections into various PGi subregions contained antero-

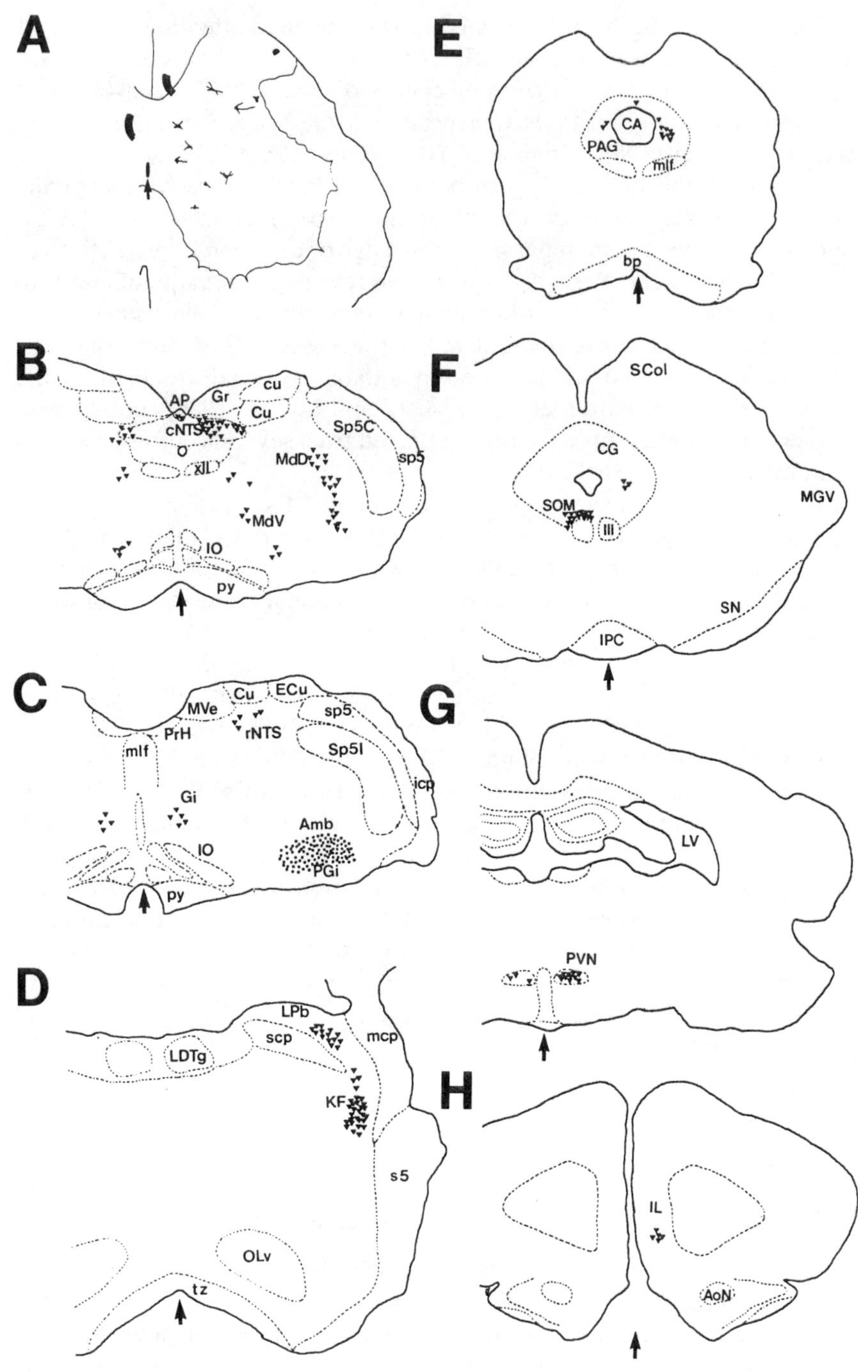
A
E
CA
PAG
mlf
bp
B
AP
Gr
cu
Cu
cNTS
Sp5C
sp5
o
xII
MdD
MdV
IO
py
F
SCol
CG
SOM
III
MGV
SN
IPC
C
Cu
ECu
MVe
sp5
PrH
rNTS
mlf
Sp5I
Gi
icp
Amb
IO
PGi
py
G
LV
D
LPb
scp
mcp
LDTg
KF
PVN
s5
H
OLv
tz
IL
AoN

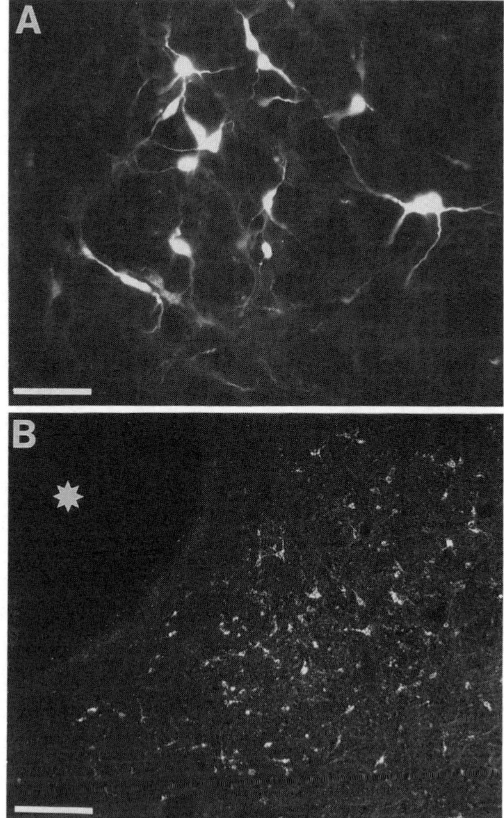

FIGURE 2.2. Photomicrographs of transverse sections illustrating retrogradely labeled neurons. **A**: An ultraviolet-illuminated epifluorescent section showing FG-labeled neurons in the caudal medullary reticular formation following an injection into PGi. Bar = 50 μm. **B**: Dark-field photomicrograph illustrating WGA-apoHRP-Gold retrograde labeling in the ventrolateral periaqueductal gray of the midbrain. Cerebral aqueduct is indicated by the star. Calibration Bar = 150 μm.

◁————————————————————————————————————————

FIGURE 2.1. Video computer-aided plots of coronal sections throughout the brain and spinal cord illustrating areas containing retrogradely labeled neurons (line drawings of neurons in the spinal cord and inverted triangles for neurons in the brain sections) following an iontophoretic injection of WGA-HRP into the PGi area. Sections are ordered from caudal to rostral (**A** to **H**) and are taken from various levels of several representative brains. Arrows indicate midline and ventral brain surface.

grade labeling within the LC. This indicates that afferents found here to PGi may interact with LC-projecting neurons, and that the neurons within PGi projecting to LC are not confined to one subregion but rather are distributed throughout the entire nucleus.

Retrogradely labeled neurons were most numerous in the brain stem and spinal cord whereas labeling in the diencephalon and telencephalon was less prominent and more variable among animals (Fig. 2.1). There were many retrogradely labeled neurons throughout the entire spinal cord, but the cervical and lumbosacral segments of the cord exhibited the greatest density of retrogradely labeled neurons (Fig. 2.1A). Figure 2.1 illustrates areas that contained the greatest number of retrogradely labeled neurons after an injection in the PGi. These areas include the caudal medullary reticular formation (MdD) just dorsal to the lateral reticular nucleus (Fig. 2.1B), the nucleus of the solitary tract (NTS; Fig. 2.1D), the lateral para-brachialis (LPB), the Kölliker-Fuse nucleus (KF; Fig. 2.1D), the peria-queductal gray (PAG; Fig. 2.1E), and the supraoculomotor nucleus of the central gray (SOM; Fig. 2.1F). This latter area is noteworthy because it has not been previously reported to innervate the ventrolateral medulla.

Areas with more moderate retrograde labeling included the contralateral PGi, the area postrema (Fig. 2.1B), the caudal raphé nuclei, the nucleus gigantocellularis (Fig. 2.1C), the medial vestibular nucleus, the accessory nucleus of the VIth and VIIth cranial nerves, the locus coeruleus, the inferior colliculus, and the region of A5 noradrenergic neurons. Certain areas of the diencephalon and telencephalon contained retrograde labeling following large injections of tracer into the PGi. Such areas included the paraventricular nucleus of the hypothalamus (Fig. 2.1G), the lateral hypothalamus, and the infralimbic cortex (Fig. 2.1H). A small number of retrogradely labeled neurons was observed in the insular cortex.

Retrograde labeling in the above-mentioned areas varied with the injection placement within PGi. Injections into the lateral division of the retrofacial PGi yielded retrogradely labeled neurons most numerously in the MdD (Fig. 2.2A). Such labeling was not as prominent following more medially placed injections. Other areas demonstrating many retrogradely labeled neurons following lateral PGi injections were the NTS (commissuralis level; Fig. 2.3A), the KF (Fig. 2.3B), and the ventromedial part of the central gray in the vicinity of the SOM (Fig. 2.4). In cases with injections placed more medially, many more retrogradely labeled neurons were found in the lateral and ventrolateral PAG (Fig. 2.2B).

Thus, the results of our retrograde tracing studies indicated that a substantial topography exists for inputs to PGi. To examine further the topography of inputs to PGi and to examine the degree of terminal arborization within subdivisions of PGi, the anterograde tracer PHA-L was iontophoretically deposited into some of these nuclei shown to contain retrogadely labeled neurons.

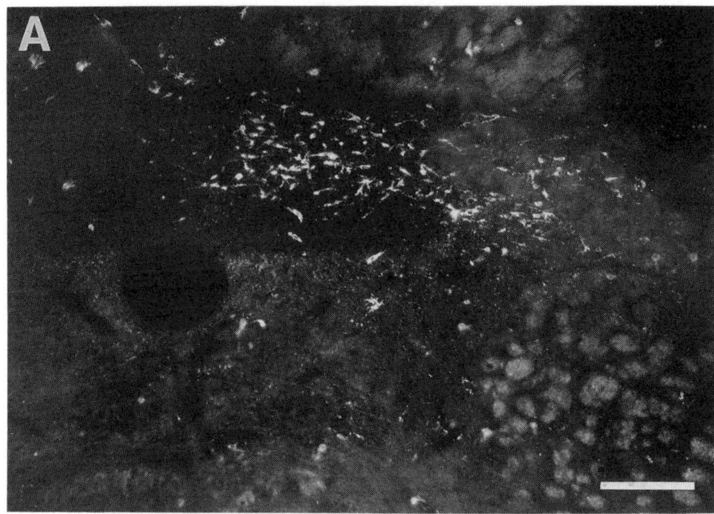

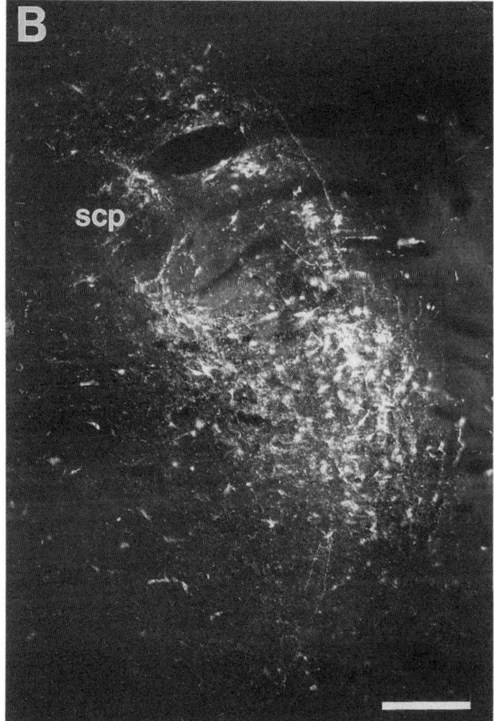


FIGURE 2.3. Dark-field photomicrographs illustrating retrogradely labeled neurons with WGA-HRP. **A**: Labeled neurons in the nucleus of the solitary tract (commissuralis level). **B**: Labeled neurons in the Kölliker-Fuse region of the lateral pons. scp: superior cerebellar peduncle. Calibration Bars = 125 $\mu$m.

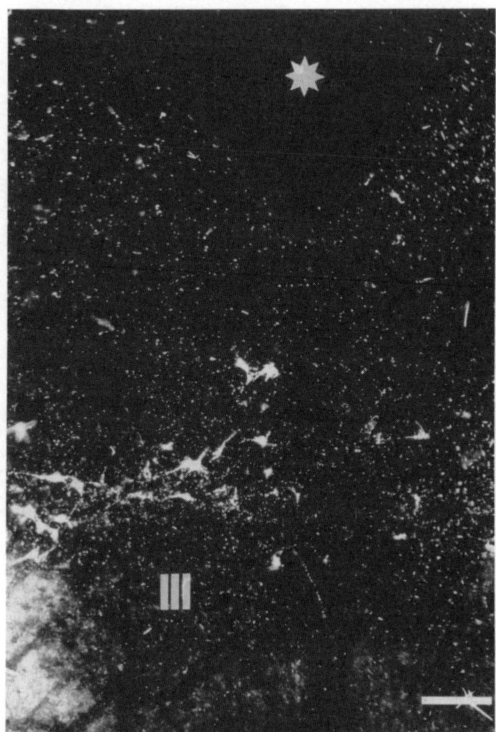

FIGURE 2.4. Dark-field photomicrograph illustrating retrogradely labeled neurons with WGA-HRP in the rostral ventromedial periaqueductal in gray the vicinity of the supraoculomotor nucleus. These neurons are located contralateral to the injection site that was placed in the lateral PGi. Cerebral aqueduct is at the star. III: oculomotor nucleus. Calibration Bar = 100 $\mu$m. (From Van Bockstaele et al., 1989.)

## Anterograde Tracing Studies

PHA-L or WGA-HRP were iontophoretically deposited into nuclei found in our retrograde tracing results to be major afferents to PGi, and the PGi area was examined for labeled fibers and terminals. In addition, using these tracers we examined projections of nuclei reported by others to project to the PGi but not found to contain retrogradely labeled neurons in our material.

One of the most prominent afferents to PGi seen with retrograde transport was the rostral ventromedial PAG, including neurons of the SOM. Injections of PHA-L into this area yielded dense anterograde labeling in the retrofacial PGi ventral to the nucleus ambiguus (Fig. 2.5A), confirming our retrograde tracing results. This was primarily a contralateral projection, with descending fibers crossing at the midbrain–pontine junction (Van Bockstaele et al., in press).

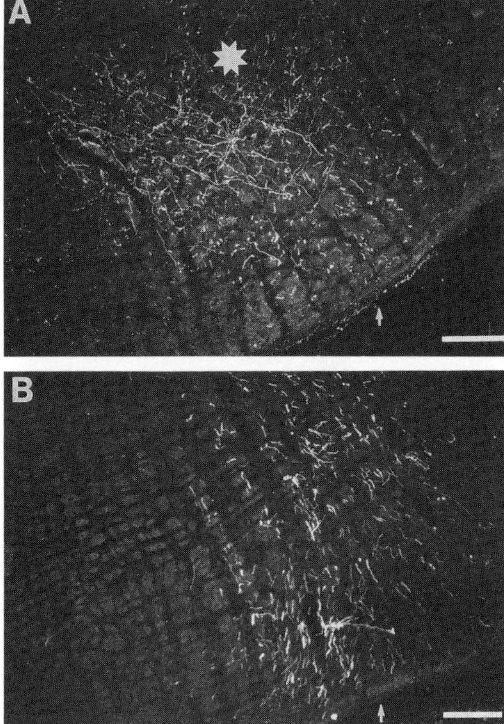

FIGURE 2.5. Dark-field photomicrographs illustrating anterograde labeling with PHA-L in PGi. **A**: PHA-L fibers in the retrofacial PGi immediately ventral to the nucleus ambiguus (at star) following an injection into the rostral ventromedial aspect of the periaqueductal gray in the vicinity of the supraoculomotor nucleus. The fibers are located predominantly in the lateral aspect of the PGi. Calibration Bar = 120 $\mu$m. **B**: PHA-L fibers in PGi at a similar level as in **A** but following an injection into the nucleus of the solitary tract (commissuralis level). Note that the bulk of the fibers are more ventrally located than the fibers in **A**. Arrows indicate ventral brain surface. Calibration Bar = 100 $\mu$m

PHA-L injections into the ventrolateral PAG yielded numerous anterogradely labeled fibers in the medial and ventral retrofacial PGi. Fibers were most dense in the raphé magnus and ventral nucleus gigantocellularis. PHA-L injections into the dorsal PAG yielded numerous anterogradely labeled fibers in the raphé magnus and in the juxtafacial portion of the PGi (Van Bockstaele et al., in press).

PHA-L injections into the caudal NTS (commissuralis level) yielded anterograde labeling in a restricted portion of the retrofacial PGi ventral to the nucleus ambiguus (Fig. 2.5B), corresponding to the nucleus rostroventrolateralis (Ross et al., 1984).

The inferior colliculus was previously reported to provide substantial innervation to the PGi (Andrezik et al., 1981), but contained only a few scattered retrogradely labeled neurons from PGi in our study. Large injections of PHA-L or WGA-HRP into the inferior colliculus yielded substantial anterograde labeling in the superior olivary nucleus and nucleus of the trapezoid body and moderate labeling in a restricted portion of the juxtafacial PGi. Similarly, both the superior colliculus and dorsal cochlear nucleus were previously reported to project to the rostral pole of the PGi (Andrezik et al., 1981). Injections into these nuclei yielded anterograde labeling in structures nearby PGi but not in PGi proper.

## *Retrograde Tracing Studies from Juxtafacial PGi*

We have recently initiated a study of the afferents to the rostral, juxtafacial PGi and the initial results are noteworthy. Iontophoretic deposits of WGA-HRP, or small pressure injections of WGA-apoHRP-Gold, into the juxtafacial PGi yielded a pattern of retrograde labeling throughout the brain that differed from that described above following injections into retrofacial PGi. Retrogradely labeled neurons were found in the MdD throughout the caudal medulla but were relatively few in number. In addition, there were only a few retrogradely labeled neurons in the caudal NTS (commissuralis level); however, at more rostral levels, retrogradely labeled neurons in NTS became more numerous. Moderate retrograde labeling was observed in the dorsal column nuclei (nucleus cuneatus and gracilis), caudal raphé nuclei (raphé magnus and pallidus), and supraolivary pontine reticular formation.

Retrogradely labeled neurons were also found in the ventrolateral, lateral, and dorsal periaqueductal gray. These were most numerous in the rostral dorsal PAG, at the level of the oculomotor and red nuclei. At this level, retrogradely labeled neurons were also present in the medial geniculate nucleus.

Our analysis of afferents to the juxtafacial PGi is still underway; in particular, several forebrain areas have not been thoroughly analyzed as possible afferents to this rostral PGi region.

## Discussion

In summary, our results indicate that diverse but functionally related brain and spinal cord areas project to the PGi. Major afferents arising from the spinal cord are located in the cervical and lumbosacral segments. When injections were restricted to the retrofacial portion of PGi, afferent nuclei were largely autonomic in nature. Many of these were restricted to the brain stem (medullary reticular formation, nucleus of the solitary tract, lateral parabrachialis, Kölliker-Fuse, periaqueductal gray). However, there were also projections from certain forebrain structures (paraventricular nucleus of the hypothalamus, lateral hypothalamus, and infralimbic cortex). A moderate number of retrogradely labeled neurons could also be found in nonautonomic areas of the brain stem (inferior colliculus, vestibular nucleus).

Many previous findings were confirmed in our study. These include afferents from the NTS, caudal raphé nuclei, PAG, and hypothalamic nuclei. Our findings also revealed some new afferents not previously described. The most prominent of these is a contralateral projection from the rostral ventromedial PAG, corresponding to the SOM.

Some of our results, however, revealed discrepancies with previous work. The nucleus of the lateral lemniscus (NLL), which was reported to be a major afferent to the PGi (Andrezik et al., 1981), was unlabeled in our studies when injections were restricted to PGi. However, when our injections extended into the facial nucleus or rostrally into the superior olivary nucleus, retrogradely labeled neurons found in the NLL were numerous. Our results indicate that the KF nucleus, which is slightly caudal and dorsal to the NLL, contains the greatest number of neurons in that region that project specifically to PGi.

Anterograde tracing studies revealed that afferents to PGi exhibit topography in their afferent terminations. Projections from the NTS (commissuralis level) and the rostral ventromedial PAG in the area of SOM target the lateral retrofacial PGi, ventral to the nucleus ambiguus, in the vicinity of spinally projecting sympathoexcitatory neurons (Ross et al., 1984) and respiratory-related neurons (Feldman, 1986), respectively. The projections from the dorsal PAG and the ventrolateral PAG preferentially innervate the medial aspect of the PGi.

## Functional Implications

Most regions projecting to the PGi are involved in autonomic control. The following lists some of the most salient features of some of the most prominent inputs.

### *Rostral Ventromedial PAG*

There is little information regarding neurons in the rostral ventromedial PAG at the level of the oculomotor nucleus. This region is rostral to the dorsal raphé nucleus and caudal to the Edinger-Westphal cell group. The location of the retrogradely labeled neurons in the rostral ventromedial PAG from PGi injections corresponds closely to a region defined as the supraoculomotor nucleus of the central gray (SOM) in the cat (Maciewicz et al., 1975) and rat (Paxinos and Watson, 1985). The rostral ventromedial PAG is a region that has not been extensively studied physiologically and the function of many of its constituent neurons remains unknown. In its most ventral aspect, the SOM has been anatomically defined as a nucleus with projections to the abducens nucleus and whose neurons are preoculo-motor in function. Many SOM neurons receive afferents from oculomotor-related areas. Studies are underway to determine if PGi-projecting neurons in this region of the central gray also innervate oculomotor nuclei, or if they may have other functional characteristics.

The dense projection from the region of the rostral ventromedial PAG to the autonomic part of the PGi implicates these PAG neurons in regulation of autonomic activities. Physiological studies are underway to examine whether these neurons influence peripheral autonomic function. Preliminary results reveal that electrical stimulation of the rostral ventromedial PAG does not have a significant effect on peripheral blood pressure. However, electrical stimulation of this area of the midbrain results in a sharp increase in respiratory activity (unpublished observations). These physiological data are consistent with the anatomical projection from this region to respiratory-related neurons in the rostral ventral medulla.

## Ventrolateral PAG

Injections of both retrograde and anterograde tracers into the ventrolateral aspect of the PGi have demonstrated projections from the PAG (Bandler, 1987; Beitz, 1982; Carrive et al., 1987; Holstege, 1988; Holstege, 1985; Van Bockstaele et al., 1989). The region of the ventrolateral PAG containing retrogradely labeled neurons has been implicated in cardiovascular regulation (Abrahams et al., 1960; Carrive et al., 1989; Carrive et al., 1987; Gauthier and Reader, 1982; Hilton and Redfern, 1986) and analgesia (Depaulis et al., 1987; Lakos and Basbaum, 1988; Morgan and Liebeskind, 1987), functions that are strongly represented within the PGi. The projection of the ventrolateral PAG neurons favors the medial aspect of the PGi, a region implicated both in cardiovascular regulation (Howe et al., 1983; Minson et al, 1987) and in pain modulation (Azami et al., 1982; Punnen et al., 1984; Satoh et al., 1979; Sun and Guyenet, 1986).

## Dorsal PAG

Neurons retrogradely labeled in the dorsal PAG coincide with regions in which electrical or chemical stimulation elicit defense behaviors (Gomita et al., 1988; Skultety, 1963). Many of the behaviors associated with defense are also accompanied by autonomic changes, perhaps via connections to the PGi. The projection from dorsal PAG neurons favors the rostral pole of the PGi, a region implicated in cardiovascular regulation, analgesia, and somatosensory integration.

## Lateral Parabrachial and Kölliker-Fuse Nuclei

The projection from neurons in the lateral pons seems to favor the lateral PGi. This has recently been confirmed and extended in a study by Herbert et al. (1990), in which anterograde tracing from the LPB and KF preferentially target the lateral aspect of the rostral ventrolateral medulla. The LPB and KF nuclei have been implicated in cardiovascular, respiratory, and pain regulation. It is possible that neurons of this region in the dorsolateral pons projecting to the rostral ventral medulla mediate some of these autonomic and nociceptive processes.

## *Nucleus of the Solitary Tract*

The projection from the NTS to the ventrolateral medulla has been well documented (Norgren, 1978; Ross et al., 1985) and is confirmed here. The projection from the caudal NTS specifically targets the lateral PGi within the nucleus rostroventrolateralis area, immediately ventral to the nucleus ambiguus in a region containing spinally projecting neurons (Hancock, 1988; Ross et al., 1985). These circuits have been implicated in mediating central responses to autonomic changes in the periphery since the target of NTS neurons involves sympathoexcitatory neurons as described above.

When injections were placed into the rostral juxtafacial PGi, a different pattern of retrograde labeling was found. One noteworthy difference is that the rostromedial PGi seems to contain an integrative relay nucleus for auditory and somatosensory inputs. An area subserving such a function was proposed in the cat. Kamiya et al. (1988) described specific projections to the rostromedial PGi from the inferior colliculus, the dorsal column nuclei, and the medial geniculate. We have confirmed these findings for rat in our preliminary studies of retrograde transport from the rostromedial PGi. We also find projections to this subregion of the rostromedial PGi from the inferior colliculus. Thus, it seems that an anatomically, and perhaps functionally, similar region exists both in the cat and rat.

Finally, it is noteworthy that neurons in the rostral ventral medulla provide the major input to the nucleus locus coeruleus (Aston-Jones et al., 1986; Guyenet and Brown, 1986; Pieribone et al., 1988). These LC-projecting neurons are broadly distributed throughout PGi but with some topographical organization. LC afferent neurons are preferentially medially located in rostral PGi and more laterally located in caudal PGi. Physiological studies have revealed that the PGi provides a predominantly excitatory input to the LC (Ennis and Aston-Jones, 1988). Thus, activation of PGi may give rise to parallel activation of both peripheral sympathetic processes and the central LC noradrenergic system. The role proposed for LC in vigilance and attention (Aston-Jones, 1988) indicates that PGi may provide a wider role than simply control of vegetative processes, including coordination of cognitive (via LC) and peripheral (via IML) systems involved in adaptive responses to environmental stimuli. It will be important for future studies to determine the sources of afferents to the PGi responsible for each of these functions, and the mechanisms whereby these processes are integrated in the PGi to provide for coordinated activities centrally and peripherally.

# References


Abrahams VC, Hilton SM, Zbrozyna A (1960): Active muscle vasodilatation produced by stimulation of the brain stem: Its significance in the defence reaction. *J Physiol* 154:491–513.

Andrezik JA, Chan-Palay V, Palay SL (1981): The nucleus paragigantocellularis lateralis in the rat: Demonstration of afferents by the retrograde transport of horseradish peroxidase. *Anat Embryol* 161:373–390.

Aston-Jones G (1988) Cellular attributes of locus coeruleus: implications for attentional processes. In: *Progress in Catecholamine Research Part B: Central Aspects*, Sandler M, Dahlstrom A, Belmaker R, eds. New York: Alan R. Liss.

Aston-Jones G, Ennis M, Pieribone VA, Nickell WT, Shipley MT (1986): The brain nucleus locus coeruleus: Restricted afferent control of a broad efferent network. *Science* 234:734–737.

Azami J, Llewelyn MB, Roberts MHT (1982): The contribution of nucleus reticularis paragigantocellularis and nucleus raphé magnus to the analgesia produced by systemically administered morphine, investigated with the microinjection technique. *Pain* 12:229–246.

Bandler R, Tork I (1987): Midbrain periaqueductal grey region in the cat has afferent and efferent connections with solitary tract nuclei. *Neurosci Lett* 74:1–6.

Beitz AJ (1982): The nuclei of origin of brain stem enkephalin and substance P projections to the rodent nucleus raphé magnus. *Neuroscience* 7:2753–2768.

Beitz AJ, Mullett AJ, Weiner LL (1983): The periaqueductal gray projections to the rat spinal trigeminal, raphé magnus, gigantocellular pars alpha and paragigantocellular nuclei arise from separate neurons. *Brain Res* 288:307–314.

Bieger D, Hopkins DA (1987): Viscerotopic representation of the upper alimentary tract in the medulla oblongata in the rat: The nucleus ambiguus. *J Comp Neurol* 262:546–562.

Carlton SM, Leichnetz GR, Young EG, Mayer DJ (1983): Supramedullary afferents of the nucleus raphé magnus in the rat: A study using the transcannula HRP gel and autoradiographic techniques. *J Comp Neurol* 214:43–58.

Carrive P, Bandler R, Dampney RAL (1989): Somatic and autonomic integration in the midbrain of the unanaesthetised decerebrate cat: A distinctive pattern evoked by excitation of neurones in the subtentorial portion of the midbrain periaqueductal grey. *Brain Res* 483:251–258.

Carrive P, Dampney RAL, Bandler R (1987): Excitation of neurones in a restricted portion of the midbrain periaqueductal grey elicits both behavioural and cardiovascular components of the defence reaction in the unanaesthetised decerebrate cat. *Neurosci Lett* 81:273–278.

Ciriello J, Caverson MM, Polosa C ( 1986): Function of the ventrolateral medulla in the control of the circulation. *Brain Res.* 11:359–391.

Dampney RAL, Moon EA (1980): Role of ventrolateral medulla in vasomotor response to cerebral ischemia. *Am J Physiol* 239:349–348.

Depaulis A. Morgan MM, Liebeskind JC (1987): GABAergic modulation of the analgesic effects of morphine microinjected in the ventral periaqueductal gray matter of the rat. *Brain Res* 436:223–228.

Ennis M, Aston-Jones G (1988): Activation of locus coeruleus from nucleus paragigantocellularis: A new excitatory amino acid pathway in brain. *J Neurosci* 8:3644–3657.

Fardin V, Oliveras JL, Besson JM (1984): Projections from the periaqueductal gray matter to the B3 cellular area (nucleus raphé magnus and nucleus reticularis paragigantocellularis) as revealed by the retrograde transport of horseradish peroxidase in the rat. *J Comp Neurol* 223:483–500.

Feldman JL (1986): Neurophysiology of breathing in mammals. In: *Handbook of Physiology: Section 1: The Nervous System: Volume IV: Intrinsic Regulatory Systems of the Brain.* Bloom FE (ed) Washington, D.C.: American Physiological Society.

Gauthier P, Reader TA (1982): Adrenomedullary secretory response to midbrain stimulation in rat: Effects of depletion of brain catecholamines or serotonin. *Can J Physiol Pharm* 60:1464–1474.

Gomita Y, Moriyama M, Ichimaru Y, Araki Y (1988): Neural systems activated by the aversive stimulation of dorsal central gray. *Jap J Pharmacol* 48:137–141.

Guertzenstein PG, Silver A (1974): Fall in blood pressure produced from discrete regions of the ventral surface of the medulla by glycine and lesions. *J Physiol (Lond)* 242:489–503.

Guyenet PG, Brown DL (1986): Nucleus paragigantocellularis lateralis and lumbar sympathetic discharge in the rat. *Am J Physiol* 250:R1081–R1094.

Guyenet PG, Young BS (1987): Projections of nucleus paragigantocellularis to locus coeruleus and other structures in rat. *Brain Res* 406:171–184.

Hancock MB (1988): Evidence for direct projections from the nucleus of the solitary tract onto medullary adrenaline cells. *J Comp Neurol* 276:460–467.

Herbert H, Moga M, Saper CS (1990): Connections of the parabrachial nucleus with the nucleus of the solitary tract and the medullary reticular formation in the rat. *J Comp Neurol* 293:540–580.

Hilton SM, Redfern WS (1986): A search for brain stem cell groups integrating the defence reaction in the rat. *J Physiol* 378:213–228.

Holstege G, Meiners L, Tan K (1985) Projections of the bed nucleus of the stria terminalis to the mesencephalon, pons, and medulla oblongata in the cat. *Exp Brain Res* 58:379–391.

Holstege G, Tan J (1988) Projections from the red nucleus and surrounding areas to the brain stem and spinal cord in the cat. An HRP and autoradiographic tracing study. *Behav Brain Res* 28:33–57.

Howe PRC, Kuhn DM, Minson JB, Stead BH, Chalmers JP (1983): Evidence for a bulbospinal serotonergic pathway in the rat brain. *Brain Res* 270:29–36.

Kamiya H, Itoh K, Yasui Y, Ino T, Mizuno N (1988): Somatosensory and auditory relay nucleus in the rostral part of the ventrolateral medulla: A morphological study in the cat. *J Comp Neurol* 273:421–435.

Lakos S, Basbaum AI (1988): An ultrastructural study of the projections from the midbrain periaqueductal gray to spinally projecting, serotonin-immunoreactive neurons of the medullary nucleus raphé magnus in the rat. *Brain Res* 443:383–388.

Li P, Lovick TA (1985): Excitatory projections from hypothalamic and midbrain defense regions to nucleus paragigantocellularis lateralis in the rat. *Exp Neurol* 89:543–553.

Loewy AD, McKellar S (1980): The neuroanatomical basis of central cardiovascular control. *Fed Proc* 39:2495–2503.

Maciewicz RJ, Kaneko CRS, Highstein SM, Baker R (1975): Morphophysiological identification of interneurons in the oculomotor nucleus that project to the abducens nucleus in the cat. *Brain Res* 96:60–65.

McAllen RM (1986): Location of neurones with cardiovascular and respiratory function, at the ventral surface of the cat's medulla. *Neuroscience* 18:43–49.

McAllen RM, Dampney AL, Goodchild AK (1987): The sub-retrofacial nucleus and cardiovascular control. In: Ciriello J, Calaresu FR, Renaud LP, Polosa C (eds.), *Organization of the Autonomic Nervous System: Central and Peripheral Mechanisms*. New York: Alan R. Liss.

Minson JB, Chalmers JP, Caon AC, Renaud B (1987): Separate area of rat medulla oblongata with populations of serotonin- and adrenaline-containing neurons alter blood pressure after L-glutamate stimulation. *J Auton Nerv Syst* 19:39–50.

Morgan MM, Liebeskind JC (1987). Site specificity in the development of tolerance to stimulation-produced analgesia from the periaqueductal gray matter of the rat. *Brain Res* 425:356–359.

Norgren R (1978). Projections from the nucleus of the solitary tract in the rat. *Neuroscience* 3:207–218.

Nosaka S, Yamomoto T, Yasunaga K (1979): Localization of vagal cardioinhibitory preganglionic neurons within rat brain stem. *J Comp Neurol* 186:79–92.

Olzewski J, Baxter D (1954): *Cytoarchitecture of the Human Brain Stem*. Basel: S. Karger.

Paxinos G, Watson C (1985): *The Rat Brain in Stereotaxic Coordinates*. New York: Academic Press.

Pieribone VA, Aston-Jones G, Bohn M (1988): Adrenergic and non-adrenergic neurons in the C1 and C3 areas project to locus coeruleus: A fluorescent double labeling study. *Neurosci Lett* 85:297–303.

Punnen S, Willette R, Krieger AJ, Sapru HN (1984): Cardiovascular response to injections of enkephalin in the pressor area of the ventrolateral medulla. *Neuropharmacology* 23:939–946.

Ross CA, Ruggiero DA, Park DH, Joh TH, Fernandez-Pardal F, Saavedra JM, Reis D (1984): Tonic vasomotor control by the rostral ventrolateral medulla: Effect of electrical or chemical stimulation of the area containing C1 adrenaline neurons on arterial pressure, heart rate, and plasma catecholamine and vasopressin. *J Neurosci* 4:474–494.

Ross CA, Ruggiero DA, Reis DJ (1985): Projections from the nucleus tractus solitarii to the rostral ventrolateral medulla. *J Comp Neurol* 242:511–534.

Satoh MA, Akaike, Takagi H (1979): Excitation by morphine and enkephalin of single neurons of nucleus reticularis paragigantocellularis in the rat: A probable mechanism of analgesic action of opioids. *Brain Res* 169:406–410.

Skultety FM (1963): Stimulation of periaqueductal gray and hypothalamus. *Arch Neurol* 8:38–50.

Sun M, Guyenet PG (1986): Effect of clonidine and γ-aminobutyric acid on the discharges of medullo-spinal sympathoexcitatory neurons in the rat. *Brain Res* 368:1–17.

Taber E (1961): The cytoarchitecture of the brain stem of the cat. I. Brain stem nuclei. *J Comp Neurol* 116:27–70.

Van Bockstaele EJ, Aston-Jones G, Pieribone VA, Ennis M, Shipley MT (in press): Subregions of the periaqueductal gray topographically innervate the rostral ventral medulla in the rat. *J Comp Neurol*

Van Bockstaele EJ, Pieribone VA, Aston-Jones G (1989): Diverse afferents converge on the nucleus paragigantocellularis in the rat ventrolateral medulla: Retrograde and anterograde studies. *J Comp Neurol* 290:561–584.

# 3
# Regulation of Autonomic Cardiovascular Function by the Rostral Ventromedial Medulla

KURT J. VARNER, ELISARDO C. VASQUEZ, STEPHEN J. LEWIS, BENEDITO H. MACHADO, CYNTHIA L. GROSSKREUTZ, JASON S. SIMON, AND MICHAEL J. BRODY

It is generally accepted that neural elements in the rostral ventral medulla (RVM) are essential for the neurogenic maintenance of arterial pressure. In recent years, the source of vasomotor tone in RVM has been ascribed to a small region in the lateral RVM lying just caudal to the posterior pole of the facial nucleus. This region, referred to as the rostral ventrolateral medulla (RVLM), contains a group of bulbospinal neurons responsible for the maintenance of sympathetic vasomotor tone in a variety of species (Barman and Gebber, 1985; Brown and Guyenet, 1985; Morrison et al., 1988; Ross et al., 1984a). These neurons are also reported to play significant roles in a number of cardiovascular and somatosympathetic reflex responses (Dampney and Moon, 1980; Granata et al., 1985; Morrison and Reis, 1989). Recent evidence suggests that the rostral medulla contains other subregions involved in the maintenance of neurogenic vasomotor tone, which also play unique roles in the tonic and reflex regulation of cardiovascular function.

Our laboratory has recently identified and begun to characterize a novel cardiovascular control region in the medial RVM, an area we have designated the rostral ventromedial medulla (RVMM). In the rat, the RVMM is centered in the gigantocellular nucleus approximately 1 mm lateral to the midline, 1.5 mm dorsal to the ventral surface, and extending from the rostral pole of the facial nucleus caudally into the ventral gigantocellular nucleus. Anatomical studies show this region to contain many bulbospinal neurons projecting to the intermediolateral nucleus in the spinal cord (Ross et al., 1984b). These bulbospinal neurons, especially those in more ventral regions, contain several transmitters including serotonin, substance P, and thyrotropin-releasing hormone (Bowker et al., 1981; Helke et al., 1986; Johansson et al., 1981; Loewy and McKellar, 1981).

In urethane-anesthetized rats bilateral inactivation of either RVMM or RVLM using microinjections of the local anesthetic lidocaine elicits equal and marked reductions in arterial pressure (Cox and Brody, 1989a; Varner et al., 1989). Combined bilateral anesthesia of RVLM and RVMM virtually eliminates the neurogenic contribution to the maintenance of arterial pressure (Varner et al., 1989). Evidence that RVMM contains the cell bodies of neurons capable of influencing cardiovascular tone is provided by microinjection studies. The microinjection of excitatory amino acids such as L-glutamate, N-methyl-D-aspartic acid (NMDA), and D,L-homocysteic acid into RVMM increases arterial pressure (Brody et al., 1990; Minson et al., 1987; Yardley et al., 1989). Conversely, microinjections of the inhibitory transmitters gamma-aminobutyric acid (GABA) or glycine into RVMM can elicit reductions in arterial pressure (Varner et al., unpublished results; Yardley et al., 1989).

Although RVLM and RVMM appear to be equally involved in the maintenance of neurogenic vascular tone in the anesthetized rat, several studies from our laboratory have shown that these two regions have different roles in the regulation of cardiovascular function. These differences are summarized below.

## Control of Regional Vascular Resistances

Cox and Brody (1989a,b) using lidocaine microinjections and electrical stimulation demonstrated that RVLM and RVMM differentially control regional vascular resistances. Local anesthesia of RVMM or RVLM elicits similar falls in renal and mesenteric vascular resistance and arterial pressure. However, the fall in hindquarter vascular resistance produced by blocking RVMM is significantly larger than that seen with block of RVLM. Electrical stimulation of RVLM and RVMM elicit equivalent graded increases in arterial pressure. However, the increase in renal vascular resistance tended to be larger with stimulation of RVLM, whereas stimulation of RVMM elicits a much greater increase in hindquarter vascular resistance. The pressor and hemodynamic responses elicited by electrical stimulation of RVLM are partially attenuated by the microinjection of lidocaine into RVMM. In contrast, responses evoked by stimulation of RVMM are not affected by inactivation of RVLM. These data indicate that the integrity of RVMM is required for the full expression of the cardiovascular responses elicited by stimulation of RVLM. A similar conclusion was reached by Minson and coworkers (1987), who demonstrated that an electrolytic lesion of a site corresponding to RVLM fails to attenuate the pressor response elicited by microinjection of L-glutamate into a more medial site.

## Influence of Respiratory Tidal Volume

The contribution of RVLM and RVMM to the maintenance of arterial pressure are differentially influenced by changes in respiratory tidal volume (Cox and Brody, 1989b). In urethane-anesthetized rats ventilated with a normal tidal volume (2.5 ml), bilateral microinjection of lidocaine into RVLM elicits marked falls in arterial pressure, vascular resistances, and renal sympathetic nerve activity (RSNA). With reduced tidal volume (1.5 ml), however, the magnitude of the decreases are significantly reduced. Attenuation of the depressor responses by a reduction in tidal volume is abolished by vagotomy and stabilization of the chest wall with pneumothoracotomy. In contrast, hemodynamic responses elicited by the microinjection of lidocaine into RVMM are not altered by changes in respiratory tidal volume. These data suggest that changes in afferent signals arising from either pulmonary stretch receptors or chest wall proprioceptors alter the control of neurogenic vasomotor activity exerted by RVLM but not RVMM. These data also indicate that there must be multiple sources of centrally derived sympathetic activity since arterial pressure and sympathetic nerve activity were normal or above normal under conditions of reduced tidal volume, yet the contribution of RVLM to this activity was significantly attenuated.

## Control of Sympathetic Nerve Discharge

Varner and colleagues (1989) showed that RVMM and RVLM differentially control the activity recorded from individual sympathetic nerves. Bilateral microinjection of lidocaine into RVMM or RVLM elicits equal reductions in arterial pressure and RSNA. In contrast, inactivation of RVLM elicits significantly larger falls in lumbar chain sympathetic nerve activity (LSNA) and splanchnic (SSNA) sympathetic nerve activity than does inactivation of the RVMM. Combined inactivation of RVLM and RVMM virtually eliminates LSNA whereas approximately 30% of RSNA and SSNA remains. The residual RSNA remaining after combined inactivation of RVMM and RVLM is eliminated by ganglionic blockade, indicating that the remaining activity represents efferent and not afferent nerve traffic.

## Control of Heart Rate

It is well known that baroreceptor reflex-mediated decreases in heart rate involve the activation of parasympathetic vagal efferent pathways to the heart. The cardiac vagal preganglionic neurons mediating these responses originate in several brain stem nuclei. Anatomical and electrophysiological studies have shown that most parasympathetic vagal preganglionic neurons originate in the nucleus ambiguus (NA), dorsal motor nucleus of the vagus (DMX), and RVLM in a variety of species (cf. Spyer, 1981). Although controversial, most cardiac vagal neurons in the rat and cat are reported to originate in the NA, not the DMX (Contreras et al., 1980; McAllen and Spyer, 1976; Spyer, 1981; Stuesse, 1982). However, Machado and Brody (1988a,b) reported that chronic bilateral chemical or electrolytic lesion of

NA and portions of RVLM reduces baroreceptor reflex-mediated bradycardia in conscious rats by only 47%. Thus, it is apparent that other sources
of parasympathetic neurons responsible for reflex-mediated reductions in
heart rate must exist. Several lines of evidence suggest that RVMM contains a substantial number of vagal preganglionic neurons.

In recent anatomical studies the retrograde tracer dyes True Blue or
Fluoro-Gold were injected into the pericardial sac. As expected, when
using a low volume of dye (20 nl, 5%) retrograde labeling is observed in the
NA and RVLM. However, when the volume of dye is increased (50–100
nl, 5%) retrogradely labeled cells are also observed in RVMM (Brody et
al., 1990). Most retrogradely labeled neurons in RVMM are concentrated
in the rostral portions of RVMM. Unilateral vagotomy virtually abolished
labeling in the ipsilateral NA, RVLM, and RVMM, whereas labeling on
the contralateral side is only slightly diminished, thus indicating that the
vast majority of the axons of these neurons course uncrossed in the vagus
nerve. Intrathoracic and intravenous injection of dye fail to produce
medullary labeling.

Immunocytochemical studies have shown neurons in the region of
RVMM to contain choline acetyltransferase (ChAT) (Brownstein and Palkovits, 1984), suggesting that some neurons in RVMM, like previously
identified parasympathetic neurons in NA or DMX, may use acetylcholine
as a transmitter.

Although equal increases in arterial pressure are elicited by electrical
stimulation of RVLM and RVMM, a significantly larger atropine-sensitive
bradycardia is elicited by stimulation of RVMM than from RVLM (Brody
et al., 1990; Grosskreutz, 1989). A similar pattern of results is observed in
response to electrical stimulation in sino-aortically deafferentated rats, suggesting that this response is not completely reflex in origin and involves the
direct activation of neural elements in RVMM (Brody et al., 1990). This
was confirmed using microinjections of NMDA. Microinjection of NMDA
into the rostral portions of RVMM (approximately 500 $\mu$m rostral to the
region producing the largest pressor responses) elicits a profound atropine-
sensitive bradycardia (up to 120 beats/min) occurring in the absence of or
preceded by 30 to 45 sec of any change in arterial pressure (Brody et al.,
1990). Sites in RVMM yielding bradycardic responses corresponded to the
location of the highest density of pericardially labeled neurons. Chemical
stimulation of caudal RVMM elicits primarily pressor responses and
associated reflex bradycardia.


## Control of Baroreceptor and Cardiopulmonary
## Reflex Function

In anesthetized rats RVLM is reported to be involved in mediating the
depressor response to baroreceptor and cardiopulmonary reflex activation

(Granata et al., 1985; Grosskreutz, 1989). Electrophysiological studies have shown bulbospinal neurons in RVLM to receive tonic baroreceptor input and decrease their discharge rate in response to baroreceptor reflex activation (Barman and Gebber, 1985; Brown and Guyenet, 1985; Morrison et al., 1988). Similarly, RVMM also appears to be involved in baroreceptor reflex function. Grosskreutz (1989) reported that acute bilateral kainic acid lesion of RVMM in urethane-anesthetized rats prevents baroreceptor reflex-mediated responses to aortic constriction. Recently, we reported that in barbiturate-anesthetized rats, NMDA-induced lesion of neurons in RVLM or RVMM blocks the development of neurogenic hypertension in response to acute sino-aortic deafferentation (Varner et al., 1990). Bilateral inactivation of RVMM or RVLM using microinjection of lidocaine in urethane-anesthetized rats attenuates cardiopulmonary reflex-mediated decreases in heart rate elicited by the intravenous injection of serotonin (5-HT) (Vasquez et al., in press).

In conscious rats RVLM and RVMM appear to differentially control baroreceptor and cardiopulmonary reflex function. In our studies chronically lesioned neurons in RVMM or RVLM with bilateral microinjections of NMDA (10–15 nmol, 100–150 nl) (Varner et al., 1990; Vasquez et al., 1990). Baroreceptor reflex function was assessed in conscious freely moving rats by examining the magnitude of reflex-mediated heart rate changes in response to changes in arterial pressure. Sigmoidal curve-fitting analysis was used to construct baroreceptor reflex curves (Lewis et al., 1989). Bilateral lesions of RVLM significantly reduce baroreceptor reflex gain and virtually abolish reflex-mediated increases in heart rate. Administration of atropine and atenolol revealed that the abolition of reflex tachycardia results from impairment of both the sympathetic activation and vagal withdrawal components of the reflex (Varner et al., 1990). In contrast, lesion of RVMM did not alter reflex gain or reflex tachycardia; rather, these lesions significantly attenuate the ability to elicit reflex bradycardia in response to increases in arterial pressure. Administration of atropine and then atenolol verified that the attenuated bradycardic responses reflect a decrease in parasympathetic vagal function (Varner et al., 1990). The initial impairment of baroreceptor reflex function in both lesion groups returns to control within 7 days postlesion.

Cardiopulmonary reflex function was assessed in conscious rats by examining the magnitude of the Bezold-Jarisch reflex-mediated decrease in heart rate in response to the intravenous administration of 5-HT, which is thought to activate directly cardiopulmonary afferent fibers. Lesions of RVLM significantly enhance the bradycardic response to 5-HT, suggesting that under normal conditions RVLM actively inhibits cardiopulmonary heart rate reflex responses. In contrast, lesions of RVMM significantly attenuate the heart rate response to 5-HT, suggesting that these lesions impair the ability to activate cardiac vagal preganglionic neurons. The bradycardic response to 5-HT in RVLM lesion rats recovers within 7 days.

However, in rats with lesions of RVMM the bradycardic responses remained attenuated 7 days after the lesion.

After 1 day, resting mean arterial pressure is significantly reduced in rats with lesions of RVLM but not in rats with lesions of RVMM (Vasquez et al., 1990). Arterial pressure returns to control levels within 7 days in rats with lesions of RVLM. Resting heart rate is not significantly different in either the RVLM or RVMM lesion groups. Similar results were obtained by Cochrane and Nathan (1989), who reported that large electrolytic lesions of RVLM in rats only temporarily (for 2 days) reduce arterial pressure. In contrast, Dormer and Bedford (1989) reported that unilateral lesions of RVLM in dogs made by microinjecting kainic acid significantly lower arterial pressure for up to 3 weeks.


## Conclusion

On the basis of our studies it is apparent that RVMM in the rat is a unique and functionally important cardiovascular control region that is functionally quite different from RVLM. The presence of multiple cardiovascular control regions, each with unique functional characteristics, raises numerous fundamental questions about the complexities of cardiovascular control under a variety of behavioral, physiological, and pathophysiological conditions.


## References

Barman SM, Gebber GL (1985): Axonal projection patterns of ventrolateral medullospinal sympathoexcitatory neurons. *J Neurophysiol* 3(6):1551–1566.

Bowker RM, Steinbusch HWM, Coulter JD (1981): Serotonergic and peptidergic projections to the spinal cord demonstrated by a combined retrograde HRP histochemical and immunocytochemical staining method. *Brain Res* 211:412–417.

Brody MJ, Varner KJ, Lewis SJ, Machado B, Grosskreutz CL, Simon JS, Rashkin J (1990): Are vagal preganglionic neurons located in rostral ventromedial medulla (RVMM) of rat? *FASEB J* 4(3):A556.

Brown DL, Guyenet PG (1985): Electrophysiological study of cardiovascular neurons in the rostral ventrolateral medulla in rats. *Circ Res* 56:359–369.

Brownstein MJ, Palkovits M (1984): Catecholamines, serotonin, acetylcholine and γ-aminobutyric acid in the rat brain. In: *Handbook of Chemical Neuroanatomy, Vol. II(1)*, Bjorklund A, Hokfelt T, eds. Amsterdam: Elsevier.

Cochrane KL, Nathan M (1989): Normotension in conscious rats after placement of bilateral electrolytic lesions in the rostral ventrolateral medulla. *J Auton Nerv Syst* 26:199–211.

Contreras RJ, Gomez MM, Norgren R (1980): Central origins of cranial nerve parasympathetic neurons in the rat. *J Comp Neurol* 190:373–394.

Cox BF, Brody MJ (1989a): Subregions of rostral ventral medulla control arterial pressure and regional hemodynamics. *Am J Physiol* 257:R635–R640.

Cox BF, Brody MJ (1989b): Mechanisms of respiration-induced changes in vasomotor control exerted by RVLM. *Am J Physiol* 257:R626–R634.

Dampney RAL, Moon EA (1980): Role of ventrolateral medulla in vasomotor response to cerebral ischemia. *Am J Physiol* 239:H349–H358.

Dormer KJ, Bedford TG (1989): Cardiovascular control by the rostral ventrolateral medulla in the conscious dog. In: *Progress in Brain Research*, Ciriello J, Caverson MM, Polosa C, eds. Amsterdam: Elsevier.

Granata AR, Ruggiero DA, Park DH, Joh TH, Reis DJ (1985): Brain stem area with C1 epinephrine neurons mediates baroreflex vasodepressor responses. *Am J Physiol* 248:H547–H567.

Grosskreutz CL (1989): *Characterization of Subregions of the Ventral Portion of the Rostral Medulla Oblongata in Neural Control of Arterial Pressure*. Doctoral thesis, University of Iowa.

Helke CJ, Sayson SC, Keeler JR, Charlton CG (1986): Thyrotropin-releasing hormone-immunoreactive neurons project from the ventral medulla to the intermediolateral cell column: Partial coexistence with serotonin. Brain Res 381:1–7.

Johansson O, Hokfelt T, Pernow B, et al. (1981): Immunohistochemical support for three putative transmitters in one neuron: Co-existence of 5 hydroxytryptamine, substance P, and thyrotropin releasing hormone-like immunoreactivity in medullary neurons projecting to the spinal cord. *Neuroscience* 6:1857–1881.

Lewis SJ, Verberne AJM, Robinson T, Beart PM, Jarrott B (1989): Excitotoxin (NMDA)-induced lesions of the central but not the basolateral nucleus of the amygdala modulate the baroreceptor heart rate reflex in conscious rats. *Brain Res* 494:232–240.

Loewy AD, McKellar S (1981): Serotonergic projections from the ventral medulla to the intermediolateral cell column in the rat. *Brain Res* 211:146 - 152.

Machado BH, Brody MJ (1988a): Effect of nucleus ambiguus lesion on the development of neurogenic hypertension. *Hypertension* 11(suppl I): I-135–I-138.

Machado BH, Brody MJ (1988b): Role of the nucleus ambiguus in the regulation of heart rate and arterial pressure. *Hypertension* 11:602–607.

McAllen RM, Spyer KM (1976): The location of cardiac vagal preganglionic motoneurons in the medulla of the cat. *J Physiol (Lond)* 258:187–204.

Minson JB, Chalmers JP, Caon AC, Renaud B (1987): Separate areas of rat medulla oblongata with populations of serotonin- and adrenalin-containing neurons alter blood pressure after L-glutamate stimulation. *J Auton Nerv Syst* 19:39–50.

Morrison SF, Milner TA, Reis DJ (1988): Reticulospinal vasomotor neurons of the rat rostral ventrolateral medulla: Relationship to sympathetic nerve activity and the C1 adrenergic cell group. *J Neurosci* 8(4):1286–1301.

Morrison SF, Reis DJ (1989): Reticulospinal vasomotor neurons in the RVL mediate the somatosympathetic reflex. *Am J Physiol* 256:R1084–R1097.

Ross CA, Ruggiero DA, Joh TJ, Park DH, Reis DJ (1984b): Rostral ventrolateral medulla: Selective projections to the thoracic autonomic cell column from the region containing C1 adrenaline neurons. *J Comp Neurol* 288:168–185.

Ross CA, Ruggiero DA, Park DH, et al. (1984a): Tonic vasomotor control by the rostral ventrolateral medulla: Effect of electrical or chemical stimulation of the area containing C1 adrenaline neurons on arterial pressure, heart rate and plasma catecholamines and vasopressin. *J Neurosci* 4(2):474–494.

Spyer KM (1981): Neural organization and control of the baroreceptor reflex. *Rev Physiol Biochem Pharmacol* 88:24–124.

Stuesse SL (1982): Origins of cardiac vagal preganglionic fibers: A retrograde transport study. *Brain Res* 236:15–25.

Varner KJ, Grosskreutz CL, Cox BF, Brody MJ (1989): Differential regulation of sympathetic nerve activity by lateral and medial subregions of the rostral ventral medulla. In: *Progress in Brain Research*, Ciriello J, Caverson MM, Polosa C, eds. Amsterdam: Elsevier.

Varner KJ, Vasquez EC, Brody MJ (1990): Chemical lesion of rostral ventrolateral (RVLM) or ventromedial (RVMM) medulla prevents neurogenic hypertension. *Soc Neurosci Abst* 16:298.

Varner KJ, Vasquez EC, Lewis SJ, Brody MJ (1990): Cardiovascular reflex effects of chronic lesions of rostral ventrolateral (RVLM) and rostral ventromedial (RVMM) medulla in rats. *FASEB J* 4(3):A557.

Vasquez EC, Varner KJ, Lewis SJ, Brody MJ (1990): Chronic N-methyl-D-aspartic acid (NMDA) lesions of neurons in rostral ventrolateral (RVLM) and rostral ventromedial medulla (RVMM). *FASEB J* 4(3):A557.

Vasquez EC, Lewis SJ, Varner KJ, Brody MJ (in press): Lesions of the rostral ventrolateral (RVLM) but not rostral ventromedial medulla (RVMM) attenuate 5-HT-induced reflex tachycardia. *FASEB J*.

Yardley CP, Andrade JM, Weaver LC (1989): Evaluation of cardiovascular control by neurons in the dorsal medulla of rats. *J Auton Nerv Syst* 29:1–12.

# 4
# Flexibility of the Map of Brainstem Neurons with Sympathetic Nerve-Related Activity

MICHAEL J. KENNEY, SUSAN M. BARMAN, BERNAT KOCSIS, AND GERARD L. GEBBER

Recent work from this laboratory (Barman and Gebber, 1987, 1989; Gebber and Barman, 1985) supports the view that medullary lateral tegmental field (LTF) neurons are contained in circuits responsible for basal sympathetic nerve discharge (SND). The naturally occurring activity of LTF neurons located in nucleus reticularis parvocellularis (R.pc.) and nucleus reticularis ventralis (R.v.) are correlated to the cardiac-related rhythm in postganglionic SND of baroreceptor-innervated cats anesthetized with diallylbarbiturate-urethane (DU) or its free-running 2-Hz to 6-Hz counterpart after baroreceptor denervation. These neurons fire earlier during the cardiac-related or 2-Hz to 6-Hz burst of SND than bulbospinal sympathoexcitatory neurons located in the rostral ventrolateral medulla (RVLM). Moreover, the axons of the earlier firing LTF neurons project to the region of the RVLM containing sympathoexcitatory neurons that innervate the thoracic spinal intermediolateral nucleus (IML). These observations have led us to propose that bulbospinal sympathoexcitatory neurons of the RVLM receive important driving inputs from the LTF (Barman and Gebber, 1987, 1989).

This chapter discusses the organization of medullary reticular circuits that control SND. We found that the map of LTF neurons with sympathetic nerve-related activity undergoes marked expansion when the animal is anesthetized with chloralose rather than with DU. Moreover, the discharge characteristics of LTF neurons in chloralose-anesthetized cats differed markedly from those of LTF neurons in DU-anesthetized cats. The anesthetic-dependent differences appear to be related to changes in forebrain and baroreceptor inputs to LTF neurons and/or the responses of these neurons to these inputs. The data support the view that the brain stem reticular network controlling SND is a flexible ensemble of neurons capable of formulating a variety of output patterns.

## Methods

Experiments were performed on baroreceptor-innervated cats anesthetized with alpha-chloralose (40–50 mg/kg, i.v.) after initial sedation with ketamine hydrochloride (10 mg/kg, im). The animals were paralyzed (gallamine triethiodide, 4 mg/kg, i.v., initial dose), artificially respired, and bilaterally pneuzmothoracotomized. As previously described (Barman and Gebber, 1987; Gebber and Barman, 1985), extracellular unit recordings were made with metal or glass microelectrodes from medullary neurons and the activity of the postganglionic inferior cardiac sympathetic nerve was recorded monophasically with bipolar platinum electrodes after capacity-coupled preamplification with a bandpass of 1 to 1000 Hz. Bursts of multiunit activity in the inferior cardiac nerve are displayed as slow waves (i.e., envelopes of spikes) when this wide bandpass is used. The frontal-parietal electroencephalogram (EEG) was recorded monophasically with a preamplifier bandpass of 1 to 1000 Hz. Brachial arterial pressure and the electrocardiogram (lead II) were recorded by using standard techniques.

The relationships among medullary unit activity, SND, the EEG, and the cardiac cycle were analyzed in the time and frequency domains. Time-domain methods included spike-triggered averaging, arterial pulse-triggered analysis, interspike interval analysis, and post-stimulus averaging (see Methods in Barman and Gebber, 1987; Gebber and Barman, 1985). Frequency-domain methods included autospectral and coherence analyses (see Methods in Gebber et al., 1990; Kocsis et al., 1990).

Baroreceptor reflex activation was accomplished by inflating the balloon-tipped end of a Fogarty embolectomy catheter placed in the thoracic aorta near the level of the diaphragm. Arterial pressure was increased proximal to the point of aortic obstruction, thus increasing afferent baroreceptor nerve activity (Barman and Gebber, 1987).

Decerebration was performed by transection of the midbrain at stereotaxic plane A3 (Huang et al., 1987). The completeness and level of transection were assessed by visual inspection of the brain at the end of each experiment. The brain stem was removed and fixed in 10% buffered formaldehyde. Frontal sections of 30-$\mu$m thickness were cut and stained with cresyl violet. The sites of brain stem unit recording were identified with reference to the bottom of the electrode tracks and the stereotaxic planes of Berman (1968).

Values in the text and tables are means ± standard errors. Means were compared by using the student's $t$ test for unpaired data. Statistical significance was indicated by $p < 0.05$.

# Results

## *Relationships among SND, EEG, and Cardiac Cycle in Chloralose-Anesthetized Cat*

Figure 4.1 depicts the relationships among SND, the EEG, and the cardiac cycle in a baroreceptor-innervated cat anesthetized with chloralose. Raw records of the three signals are shown in panel A. The results obtained with frequency-domain analysis are shown in panel B. Most of the power in the autospectra of SND and the EEG was contained below 6 Hz, whereas the autospectra of the arterial pulse (AP) contained a sharp peak at the frequency (4.1 Hz) of the heart rate. Each of the coherence functions (i.e., normalized cross-spectra) shows how linear correlation of two of the signals varies as a function of frequency. A coherence value of 1.0 indicates perfect coherence between two signals whereas a value of zero signifies the lack of a relationship. If the coherence value is significantly different from zero (see below) but less than unity, one or more of three situations exists (Bendat and Piersol, 1966): 1) the two signals have common and uncommon sources, 2) noise is present in the signals, or 3) the system relating the two signals is not linear. In the experiment illustrated in Fig. 4.1, SND and the EEG were related at frequencies between 1.5 and 5 Hz. The peak coherence value was 0.24 at 3.7 Hz. This relationship reflects a descending influence of forebrain delta slow wave generators on SND (Kenney et al., 1990). SND also contained a cardiac-related component as shown by the peak at 4.1 Hz in the AP → SND coherence function. The AP → EEG coherence function shows that these signals were not related.

The relationships among the three signals in chloralose-anesthetized cats (as reflected by peak coherence values) are summarized in Table 4.1. The 95% confidence intervals of Benignus (1969, 1970) were used as a test of zero coherence in individual experiments. According to Benignus, coherence values of 0.04 (32–63 windows averaged) and 0.02 (>64 windows) signify a statistically significant relationship between two signals. Table 4.1 shows that SND was related to the EEG in chloralose-anesthetized cats. In contrast, these two signals are unrelated when the animal is anesthetized with DU (Gebber et al., 1990; see Table 4.1). Table 4.1 also shows that the cardiac-related component of SND is weaker in chloralose-anesthetized cats than in DU-anesthetized cats (Gebber et al., 1990). This was the case even though mean arterial pressure in chloralose-anesthetized cats (118 ± 8 mm Hg) was the same as in DU-anesthetized cats (117 ± 6 mm Hg). The EEG and arterial pressure were unrelated in chloralose-anesthetized or DU-anesthetized cats (Gebber et al., 1990) (Table 4.1).

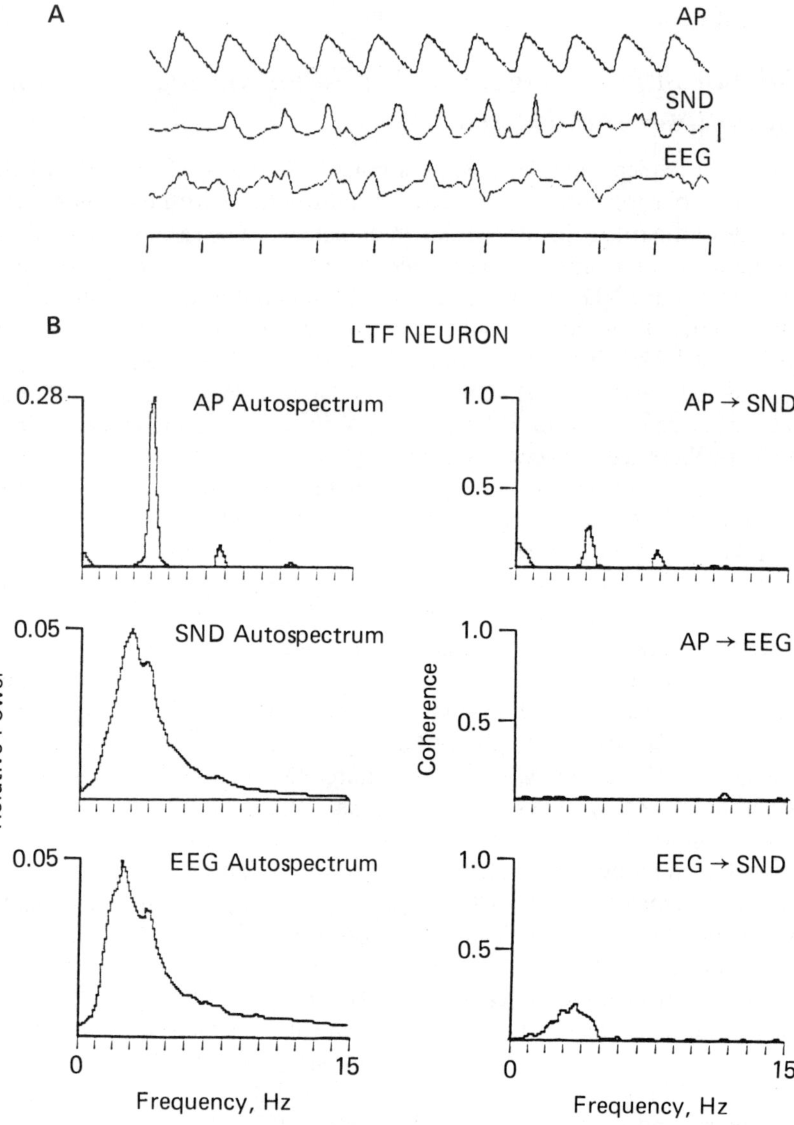


FIGURE 4.1. Relationships among arterial pulse (AP), inferior cardiac sympathetic nerve discharge (SND), and frontal-parietal cortical activity (EEG) in a chloralose-anesthetized cat. **A**: Oscilloscopic records. Vertical calibration (amplified signals) is 90 mV for SND and 55 mV for EEG. Time base is 300 msec/division. **B**: Records in left column show autospectrum of each signal. The values of relative power when multiplied by 100 equal the percentage of total power in the bin containing the peak frequency. Records in right column are coherence functions. The spectra are based on 155 5-sec windows. Frequency resolution is 0.2 Hz/bin in this and subsequent figures. The 95% confidence interval signifying a coherence value significantly different from zero is 0.02.

TABLE 4.1. Relationships among sympathetic nerve discharge (SND), frontal-parietal cortical activity (EEG), and the arterial pulse (AP) in chloralose-anesthetized and diallylbarbiturate-urethane (DU)-anesthetized cats.

| | | EEG → SND | AP → SND[a] | AP → EEG |
|---|---|---|---|---|
| A. | Chloralose anesthesia (n = 34) | | | |
| | Peak coherence value | 0.17 ± 0.02 | 0.29 ± 0.04 | 0 |
| | Peak coherent frequency, Hz | 2.37 ± 0.24 | 3.40 ± 0.17 | — |
| B. | DU anesthesia (n = 16) | EEG → SND | AP → SND[a] | AP → EEG |
| | Peak coherence value | 0 | 0.90 ± 0.10[b] | 0 |
| | Peak coherent frequency, Hz | — | 3.34 ± 0.17 | — |

[a] Mean arterial pressure was not significantly different in chloralose-anesthetized and DU-anesthetized cats (see text).
[b] Significantly different ($p < 0.05$) from corresponding value in chloralose-anesthetized cats.
0 indicates that the peak coherence value in individual experiments was not significantly different from zero.
The data from DU-anesthetized cats are from Gebber et al. (1990).

## Medullary Neurons with Sympathetic Nerve-Related Activity in Chloralose-Anesthetized Cats

In chloralose-anesthetized cats, the naturally occurring discharges of 129 of 261 neurons located in the medullary LTF and adjoining nucleus reticularis gigantocellularis (R.gc.) were correlated to inferior cardiac SND and the frontal-parietal EEG. Figure 4.2 shows the results obtained with time-domain analyses for two such neurons. The spike-triggered averages in panels IA and IIA show SND and cortical activity that preceded and followed unit discharge at zero lag. Unit activity was considered to be related to SND or the EEG when the amplitude of the peak closest to zero lag in the spike-triggered average was at least three times that of the largest deflection appearing in the "dummy" average of the same signal. "Dummy" averages of SND and the EEG (not shown in Fig. 4.2) were constructed using a random series of triggers in place of the unit spike train. On average, peak activity in the inferior cardiac nerve was reached 115 ± 5 msec (n = 47) after the discharges of rostral LTF and adjacent R.gc. neurons, and 107 ± 3 msec (n = 82) after the discharges of caudal LTF neurons (anatomical distributions to be described). These values were not significantly different from each other or from that reported for caudal LTF neurons in DU-anesthetized cats (Barman and Gebber, 1987; Gebber and Barman, 1985). The cortical event correlated to LTF unit activity usually began before the reference spike used to construct the average. This was the case for both examples in Figure 4.2 where the peak of the cortical event was almost coincident with LTF unit spike occurrence.

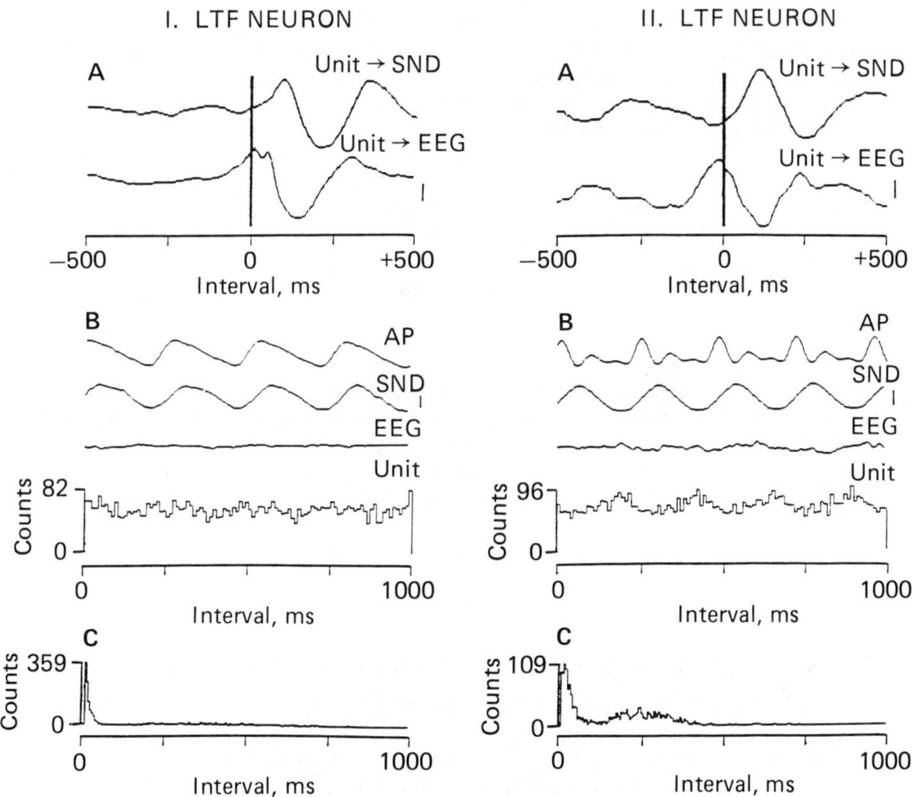


FIGURE 4.2. Time-domain relationships among rostral lateral tegmental field (LTF) unit activity, SND, EEG, and AP. I and II show data for different LTF neurons. Data in I are from same experiment illustrated in Fig. 4.1. **IA, IIA**: Spike-triggered averages of SND and EEG (1509 reference spikes in IA, 1726 reference spikes in IIA). Bin width, 5 msec. Vertical calibration (amplified signals) is 90 mV (IA) and 110 mV (IIA) for SND and 50 mV (IA) and 65 mV (IIA) for EEG. **IB, IIB**: Arterial pulse-triggered averages of AP, SND, EEG, and histogram of LTF unit spike occurrences (1760 reference pulses in IB and 1335 reference pulses in IIB). Bin width is 5 msec for averages and 10 msec for histograms. Vertical calibration is 110 mV (IB) and 190 mV (IIB) for SND and EEG. **IC, IIC**: Interspike interval histograms for LTF neurons. Number of counts is 2420 in IC and 1722 in IIC. Bin width, 5 msec.

Arterial pulse-triggered averaging (Fig. 4.2IB, IIB) revealed a cardiac-related component in SND. This was not unexpected in view of the results obtained with coherence analysis (Table 4.1). Nevertheless, less than 10% of the LTF and R.gc. neurons with sympathetic nerve-related activity exhibited cardiac-related discharges. In such cases, the relationship was weak. That is, the cardiac-related peak in the arterial pulse-triggered histogram of unit activity barely rose above background level (Fig. 4.2IIB).

LTF and R.gc. neurons in chloralose-anesthetized cats fired in high frequency bursts with interspike intervals as short as 3 to 10 msec. The bursts were manifested by a peak close to the origin of the interspike interval histograms for these neurons (Fig. 4.2IC, IIC). The high frequency bursts generated by LTF and R.gc. neurons were irregularly spaced, that is, these neurons missed firing in a variable number of cycles of SND. This was

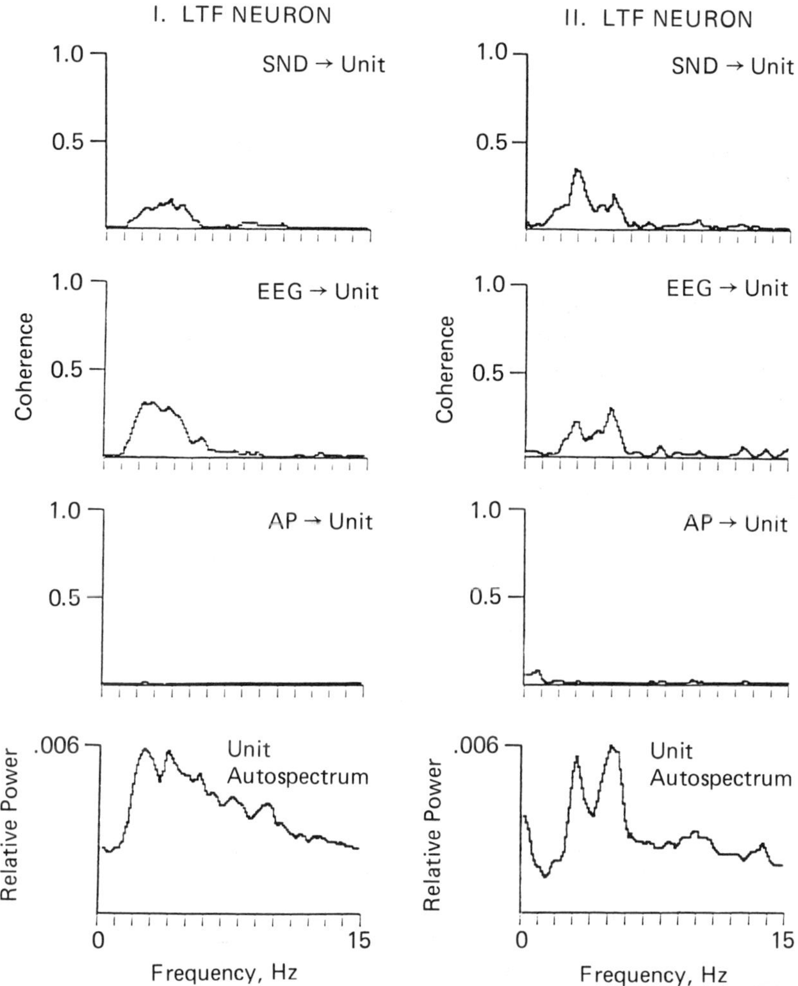


FIGURE 4.3. Frequency-domain relationships among rostral LTF unit activity, SND, EEG, and AP. Data in I, II are for same neurons in Fig. 4.2I, II. Coherence functions are based on 155 (**I**) and 62 (**II**) 5-sec windows. The 95% confidence interval signifying a coherence value significantly different from zero is 0.02. Bottom trace in **I**, **II** is LTF unit autospectrum based on same number of windows as for corresponding coherence functions.

indicated by the long-tailed densities in the interspike interval histograms.

Coherence analysis was used to quantify the linear relationships among LTF or R.gc. unit activity, SND, the EEG, and the cardiac cycle. Examples are shown in Figure 4.3. LTF or R.gc. unit activity cohered to both SND and the EEG at frequencies between 1.5 and 6 Hz. In no case did coherence analysis reveal a relationship between LTF or R.gc. unit activity and the arterial pulse. The bottom panels in Figure 4.3 I and II show the autospectra of medullary unit activity. Note that peak power in the autospectra occurred in the frequency range over which unit activity cohered to SND and the EEG.

Table 4.2 summarizes the results obtained with coherence analysis for 34 LTF and R.gc. neurons in chloralose-anesthetized cats. The strength of the relationship between medullary unit activity and SND was not significantly different from that between unit activity and the EEG. The results for caudal LTF, rostral LTF, and R.gc. neurons were pooled since there was no indication that anatomical location dictated the strength of the relationships. Table 4.2 contains information from a previous study on caudal LTF neurons with sympathetic nerve-related activity in DU-anesthetized cats (Gebber et al., 1990). The activity of these neurons, unlike that of LTF and R.gc. neurons in chloralose-anesthetized cats, cohered to the arterial pulse but not to the EEG. LTF unit activity tended to be more strongly related to SND in DU-anesthetized than in chloralose-anesthetized cats. The coherence of LTF unit activity and SND in DU-anesthetized cats was strongest at the frequency of the heart rate.

Recordings were made from five RVLM neurons with sympathetic nerve-related activity in two baroreceptor-innervated cats anesthetized

TABLE 4.2. Relationships among medullary unit activity (LTF and R.gc.), sympathetic nerve discharge (SND), cortical activity (EEG), and the arterial pulse (AP) in chloralose-anesthetized and diallylbarbiturate-urethane (DU)-anesthetized cats.

| A. | Chloralose anesthesia (n = 34) | | | |
| --- | --- | --- | --- | --- |
| | | SND → Unit | EEG → Unit | AP → Unit |
| | Peak coherence value | $0.18 \pm 0.02$ | $0.21 \pm 0.02$ | 0[a] |
| | Peak coherent frequency, Hz | $2.98 \pm 0.22$ | $3.14 \pm 0.34$ | — |
| B. | DU anesthesia (n = 9) | | | |
| | | SND → Unit | EEG → Unit | AP → Unit |
| | Peak coherence value | $0.31 \pm 0.11$ | 0 | $0.34 \pm 0.11$ |
| | Peak coherent frequency, Hz | $3.29 \pm 0.20$ | — | $3.29 \pm 0.20$ |

[a] Post-R wave histograms of unit activity occasionally showed a weak cardiac relationship even though the AP → unit coherence value was not significantly different from zero.
0 indicates that the peak coherence value in individual experiments was not significantly different from zero.
The data from DU-anesthetized cats are from Gebber et al. (1990).

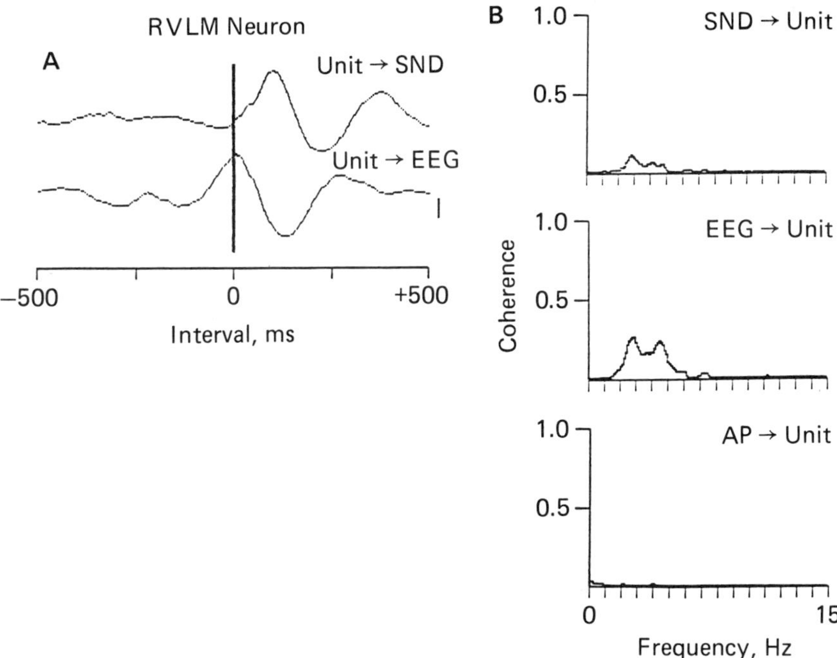


FIGURE 4.4. Time-domain and frequency-domain relationships among SND, EEG, AP, and discharges of a neuron in rostral ventrolateral medulla (RVLM). A: Spike-triggered average of SND and EEG (1278 reference spikes). Bin width, 5 msec. Vertical calibration (amplified signals) is 45 mV for SND and 30 mV for EEG. B: Coherence functions based on 102 5-sec windows. The 95% confidence interval signifying a coherence value significantly different from zero is 0.02.

with chloralose. These neurons were located in the region of the RVLM that contains sympathoexcitatory neurons with spinal axons innervating the thoracic IML (Barman and Gebber, 1985). Like LTF and R.gc. neurons in chloralose-anesthetized cats, the discharges of RVLM neurons cohered to SND and the EEG in the 2-Hz to 6-Hz band and had little or no cardiac-related activity. Similarly, they also fired in high frequency bursts that were irregularly spaced. The spike-triggered averages and coherence functions in Figure 4.4 depict the relationships among the discharges of one of these RVLM neurons, SND, the EEG, and the cardiac cycle.

## Anatomical Distribution of Medullary LTF and R.gc. Neurons

The anatomical distribution of LTF and R.gc. neurons with sympathetic and cortical-related activity in chloralose-anesthetized cats is shown in Figure 4.5. Such neurons were distributed in the LTF (R.pc. and R.v.) from

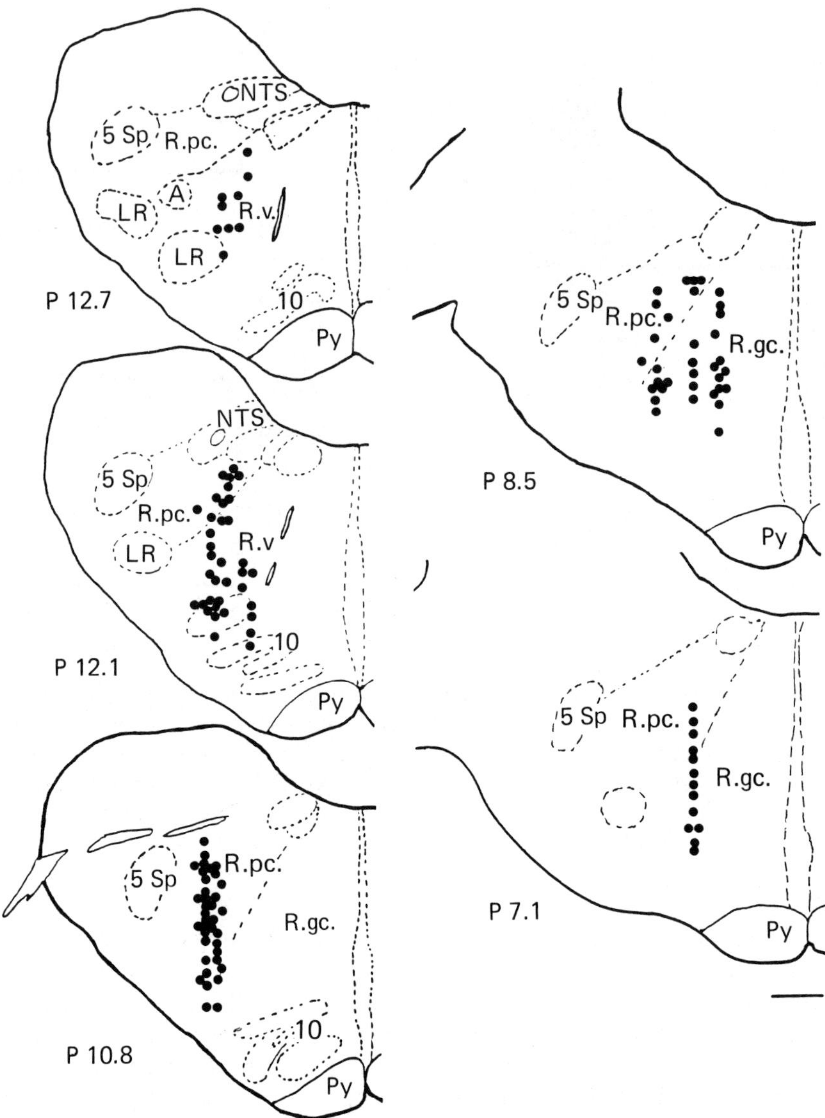



FIGURE 4.5. Anatomical distribution of LTF and R.gc. neurons with sympathetic nerve-related activity in chloralose-anesthetized cats. A, nucleus ambiguus; IO, inferior olive; LR, lateral reticular nucleus; NTS, nucleus of tractus solitarius; Py, pyramid; R.gc., nucleus reticularis gigantocellularis; R.pc., nucleus reticularis parvocellularis; R.v., nucleus reticularis ventralis; 5Sp, spinal nucleus of trigeminal nerve. Calibration is 1 mm.

a level just rostral to the obex (stereotaxic plane P12.7) to the ponto-medullary border (P7.1). In addition, neurons with sympathetic nerve-related activity were found in R.gc. between P8.5 and P7.1. In this chapter the LTF is partitioned into caudal (left side of Fig. 4.5) and rostral (right side of Fig. 4.5) divisions. The map of LTF and R.gc. neurons with sympathetic nerve-related activity in chloralose-anesthetized cats is quite different from that in DU-anesthetized cats. In DU-anesthetized cats, LTF neurons with sympathetic nerve-related activity are located only in the caudal division (Gebber and Barman, 1985). Moreover, the R.gc. did not contain neurons with sympathetic nerve-related activity in DU-anesthetized cats.

Whereas 47 of 97 neurons in the rostral LTF and adjoining R.gc. had sympathetic nerve-related activity in chloralose-anesthetized cats with an intact neuraxis, only 2 of 65 neurons in these regions had sympathetic

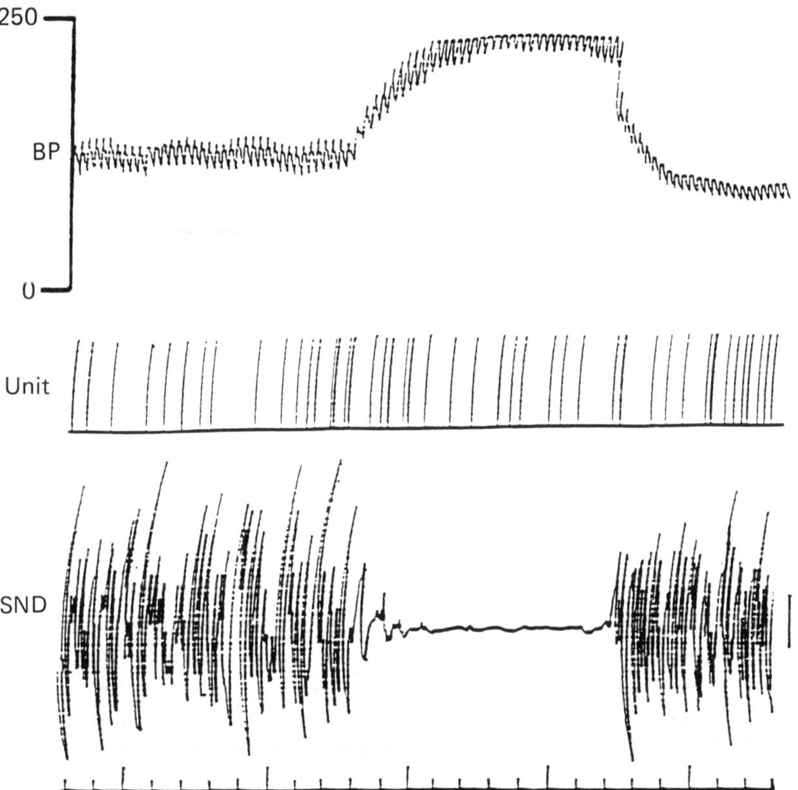


FIGURE 4.6. Baroreceptor reflex responses during rise in blood pressure proximal to aortic obstruction. Traces show (top to bottom) brachial arterial pressure (BP; mm Hg), standardized pulses derived from LTF unit action potentials and inferior cardiac SND. Vertical calibration is 100 $\mu$V. Time base is 1 sec/division.

nerve-related activity in chloralose-anesthetized decerebrate cats (four experiments).

## *Responses of LTF and R.gc. Neurons to Baroreceptor Reflex Activation*

Although LTF and R.gc. neurons with sympathetic nerve-related activity showed little or no cardiac-related activity in chloralose-anesthetized cats, 31 of 52 caudal LTF neurons responded to baroreceptor reflex activation. Their firing rates were either decreased ($3.4 \pm 0.7$ Hz to $1.2 \pm$

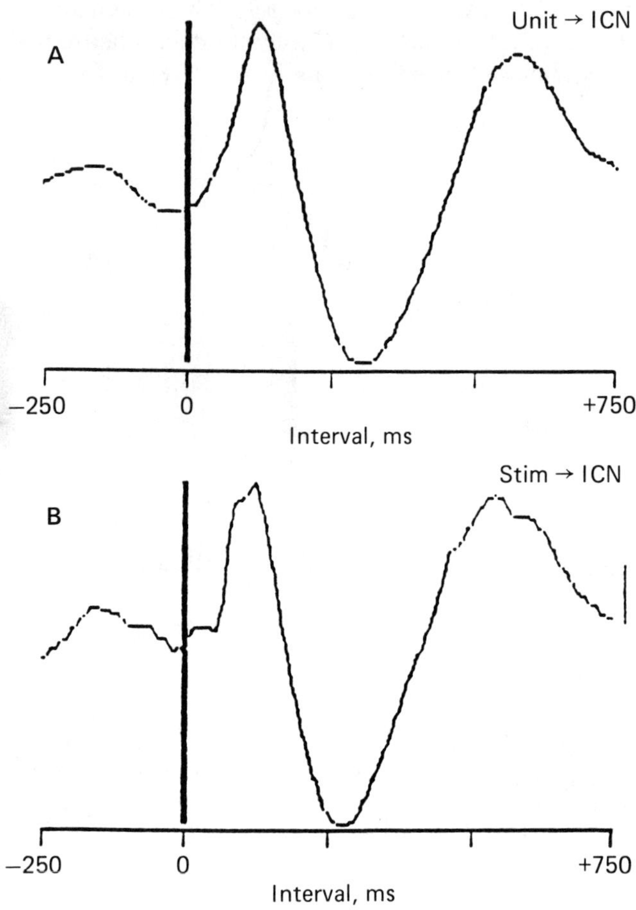


FIGURE 4.7. Spike-triggered and stimulus-triggered averages of inferior cardiac SND. **A**: Spike-triggered average (301 reference spikes) for a rostral LTF neuron. **B**: Stimulus-triggered average (75 reference stimuli). Stimulus (30 $\mu$A, 1 msec) was applied once every 2 sec at site of LTF unit recording. Bin width, 1 msec. Vertical calibration (amplified signals) is 110 mV for A and 100 mV for B.

0.5 Hz; n = 21) or increased (2.4 ± 0.4 Hz to 4.5 ± 0.8 Hz; n = 10) during
the reflex inhibition of SND accompanying the rise in blood pressure
produced by aortic obstruction. There was no anatomical segregation of
caudal LTF neurons on the basis of their response (or lack thereof) to
baroreceptor reflex activation. Only 2 of 15 rostral LTF and adjacent R.gc.
neurons with sympathetic nerve-related activity responded to baroreceptor
reflex activation. An example of a nonresponding rostral LTF neuron is
shown in Figure 4.6.

## Microstimulation of Rostral LTF and Adjoining R.gc

We compared the changes in inferior cardiac SND accompanying naturally
occurring rostral LTF or R.gc. unit activity with that produced by microstimulation at the site of unit recording. Single shocks (<40 $\mu$A) were
applied once every 2 sec through the recording microelectrode and the
sympathetic nerve responses produced by 75 such stimuli were averaged.
Microstimulation of rostral LTF and R.gc. recording sites invariably in-

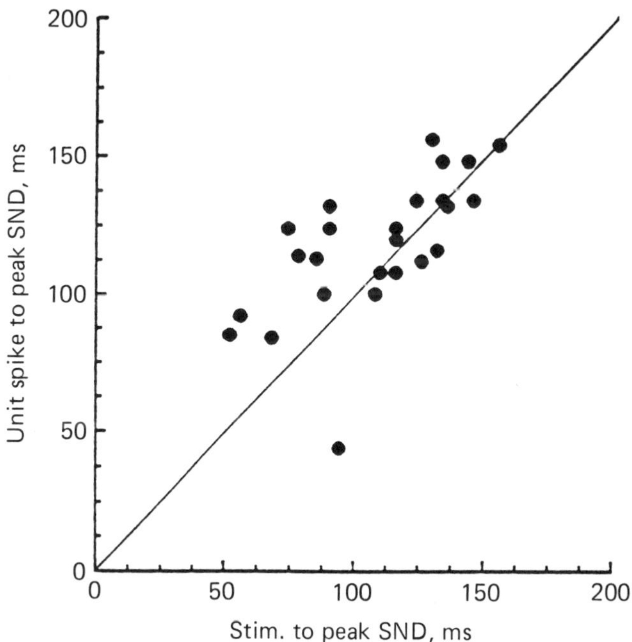


FIGURE 4.8. Comparison of changes in inferior cardiac SND accompanying rostral
LTF or R.gc. unit spike occurrence and those following an electrical stimulus applied at site of unit recording. Interval between unit spike occurrence and first peak
to right of zero lag in spike-triggered average of SND is plotted against that between stimulus and peak increase in SND (measured from stimulus-triggered average). The identity line appears in the plot.

creased SND. The results of one such experiment are illustrated in Figure 4.7. The contour of the sympathetic nerve response and its temporal relationship to the electrical stimulus were very similar to those of the sympathetic nerve waveform locked to spontaneously occurring LTF unit activity. The interval between unit spike occurrence and peak SND (measured from spike-triggered average) is plotted against that between the electrical stimulus and the peak of the increase in SND (measured from poststimulus average) in Figure 4.8. Each of the 25 data points represents a different unit recording site. The product-moment correlation-coefficient ($r = 0.66$) revealed that the two intervals were significantly related ($p < 0.001$).

## Neurons in Other Brain Stem Regions

As demonstrated with spike-triggered averaging, only 1 of 19 spontaneously active neurons in the midbrain periaqueductal gray and 1 of 14 neurons in the red nucleus (stereotaxic planes, A2–A3) of five chloralose-anesthetized cats had sympathetic nerve-related activity. On the other hand, 11 of 20 neurons located in the midbrain reticular formation between the periaqueductal gray and red nucleus had sympathetic nerve-related activity. The interval between the discharges of these 11 midbrain reticular neurons and peak SND was $119 \pm 8$ msec, a value not significantly different from those for caudal LTF or rostral LTF and adjacent R.gc. neurons.

## Discussion

The results of the current study demonstrate that the anatomical and functional features of the map of medullary reticular neurons with sympathetic nerve-related activity are altered when DU anesthesia is replaced by chloralose anesthesia. The following changes were noted. 1) The region containing such neurons was expanded from the caudal LTF and RVLM in DU-anesthetized cats into the rostral LTF and adjoining R.gc. of chloralose-anesthetized cats. 2) The percentage (49%) of LTF and R.gc. neurons with sympathetic nerve-related activity in chloralose-anesthetized cats exceeded that (28%) (Gebber and Barman, 1985) in the caudal LTF of DU-anesthetized cats. 3) In chloralose-anesthetized cats, LTF and R.gc. neurons had cortical-related and sympathetic nerve-related activity but little or no cardiac-related activity. Such was also the case for the few RVLM neurons sampled in the current study. In contrast, LTF and RVLM neurons with sympathetic nerve-related and cardiac-related activity in DU-anesthetized cats did not have cortical-related activity (Gebber et al., 1990). These relationships generally reflected those among SND, cortical activity, and the cardiac cycle (see Table 4.1). That is, SND and cortical activity were related in chloralose-anesthetized cats but not in DU-anesthetized cats with intact baroreceptor nerves (Barman and Gebber, 1981). Moreover, SND was more weakly correlated to the cardiac cycle in chloralose- than in DU-anesthetized cats. 4) LTF and RVLM neurons with sympathetic nerve-related activity in chloralose-anesthetized cats fired in high frequency bursts whereas their counterparts in DU-anesthetized cats (Gebber et al., 1990) rarely fired more than once in a cardiac cycle.

The expansion in number and anatomical distribution of medullary neurons with sympathetic nerve-related activity in chloralose-anesthetized cats is presumed to reflect at least two factors. The first factor is the forebrain-dependent component of SND that is prominent in chloralose-anesthetized but not in DU-anesthetized cats (Huang et al., 1987). Under chloralose anesthesia, LTF and R.gc. neurons may develop increased sensitivity to their forebrain inputs, thus accounting for their cortical-related and a variable proportion of their sympathetic nerve-related activity. Alternatively, or in addition, the level of activity in the forebrain inputs to LTF and R.gc. neurons may be higher in chloralose-anesthetized than in DU-anesthetized cats. It would not be surprising if the number and anatomical distribution of medullary neurons with sympathetic nerve-related activity were increased under these conditions. Our proposal (Kenney et al., 1990) that the coherence of SND to cortical activity reflects descending influences of forebrain delta slow wave generators is reinforced by the virtual absence of neurons with sympathetic nerve-related activity in the rostral LTF and adjoining R.gc. after decerebration in chloralose-anesthetized cats.

Impairment of baroreceptor reflex function may be a second factor involved in explaining the increase in number and anatomical distribution of medullary neurons with sympathetic nerve-related activity in chloralose-anesthetized cats. Although SND was effectively inhibited during the rise in blood pressure produced by aortic obstruction in chloralose-anesthetized cats, the cardiac-related component in SND was weak in the same preparations and few LTF and R.gc. neurons had cardiac-related activity. The latter two observations are consistent with the ability of chloralose to attenuate some types of central synaptic inhibition (Biscoe and Krnjevic, 1963; Marginelli et al., 1983).

There are at least three ways to explain the temporal relationship between rostral LTF or R.gc. unit activity and SND in chloralose-anesthetized cats. First, the relationship might reflect a role of such neurons in controlling SND. Second, inputs from the forebrain might act to synchronize the discharges of "nonsympathetic" rostral LTF and R.gc. neurons to sympathetic neurons located in other brain stem regions (e.g., caudal LTF, RVLM). Third, cross-talk between medullary neurons contained in different functional circuits might have resulted from chloralose-induced impairment of central inhibition. In the latter two cases, reticular circuits with different targets would function as a unit. The results obtained with microstimulation support the first possibility. We found that the interval between rostral LTF or R.gc. unit discharges and peak activity in the inferior cardiac nerve was correlated to that between an electrical stimulus applied to the site of unit recording and the peak of the evoked increase in SND. Moreover, the contour of the sympathetic nerve waveform correlated to rostral medullary unit firing was similar to that of the electrically evoked increase in SND. On this basis, we propose that at least some of the rostral LTF and adjoining R.gc. neurons with sympathetic nerve-related activity were contained in circuits that control SND. It is also worth noting that microinjection of homocysteic acid into the rostral LTF of the cat elicits pressor responses greater than 80 mm Hg (Lin et al., 1989).

Whereas the firing rate of most caudal LTF neurons was changed when blood pressure was raised by aortic obstruction in chloralose-anesthetized cats, only 2 of 15 rostral LTF and adjacent R.gc neurons with sympathetic nerve-related activity responded. Since SND was completely inhibited during baroreceptor reflex activation, the actions exerted by nonresponding LTF and R.gc. neurons in sympathetic circuits must have been gated at an output stage.

The midbrain periaqueductal gray and red nucleus were essentially devoid of neurons with sympathetic nerve-related activity in chloralose-anesthetized cats. In contrast, approximately 50% of the reticular neurons sampled at the same midbrain level showed sympathetic nerve-related activity. Microinjection of excitatory amino acids into the midbrain reticular formation is known to alter blood pressure and vascular resistance (Hilton and Redfern, 1986; Tan et al., 1983). Thus, the possibility exists that under chloralose anesthesia, the distribution of brain stem reticular neurons contributing to SND extends rostrally beyond the pontomedullary border.


## Summary

The results of the current study are consistent with the view that the brain stem reticular network controlling SND is a flexible ensemble of neurons capable of formulating a variety of output patterns. As such, the network can assume different anatomical configurations and functional characteristics. The different states of the network observed under chloralose versus DU anesthesia appear to be related to changes in forebrain and baroreceptor inputs to LTF and R.gc. neurons and/or the responses of these neurons to these inputs.

Our results are reminiscent of those from studies on the primary somatosensory cortex (Kaas et al., 1983; Rasmusson, 1982; Wall, 1988) and visual cortex (Kaas et al., 1990) in adult mammals. These studies demonstrated that the somatotopic map of the hand region and retinotopic maps of areas 17 and 18 change when their inputs are altered. Thus, brain maps are not fixed entities in the adult.

*Acknowledgments.*  The authors are grateful to Ms. Diane Hummel for typing the manuscript and to Ms. Afsar Sokhansanj and Mr. Sheng Zhong for technical assistance. This study was supported by National Heart, Lung, and Blood Institute grants HL13187 and HL33266.

# References


Barman SM, Gebber GL (1981): Brain stem neuronal types with activity patterns related to sympathetic nerve discharge. *Am J Physiol* 240:R335–R347.

Barman SM, Gebber GL (1985): Axonal projection patterns of ventrolateral medullospinal sympathoexcitatory neurons. *J Neurophysiol* 53:1551–1566.

Barman SM, Gebber GL (1987): Lateral tegmental field neurons of cat medulla: A source of basal activity of ventrolateral medullospinal sympathoexcitatory neurons. *J Neurophysiol* 57:1410–1424.

Barman SM, Gebber GL (1989): Basis for the naturally occurring activity of rostral ventrolateral medullary sympathoexcitatory neurons. *Prog Brain Res* 81:117–129.

Bendat JS, Piersol AG (1966): *Measurement and Analysis of Random Data.* New York: John Wiley & Sons.

Benignus VA (1969): Estimation of the coherence spectrum and its confidence interval using the Fast Fourier Transform. *IEEE Trans Audio Electroacoust* AU-17:145–150.

Benignus VA (1970): Correction to "Estimation of the coherence spectrum and its confidence interval using the Fast Fourier Transform." *IEEE Trans Audio Electroacoust* AU-18:320.

Berman AL (1968): *The Brain Stem of the Cat. A Cytoarchitectonic Atlas with Stereotaxic Coordinates.* Madison: University of Wisconsin Press.

Biscoe TN, Krnjevic K (1963): Chloralose and the activity of Renshaw cells. *Exp Neurol* 8:395–405.

Gebber GL, Barman SM (1985): Lateral tegmental field neurons of cat medulla: A potential source of basal sympathetic nerve discharge. *J Neurophysiol* 54:1498–1512.

Gebber GL, Barman SM, Kocsis B (1990): Coherence of medullary unit activity and sympathetic nerve discharge. *Am J Physiol* 259:R561– R571.

Hilton SM, Redfern WS (1986): A search for brain stem cell groups integrating the defence reaction in the rat. *J Physiol (Lond)* 378:213–228.

Huang Z-S, Gebber GL, Barman SM, Varner KJ (1987): Forebrain contribution to sympathetic nerve discharge in anesthetized cats. *Am J Physiol* 252:R645–R652.

Kaas JH, Krubitzer LA, Chino YM, Langston AL, Polley EH, Blair N (1990): Reorganization of retinotopic cortical maps in adult mammals after lesions of the retina. *Science* 248:229–231.

Kaas JH, Merzenich MM, Killackey HP (1983): The reorganization of somatosensory cortex following peripheral nerve damage in adult and developing mammals. Annu Rev Neurosci 6:325–356.

Kenney MJ, Gebber GL, Barman SM, Kocsis B (1990): Forebrain rhythm generators influence sympathetic activity in anesthetized cats. *Am J Physiol* 259: R572–R578.

Kocsis B, Gebber GL, Barman SM, Kenney MJ (1990): Relationships between activity of sympathetic nerve pairs: Phase and coherence. *Am J Physiol* 259:R549–R560.

Lin AMY, Wang Y, Kuo JS, Chai CY (1989): Homocysteic acid elicits pressor responses from ventrolateral medulla and dorsomedial medulla. *Brain Res Bull* 22:627–631.

Margnelli M, Marini G, Sotgiu ML (1983): The effect of $\alpha$-chloralose on inhibitory processes in the thalamic ventrobasal complex and in the spinal cord. In: *Somatosensory Integration in the Thalamus*, Macchi G, Rustioni A, Spreafico R, eds. Amsterdam: Elsevier.

Rasmusson DD (1982): Reorganization of raccoon somatosensory cortex following removal of the fifth digit. *J Comp Neurol* 205:313–326.

Tan E, Goodchild AK, Dampney RAL (1983): Intense vasoconstriction and bradycardia evoked by stimulation of neurones within the midbrain ventral tegmentum of the rabbit. *Clin Exp Pharmacol Physiol* 10:305–309.

Wall JT (1988): Variable organization in cortical maps of the skin as an indication of lifelong, adaptive capacities of circuits in the mammalian brain. *Trends Neurosci* 11:549–557.

# 5
# Imidazole Receptors and their Endogenous Ligand in the Rostral Ventrolateral Medulla: Relationship to the Action of Clonidine on Arterial Pressure

DONALD J. REIS, PAUL R. ERNSBERGER, AND MARY P. MEELEY

Over the past few years there has been increasing awareness that a restricted region of the brain residing in the rostral and ventrolateral medulla oblongata (RVL) contains neurons that act tonically to maintain a resting level of arterial pressure (AP) and to integrate many cardiovascular reflexes (Reis et al., 1988, 1989). Interestingly, this area appears to share pharmacological characteristics with the adjacent ventral surface of the medulla (VSM), a region that respiratory physiologists and neuropharmacologists, notably Feldberg and associates (Feldberg, 1986), have defined as a chemically sensitive area wherein neurotransmitters and drugs, including centrally active antihypertensive agents related to clonidine (Bousquet and Schwartz, 1983), act to control AP.

Several years ago Bousquet et al. (1984; see Bousquet et al., 1989) suggested, on indirect grounds, that the antihypertensive actions of clonidine related more to its structure as an imidazole than to its actions as an $\alpha_2$-adrenergic agonist. If indeed this hypothesis was correct, what was the evidence for imidazole receptors in this region? And, if imidazole receptors were of importance, what was their natural ligand? Could it be a purported substance isolated from brain by Atlas and Burstein (1984), clonidine-displacing substance (CDS), which they originally believed was a noncatecholaminergic agent binding to the $\alpha_2$-adrenergic receptor?

Over the past several years, we have been interested in the neurobiology of that region of the RVL involved in cardiovascular control. In particular, we have sought to: 1) assess whether the RVL is the central site of action of clonidine, 2) establish, by ligand binding methods, if the RVL truly contains imidazole receptors and if these are relevant to the hypotensive actions of clonidine and associated imidazoles, and 3) determine if CDS is present in RVL and possibly interacts with the receptors that recognize clonidine.

# The C1 Area of Rostral Ventrolateral Medulla:
# A Site of Action of Clonidine

Several years ago we proposed (Ross et al., 1984) that the critical region in RVL involved in AP control corresponded to an area of the brain stem populated by a subset of catecholamine neurons synthesizing adrenaline (the C1 group). Recent anatomical studies have further defined the cardiovascular active zone as a subregion of a distinct brain stem nucleus that we have termed the rostral ventrolateral reticular nucleus (RVL) (Ruggiero et al., 1989). The RVL lies caudal to the VIIth nerve nucleus, is just beneath the nucleus ambiguus, and is subjacent to the ventricular surface (Fig. 5.1). The RVL has two other characteristic features: in its ventral half it contains a nest of adrenergic neurons of the C1 group and it is heavily innervated by projections from the nucleus tractus solitarii (NTS) (Fig. 5.1). Functional studies, moreover, have defined the active zone of the RVL as overlapping exactly the adrenergic neuronal region, and it is this cardiovascularly active subarea of RVL we have termed the C1 area.

Functionally (see Reis et al., 1988, 1989 for review), neurons of the C1 area are tonically active and sympathoexcitatory: electrical or chemical stimulation of the region will elevate sympathetic nerve activity and AP. In contrast, bilateral lesions or pharmacological inactivation will profoundly reduce AP. The cardiovascularly active zone of the C1 area in rat is about

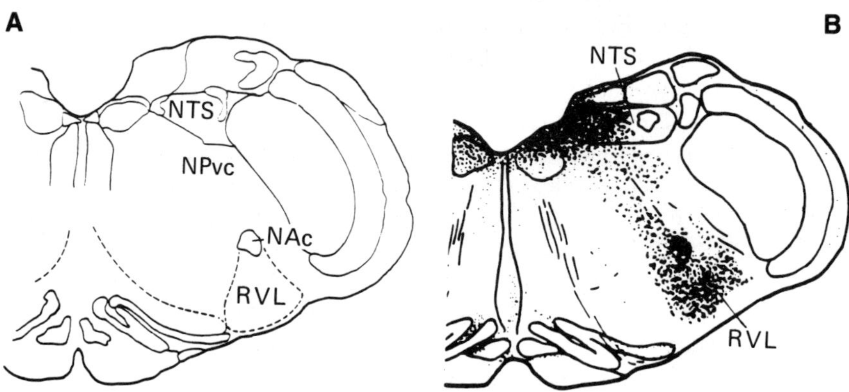


FIGURE 5.1. **A**: Camera lucida drawings of coronal sections through the rostral ventrolateral medulla demonstrating the neuroanatomical boundaries of nucleus reticularis rostroventrolateralis (nucleus RVL). Note that the apex of nucleus RVL is formed by the compact division of the nucleus ambiguus (also sometimes referred to as the retrofacial nucleus). **B**: A terminal field in the nucleus RVL derived from cells in cardiopulmonary subdivisions of the nucleus of the solitary tract (NTS). Processes in the nucleus RVL were labeled by anterograde transport of a cocktail of tritiated amino acids injected into the NTS at the level of the calamus scriptorius. (From Ruggiero et al., 1989, with permission.)

400 $\mu$m in length (Ruggiero et al., 1989) and contains neurons that descend into the spinal cord to innervate monosynaptically and bilaterally preganglionic sympathetic neurons of the intermediolateral columns (Milner et al., 1989; Reis et al., 1988, 1989; Ruggiero et al., 1989). In rat, only 200 to 300 neurons innervate the cord, of which 70% to 80% contain PNMT (Cravo et al., 1989). Thus, few neurons appear responsible for exerting potent and widespread actions on AP.

Electrophysiologically, reticulospinal neurons of the C1 area (identified by antidromic activation from the intermediolateral columns) are tonically active, fire in rhythmic relationship to and in advance of sympathetic preganglionic neurons, are inhibited by baroreceptors, and discharge in aggregate with a rhythmicity linked to the cardiac cycle that they then impose on sympathetic nerves (reviewed in Reis et al., 1988). It is likely these neurons fire as a group in relative synchrony and, through highly collateralized axons in the spinal cord, activate wide fields of preganglionic sympathetic neurons.

Neurons of the C1 area are critical in the expression of a number of reflexes acting on AP. Interference with the C1 area will block arterial baroreceptor and other cardiopulmonary reflexes, the reflex elevations of AP associated with pain, exercise, and emotional behaviors (LeDoux et al., 1988; Reis et al., 1988, 1989).

The C1 area of the RVL also appears to be the site at which neurotransmitters or drugs applied to the VSM act to modify AP (Feldberg, 1986). This contention is supported by the evidence (Benarroch et al., 1986) that: 1) the most sensitive zone for eliciting an elevation of AP with topical application of the excitatory amino acid L-glutamate overlies the glycine sensitive area of Feldberg (1986), 2) this zone precisely overlies the C1 area, 3) the pharmacological profile with respect to the actions of topically applied agents in elevating or reducing AP are identical to those elicited in cat from the glycine-sensitive area (Feldberg, 1986), 4) the region for the lowest threshold for eliciting a sympathetic response by electrical or chemical stimulation lies beneath the VSM within the C1 area, 5) unilateral lesions of the descending pathway, over which C1 area neurons project to the spinal cord, will block AP responses to application of drugs to the ipsilateral but not contralateral VSM (Ruggiero et al., 1989), and 6) adrenergic neurons of the C1 area send processes to lie in immediate apposition to the VSM and, hence, are accessible to the action of drugs applied to this zone.

Although neurons of the C1 area, mostly adrenergic, descend to innervate monosynaptically preganglionic sympathetic neurons (Milner et al., 1988; Morrison et al., 1989), the identity of the excitatory neurotransmitter released from them is still not known. It does not appear to be adrenaline. Recently, evidence has accrued to suggest that the excitatory amino acid L-glutamate may mediate the effect (Morrison et al., 1989). Thus the IML and the dorsal horns are heavily innervated by immunoreactive glutamatergic fibers and that following spinal cord transection, the innervation of the IML (but not that of the dorsal horn) disappears. This finding is consistent with the view that the innervation of the IML arises from supraspinal sources whereas those of the dorsal horn, as well known, are largely segmental. Second, the IML contains glutamate receptors and, finally, the discharge of electrophysiologically identified preganglionic neurons elicited by single-shock stimulation of RVL can be blocked by the iontophoretic application of the nonselective glutamate antagonist, kynurenic acid. At present, it is not known whether or not glutamatergic and adrenergic fibers innervating the IML arise from distinct neurons or whether or not the transmitters are colocalized. Investigations are currently underway to distinguish between these possibilities.

The RVL is innervated by multiple inputs from other areas of the brain and spinal cord (Ruggiero et al., 1989). Among these are dense projections from spinal afferents, from the NTS, and from a sympathoinhibitory area in the caudal ventrolateral medulla (CVL) (Blessing and Li, 1989; Blessing et al., 1984). It is through these pathways that the RVL is engaged to mediate a number of reflex responses. However, interposed neurons may well play a role. For example, it is now well recognized that the RVL is critical in the expression of baroreceptor reflexes (Granata et al., 1985). Whereas originally believed that the response may be mediated directly, there is evidence now that the pathway from NTS to RVL includes interposed neurons in the CVL (Gordon, 1987). This neuron is conceivably GABAergic (Blessing and Li, 1989; Cravo et al., 1989) and inhibits the tonic activity of RVL neurons, thereby reducing preganglionic sympathetic nerve activity. Other cardiovascular reflexes, including those arising from cardiopulmonary receptors innervated by the Xth cranial nerve, arterial chemoreceptor reflexes, somatosympathetic reflexes arising from pain fibers to skin, that part of the elevation of AP in exercise initiated from skeletal muscle, and some of the activation of AP associated with conditioned emotional responses, all depend on the integrity of neurons of the RVL (LeDoux et al., 1988; Reis et al., 1988).

The RVL has also been investigated with respect to its pharmacological characteristics. The microinjection of a number of agents into the RVL or by application to the surface has demonstrated that the area is sensitive to a number of these substances. Thus, L-glutamate, acetylcholine, angiotensin II, or CRF may all elevate AP when applied to the RVL whereas gamma-aminobutyric acid (GABA), enkephalin, and $\beta$-endorphin may also be inhibitory (see Reis et al., 1989). Some of these agents exert tonic regulatory control: for example, the application locally of the GABA antagonist bicuculline results in profound elevations of blood pressure (Ross et al., 1984), demonstrating that GABA is continuously released to modulate the excitability of C1 adrenergic neurons. In contrast, direct or indirect blockade of acetylcholine in the RVL will result in a fall of AP, demonstrating that this transmitter is tonically excitatory and acts on muscarinic receptors within that region. Indeed, from the pharmacological point of view some of the local receptors in RVL may be responsible for mediating systemic actions of drugs that act through selective transmitter systems. Thus, the elevation of AP resulting from systemic neostigmine will be blocked by local microinjection of scopolamine into the RVL (Giuliano et al., 1989).

Careful immunocytochemical analysis of the RVL has demonstrated that many of these agents are part of intrinsic neurotransmitter systems. Studies by Milner et al. (1989) have demonstrated by electron microscopic immunocytochemistry that local neurons in the region contain GABA, enkephalin, substance P, acetylcholine, and catecholamines and that many of these make direct synaptic contact with adrenergic neurons of the C1 area. One exception are cholinergic neurons and/or processes that, although abundant, make few contacts with C1 adrenergic neurons but rather seem to synapse on other neurons in the region, possibly GABAergic. This fact raises the possibility that the excitatory action of acetylcholine in RVL results from inhibition of a GABAergic inhibitory neuron rather than direct excitation and emphasizes the point that it is not always possible to ascertain by the microinjection of an agent into this region whether it is acting as an agonist or antagonist of other intrinsic networks.

The C1 area of RVL also appears to be the site of the hypotensive actions of clonidine and related compounds, including the oxazoline rilmenidine. Two lines of evidence support the contention. First, microinjection of clonidine, rilmenidine, and other substances into the RVL will elicit a dose-dependent fall of AP. The response in rat appears to be anatomically highly restricted to this region, the response is dose-dependent, and the doses eliciting maximal responses are an order of magnitude less than those required for eliciting the response by peripheral administration. Moreover, systemic administration of the maximal dose in the anesthetized rat fails to have an action on AP (Gomez et al., 1990). Second, as will be described below, there is evidence that the microinjection into the RVL of idazoxan, an agent competing with both $\alpha_2$-adrenergic and imidazole receptors, will block the systemic actions of clonidine and rilmenidine (Gomez et al., 1990).

## Imidazole Receptors and the RVL

To determine the identity of the receptor(s) in RVL that might be responsible for the hypotensive actions of the drug, we examined the binding characteristics of the clonidine analogue $^3$H-p-aminoclonidine ($^3$H-PAC) to membranes of the bovine ventrolateral medulla (VLM) and, for comparison, the frontal cortex. While autoradiographic studies by Unnerstall et al. (1984) demonstrated this ligand could bind to a region corresponding to the RVL in rat brain, this interaction was assumed to be exclusively to $\alpha_2$-adrenergic receptors.

We observed that binding of [3H]-PAC to membranes of VLM and frontal cortex as specific, saturable, of high affinity, and reversible (Ernsberger et al., 1987). Scatchard analysis indicated that [3H]-PAC bound to two sites in both regions, the higher with a $K_d$ in the 0.5 to 1.0 nM range and the second in the range of 15 to 40 nM.

Competition studies using a range of ligands indicated that whereas clonidine could completely displace [3H]-PAC from VLM membranes (Fig. 5.2), norepinephrine and other phenylethylamines could displace only approximately 70% of [3H]-PAC binding in this tissue. The potency order characteristics of such displacement were consistent with the receptor being an $\alpha_2$-adrenergic receptor. However, even in the presence of high concentrations of norepinephrine, clonidine could still fully displace [3H]-PAC (Fig. 5.2). These observations indicated the presence of some recep-

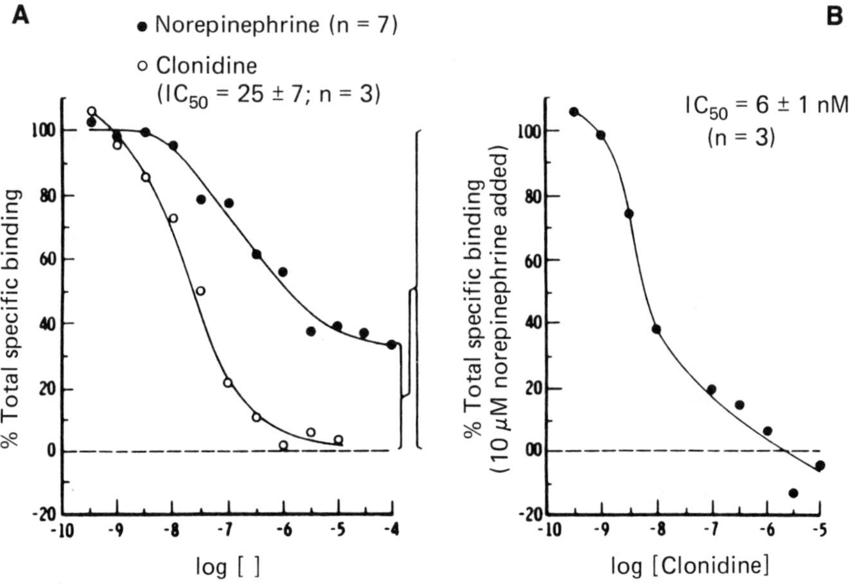


FIGURE 5.2. Inhibition of [3H]p-aminoclonidine binding to distinct subpopulations of sites in ventrolateral medulla membranes. Bovine ventrolateral medulla membranes were incubated for 40 min at 25°C with 1.0 nM [3H]PAc and 9-12 concentrations of competing drug. Ordinate: percent of total specific [3H]PAC binding as defined in parallel incubations in the presence of 10 μM phentolamine. Abscissa: log molar concentration of test compound. A: Inhibition by clonidine and (−)-norepinephrine. B: Inhibition by clonidine in the presence of 10 μM (−)-norepinephrine. Total binding in B refers to that remaining with 10 μM norepinephrine added to the incubation medium. Values represent the means of 3–7 experiments, each performed in triplicate. (From Ernsberger et al., 1987, with permission.)

tor other than the $\alpha_2$-adrenergic one to which clonidine was binding in the VLM.

A number of imidazoles, such as imidazole-4-acetic acid (IAA) or cimetidine, could displace approximately 30% of binding with a very high affinity in membranes of the VLM. This demonstrated the presence of an imidazole receptor. On the other hand, there was very little displacement from membranes of the frontal cortex where it appeared that most of the binding of clonidine and like compounds was to $\alpha_2$-adrenergic receptors. In support of the evidence for an imidazole receptor representing the remaining nonadrenergic component was the finding that masking studies in which cold norepinephrine or IAA were used to mask, respectively, $\alpha_2$-adrenergic receptors or imidazole receptors, all of the binding could be quantitatively accounted for by these two classes of receptors.

Using the masking technique or by comparing binding between frontal cortex ($\alpha_2$-adrenergic receptors only) and VLM ($\alpha_2$-adrenergic and imidazole receptors), it was then possible to assess the binding characteristics of a number of imidazoles and or adrenergic ligands with respect to their relative binding to either receptor class. In brief, it was evident that clonidine and other imidazolines as well oxazolines including rilmenidine bound potently to both classes of receptors and that catecholamines recognized only the $\alpha_2$-adrenergic receptor, whereas imidazoles including IAA, cimetidine, and histamine bound principally to the imidazole receptor. Of relevance was the fact that nonimidazole ligands for histamine receptors failed to interact with either receptor class as did a wide range of other putative neurotransmitters.

Having demonstrated that in RVL clonidine was binding to both $\alpha_2$-adrenergic and imidazole receptors, the question then arose, which was responsible for mediating hypotension? Two lines of evidence strongly suggest it is the imidazole receptor. First, there was an extremely close correlation between hypotension produced by microinjection of drugs in RVL and binding to imidazole but not adrenergic receptors (Fig. 5.3). Second, the microinjection of idazoxan, an agent binding to both receptors, could reverse the hypotension elicited by the systemic action of clonidine or rilmenidine (Ernsberger et al., 1990b; Gomez et al., 1990), but local administration of the selective $\alpha_2$-adrenergic antagonist SKF-86466 had no effect (Fig. 5.4). It should be noted, however, that some adrenergic agents injected into RVL may lower AP, and clearly adrenergic receptors in the region may contribute to AP control although the regulation may be complex.

The actions of clonidine in RVL, however, are probably complex. The mechanism could be direct to inhibit the discharge of RVL neurons or indirect (e.g., by exciting inhibitory, possibly GABAergic interneurons or by inhibiting neurons themselves inhibiting GABA neurons). It is also unclear whether the binding of clonidine in RVL is to neurons expressing one class of receptor or that both are expressed together.

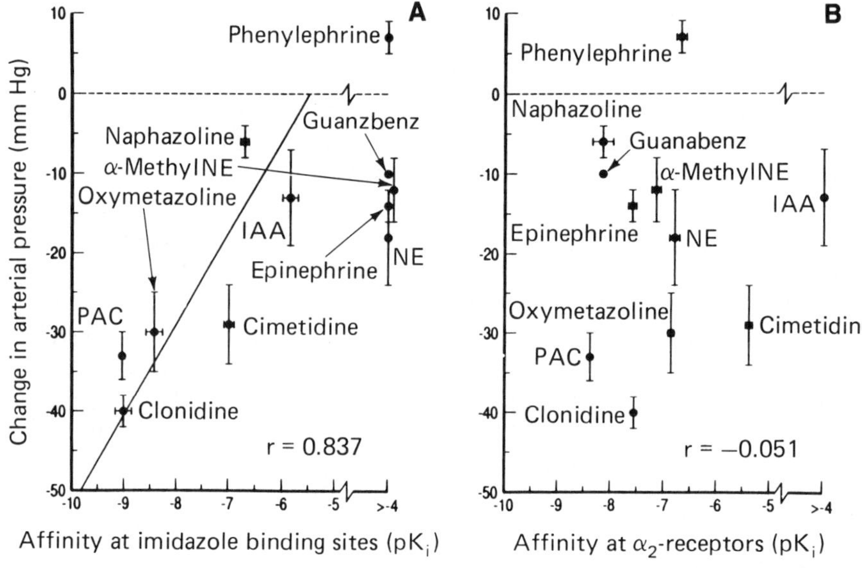



FIGURE 5.3. Relationship between vasodepressor potency and binding affinity at imidazole binding sites **A** or $\alpha_2$-adrenergic receptors **B** for a series of clonidinelike compounds. Ordinate: maximum fall in AP elicited by bilateral microinjection of the test compound (1 nmol in 50 nl) into the RVL in urethane-anesthetized, paralyzed, and ventilated rats. Abscissa: binding affinity at imidazole binding sites (**A**) or $\alpha_2$- adrenergic receptors in the RVL (**B**). As shown in (**A**), the fall in AP elicited by a standard dose microinjected within the RVL was directly related to imidazole binding site affinity for those compounds with significant affinity at imidazole sites ($K_i < 0.1$ mM). The fall in AP was unrelated to $\alpha_2$-receptor affinity (**B**). (From Ernsberger et al., 1990b, with permission.)

We therefore sought to establish whether the imidazole and adrenergic receptors could be independently expressed. By examining binding in several cell and tissue lines and also seeking anatomical heterogeneity in tissues, we have found that the two classes of receptor may be independently expressed. Thus, we have found that whereas the neuroblastoma-glial hybrid cells, the NG-108-15 line, expressed both receptors, astroglial cells expressed only $\alpha_2$-adrenergic receptors while in the adrenal chromaffin cells only imidazole receptors were expressed (Emsberger et al., 1989a,b). Moreover, in kidney, which contains both receptors (Emsberger et al., 1990a; Parini et al., 1989), the intrarenal distribution differs. The fact that the two receptors are independently expressed and probably anatomically distinct entities in kidney has recently been demonstrated by several other groups (Michel et al., 1990; Parini et al., 1989).

In summary, the evidence demonstrates that in RVL clonidine and other hypotensive imidazol(in)es as well as oxazolines lower AP primarily by interacting with imidazole receptors. However, the possibility that an in-

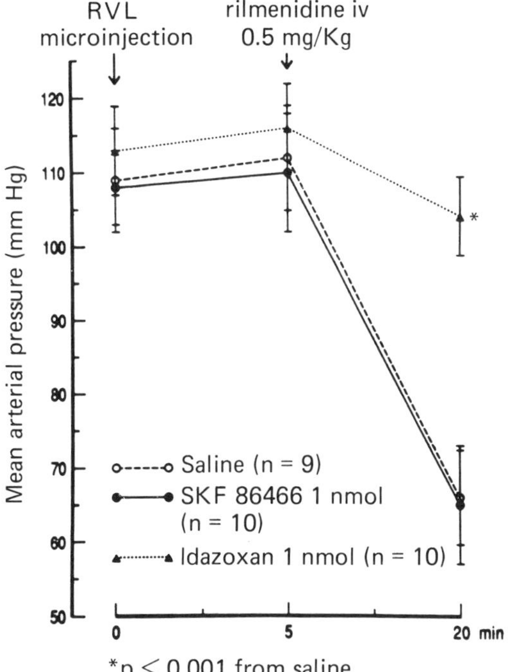



FIGURE 5.4. Effect of antagonists microinjected into RVL on the vasodepressor response elicited by intravenous injection of rilmenidine. The rats received bilateral microinjection of saline, SKF 86466, or idazoxan into RVL and 5 min later 0.5 mg/kg of rilmenidine was injected. Idazoxan blocks the hypotensive effect of rilmenidine. $^*p < 0.001$ idazoxan vs. saline. o = saline (n = 10); ● = 1 nmol SKF 86466 (n = 9); Δ = 1 nmol idazoxan (n = 10). (From Gomez et al., 1990, with permission.)

teraction with $\alpha_2$-adrenergic receptors for some drugs may also contribute to the associated hypotension cannot be ruled out.

## Clonidine-Displacing Substance in Brain

The identification of imidazole receptors in the RVL raises the question as to the identity of the ligand with which this receptor would interact. In 1984, Atlas and Burstein (1984) identified a substance in bovine brain that competed with the binding of clonidine, rauwolscine, and yohimbine to membranes of rat brain and human platelets. The material, a noncatecholamine of low molecular weight and not susceptible to peptide digestion, was termed clonidine-displacing substance (CDS). It was believed to represent a natural ligand selective for $\alpha_2$-adrenergic receptors and not binding to $\beta$-adrenergic or $\alpha_1$-adrenergic receptors. CDS was also believed to be bioactive on the grounds that, like clonidine, it inhibited the electrically stimulated rat vas deferens (Diamant and Atlas, 1986). The effect, however, was considered to reflect an action on $\alpha_2$-adrenergic receptors since it was reversed by two $\alpha_2$-adrenergic antagonists, yohimbine and phentolamine.

The studies of Atlas and Burstein (1984) suggested that CDS interacted with only $\alpha_2$-adrenergic receptors. We sought to determine if CDS, like clonidine, also interacted with imidazole receptors in RVL. Isolating CDS from bovine brain, we were first able to confirm the observations of Atlas and Burstein (1984) of the presence of a substance of low molecular weight ($< 500$ Da) in homogenates of bovine ventral medulla (Meeley et al., 1986a) capable of displacing $^3$H-PAC from brain membranes. We were able to show, moreover, that CDS, like clonidine, bound not only to $\alpha_2$-adrenergic but also to imidazole receptors in the RVL (Ernsberger et al., 1988; Meeley et al., 1986b). The affinity of CDS for imidazole receptors was substantially greater than that for $\alpha_2$-adrenergic receptors. The inhibition was competitive and heterogeneous but differed in some respects from that of clonidine. The interaction of CDS with both classes of receptors has been now demonstrated to occur in kidney as well (Coupry et al., 1990; Ernsberger et al., 1990a; Parini et al., 1989).

Further evidence to support the contention that CDS, like clonidine, binds to both imidazole and $\alpha_2$-adrenergic receptors has been obtained by examining the interaction of CDS with polyclonal antibodies raised against **p**-amino clonidine, a model of a native receptor (Meeley et al., 1988a,b, 1989). We have demonstrated that such antibodies recognize, with high affinity, clonidine, PAC, and several other clonidinelike compounds that contain a phenyl and imidazole ring, but that compounds without both structures (e.g., epinephrine or histamine) fail to interact with the antibodies. Of relevance were the observations that CDS exhibited a dose-dependent high affinity binding with the antiserum and that the antiserum was capable of immunoprecipitating CDS. The experiment, therefore, not only suggested that structurally CDS shared with clonidine a number of determinants but that CDS was in all probability a biologically unique molecule containing within its structure imidazol(in)e and phenyl ring systems.

Seeking to establish further the nature of the receptors with which CDS may interact, we began to investigate other biological functions of the substance hoping to define a biological system that would permit examination of the pharmacology of CDS. By reviewing a number of classic bioassay systems, we discovered that CDS was capable of producing a dose-dependent contraction of the rat gastric fundus (Emsberger et al., 1991; Felsen et al., 1987). The contractile response was relatively selective in that other gastrointestinal or vascular smooth muscle preparations failed to show a comparable response. The response appeared to reflect a direct action of CDS on smooth muscle because it was not blocked by tetrodotoxin, was dependent on $Ca^{++}$ channel activation, and so far has appeared pharmacologically unique since antagonists of agents known to contract stomach strips failed to block the action of CDS, and desensitization to gastric peptides of interest did not attenuate the response to CDS (Ernsberger et al., 1991).

By use of combined bioassay using the rat gastric fundus, a radioimmunoassay with anti-PAC antibodies and receptor assays with $^3$H-PAC, we have begun to examine the distribution of purported CDS in rat brain, other organs, and in some cell lines. In brain, CDS has a distribution appropriate to that of a neurotransmitter: it is synaptosomal and unequally distributed, being highest in hypothalamus and lowest within the cerebellum. It is also found in peripheral tissues of rat including stomach, heart, and adrenal gland (Hensley et al., 1989) and, as first described by Atlas and associates (Kreisberg et al., 1987), is present in serum, thus raising the prospect that CDS may be a hormone. CDS has also been detected in the neuroblastoma-glial hybrid NG-108-15 cell line (Ernsberger et al., 1989a), indicating that line may be a useful future tool for illuminating the molecular biology of the substance. Future studies on the biology of CDS will depend on the isolation and characterization of the molecule's structure.

## Summary and Conclusions

1. Neurons within the C1 area of the rostral ventrolateral medulla are critical for the maintenance of resting and reflex control of AP.
2. The C1 area also appears to mediate the hypotensive actions of clonidine and comparable agents including the oxazoline rilmenidine.
3. In RVL clonidine and like agents bind to $\alpha_2$-adrenergic receptors as well as to a class of receptors recognizing imidazol(in)es.
4. The facts that: 1) the hypotensive potency of a number of centrally acting agents highly correlates with binding affinity to imidazole and not $\alpha_2$-adrenergic receptors, and 2) the microinjection of selective $\alpha_2$-adrenergic antagonists in the RVL fails to alter the hypotensive actions of systemic clonidine or rilmenidine, while microinjection of idazoxan does, indicates that the hypotensive actions of clonidine and comparable agents are due to an interaction with the imidazole receptors in that brain area.
5. An endogenous agent, probably nonpeptidergic and of low molecular weight, CDS, which can be isolated from synaptosomes of bovine ventral medulla, may be an endogenous ligand and like clonidine binds to both imidazole and $\alpha_2$-adrenergic receptors in membranes of RVL.
6. Clonidine and associated agents therefore appear to lower AP by interacting with imidazole receptors in the RVL whose native ligand may be CDS. CDS may be an important regulator in brain of AP in health and possibly hypertensive disease.

# References


Atlas D, Burstein Y (1984): Isolation and partial purification of a clonidine-displacing endogenous brain substance. *Eur J Biochem* 144:287–293.

Benarroch EE, Granata AR, Ruggiero DA, Park DH, Reis DJ (1986): Neurons of the C1 area mediate cardiovascular responses initiated from ventral medullary surface. *Am J Physiol (Regulatory)* 250(5 Pt 2):R932–R945.

Blessing WW, Li YW. (1989): Inhibitory vasomotor neurons in the caudal ventrolateral region of the medulla oblongata. In: *Progress in Brain Research 81*, Ciriello J, Polosa C, Caverson M, eds. Amsterdam: Elsevier, pp. 83–97.

Blessing WW, Sved AF, Reis DJ. (1984): Arterial pressure and plasma vasopressin: Regulation by neurons in the caudal ventrolateral medulla of the rabbit. In *Clinical and Experimental Hypertension, Part A: Theory and Practice* A6(Nos. 1 & 2). New York: Marcel Dekker, pp. 149–156.

Bousquet P, Feldman J, Schwartz J (1984): Central cardiovascular effects of alpha adrenergic drugs: differences between catecholamines and imidazolines. *J Pharmacol Exp Ther* 230(1):232–236.

Bousquet P, Feldman J, Tibirica E, et al. (1989): New concepts on the central regulation of blood pressure. Alpha-2-adrenoceptors and "imidazoline receptors." *Am J Med* 87:10S–13S.

Bousquet P, Schwartz J (1983): Alpha-adrenergic drugs. Pharmacological tools for the study of the central vasomotor control. *Biochem Pharmacol* 32(9):1459–1465.

Coupry I, Atlas D, Podevin RA, Uzielli I, Parini A (1990): Imidazoline-guanidinium receptive site in renal proximal tubule: Asymmetric distribution, regulation by cations and interaction with an endogenous clonidine displacing substance. *J Pharmacol Exp Ther* 252(1):293–299.

Cravo SL, Morrison SF, Reis DJ (1989): Caudal ventrolateral medulla (CVL): A source of tonic and baroreceptor-mediated sympathoinhibition. *Soc Neurosci Abstr* 15:594.

Diamant S, Atlas D (1986): An endogenous brain substance, CDS (clonidine-displacing-substance), inhibits the twitch response of rat vas deferens. *Biochem Biophys Res Commun* 134(1):184–190.

Ernsberger P, Evinger MJ, Meeley MP, Feinland G, Reis DJ (1989a): Adrenal chromaffin cells express imidazole receptors which bind clonidine and an endogenous clonidine-displacing substance. *Soc Neurosci Abstr* 15:683.

Ernsberger P, Felsen D, Meeley MP, Reis DJ (1991): An endogenous clonidine-displacing substance elicits a specific contractile response in rat stomach. *J. Neural Trans.* (submitted).

Ernsberger P. Feinland G, Meeley MP, Reis DJ (1990a): Characterization and visualization of clonidine-sensitive imidazole sites in rat kidney which recognize clonidine-displacing substance. *Am J Hypertens* 3:90–97.

Ernsberger P. Giuliano R. Willette RN, Reis DJ (1990b): Role of imidazole receptors in the vasodepressor response to clonidine analogs in the rostral ventrolateral medulla. *J Pharmacol Exp Ther* 253(1):408–418.

Ernsberger PR, Meeley MP, Mann JJ, Reis DJ (1987): Clonidine binds to imidazole binding sites as well as alpha$_2$-adrenoceptors in the ventrolateral medulla. *Eur J Pharmacol* 134(1):1–14.

Ernsberger P, Meeley MP, Reis DJ (1988): An endogenous substance with clonidine-like properties: Selective binding to imidazole sites in the ventrolateral medulla. *Brain Res* 441:309–318.

Ernsberger P, Meeley MP, and Reis DJ (1989b): Neuroblastoma-glioma hybrid cells contain clonidine-displacing substance. *Eur J Pharmacol* 174:135– 138.

Feldberg W (1986): Honorary plenary lecture: History of in vivo analysis of brain functions elicited from its inner and outer surfaces. *Ann NY Acad Sci* 473:1–20.

Felsen D, Ernsberger P, Meeley MP, Reis DJ (1987): Clonidine-displacing substance is biologically active on smooth muscle. *Eur J Pharmacol* 142:453–455.

Giuliano R. Ruggiero DA, Morrison S, Ernsberger P, Reis DJ (1989): Cholinergic regulation of arterial pressure by the C1 area of the rostral ventrolateral medulla. *J Neurosci* 9(3):923–942.

Gomez RE, Ernsberger P, Feinland G, Reis DJ (1990): Rilmenidine lowers arterial pressure via imidazole receptors in brainstem C1 area. *Eur J Pharmacol* (submitted).

Gordon FJ (1987): Aortic baroreceptor reflexes are mediated by NMDA receptors in caudal ventrolateral medulla *Am J Physiol* 252(3 Pt. 2):R628 – R633.

Granata AR, Ruggiero DA, Park DH, Joh TH, Reis DJ (1985): Brain stem area with C1 epinephrine neurons mediates baroreflex vasodepressor responses. *Am J Physiol (Heart 17)* 248:H547–H567.

Hensley ML, Meeley MP, McCauley PM, Ernsberger P, Reis DJ (1989): Clonidine-displacing substance is present in peripheral tissues of the rat. *Am J Hypertens* 2:917–919.

Kreisberg GA, Diamant S, Diamant YZ, Atlas D (1987): Raised levels of an endogenous nonadrenergic substance in the serum of pregnancy-induced hypertension patients. *Isr J Med Sci* 23(12):1194–1197.

LeDoux JE, Iwata J, Cicchetti P, Reis DJ (1988): Different projections of the central amygdaloid nucleus mediate autonomic and behavioral correlates of conditioned fear. *J Neurosci* 8:2517–2529.

Meeley MP, Emsberger PR, Granata AR, Reis DJ (1986a): An endogenous clonidine-displacing substance from bovine brain: Receptor binding and hypotensive actions in the ventrolateral medulla. *Life Sci* 38:1119–1126.

Meeley MP, Ernsberger P, McCauley PM, Reis DJ (1988a): Clonidine-specific antibodies as models for imidazole and $\alpha_2$-adrenergic receptor binding sites: Implications for the structure of clonidine-displacing substance. *J Hypertens* 6(suppl 4):S490–S493.

Meeley MP, Ernsberger PR, Reis DJ (1986b): An endogenous substance with clonidine-like receptor binding selectivity: The brain's own clonidine? *J Hypertens* 4(suppl 6):S257–S259.

Meeley MP, Towle AC, Ernsberger P, et al. (1989): Clonidine-specific antisera recognize an endogenous clonidine-displacing substance in brain. *Hypertension* 13:341–351.

Meeley MP, Towle AC, Ernsberger P, Reis DJ (1988b): A specific antiserum recognizes clonidine-displacing substance: Implications for the structure of the brain's own clonidine. *Neurosci Lett* 84:84–90.

Michel MC, Regan JW, Gerhardt MA, Neubig RR, Insel PA, Motulsky HJ (1990); Nonadrenergic [$^3$H]idazoxan binding sites are physically distinct from alpha 2-adrenergic receptors. *Mol Pharmacol* 37(1):65–8.

Milner TA, Morrison SF Abate C, Reis DJ (1988): Phenylethanolamine N-methyltransferase containing terminals synapse directly on sympathetic preganglionic neurons in the rat. *Brain Res* 448:205–222.

Milner TA, Pickel VM, Morrison SF, Reis DJ (1989): Adrenergic neurons in the rostral ventrolateral medulla: Ultrastructure and synaptic relations with other transmitter-identified neurons. In: *Progress in Brain Research 81*, Ciriello J, Polosa C, Caverson M, eds. Amsterdam: Elsevier, pp. 29–47.

Morrison SF, Ernsberger P, Milner TA, Callaway J, Gong A, Reis DJ (1989): A glutamate mechanism in the intermediolateral nucleus mediates sympathoexcitatory responses to stimulation of the rostral ventrolateral medulla. In: *Progress in Brain Research 81*, Ciriello J, Polosa C, Caverson M, eds. Amsterdam: Elsevier, pp. 159–169.

Parini A, Coupry I, Graham RM, Uzielli I, Atlas D, Lanier SM (1989): Characterization of an imidazoline/guanidinium receptive site distinct from the alpha 2-adrenergic receptor. *J. Biol Chem* 264(20):11874–11878.

Reis DJ, Morrison SM, Ruggiero D (1988): The C1 area of the brainstem in tonic and reflex control of blood pressure. *Hypertension* 11(2 Pt 2):I8–I13.

Reis DJ, Ruggiero DA, Morrison SF (1989): The C1 area of the rostral ventrolateral medulla oblongata. A critical brainstem region for control of resting and reflex integration of arterial pressure. *Am J Hypertens* 2(12 Pt 2):363S–374S.

Ross CA, Ruggiero DA, Park DH, et al. (1984): Tonic vasomotor control by the rostral ventrolateral medulla: Effect of electrical or chemical stimulation of the area containing C1 adrenaline neurons on arterial pressure, heart rate, and plasma catecholamines and vasopressin. *J Neurosci* 4(No. 2):474–494.

Ruggiero DA, Cravo S, Arango V, Reis DJ (1989): Central control of the circulation by the rostral ventrolateral reticular nucleus: Anatomical substrates. In: *Progress in Brain Research 81*, Ciriello J, Polosa C, Caverson M, eds. Amsterdam: Elsevier, pp. 49–79.

Unnerstall JR, Kopajtic T, Kuhar MJ (1984): Distribution of alpha-2 agonist binding sites in the rat and human central nervous system: Analysis of some functional anatomic correlates of the pharmacological effects of clonidine and related adrenergic agents. *Brain Res Rev* 7:69–101.

# 6
# The Role of the Rostral Ventrolateral Medulla in the Synchronization of Respiratory and Sympathetic Functions

STANISLAW BARADZIEJ AND ANDRZEJ TRZEBSKI

## Introduction

Neurons in the rostral ventrolateral medulla (RVLM) that project to spinal sympathetic preganglionic neurons mediate and/or generate tonic sympathetic activity and integrate circulatory reflexes, and therefore represent the main supraspinal sympathoexcitatory common pathway (McAllen, 1986; Morrison et al., 1988; Sun et al., 1988, for references Ciriello et al., 1989). The dorsal border of the RVLM in the rat is situated in close proximity to the compact and semicompact divisions of the nucleus ambiguus (Ruggiero et al., 1989), the region which contains respiratory-related propriobulbar neurons (Saether et al., 1987). The anatomical proximity of sympathoexcitatory and respiratory neurons strongly suggests that this region may be a site of respiratory-sympathetic integration. Respiratory-modulated sympathoexcitatory neurons have been reported within the RVLM in the rat (Haselton and Guyenet, 1989). Our previous studies in the rat have shown that glutamate microinjections applied ventrally into the rostral compact division of the nucleus ambiguus reversibly change the timing and pattern of respiratory-sympathetic synchronization within the respiratory cycle (Baradziej and Trzebski, 1989). The present study provides further evidence that the ventral and medial border of the pars compacta of the nucleus ambiguus (para-ambigual area, PA Fig. 6.1) is critically involved in the generation of respiratory-related periodicities of the sympathetic discharge. Furthermore, our results indicate that this part of the RVLM plays a critical role in the generation of other sympathetic rhythmicities.

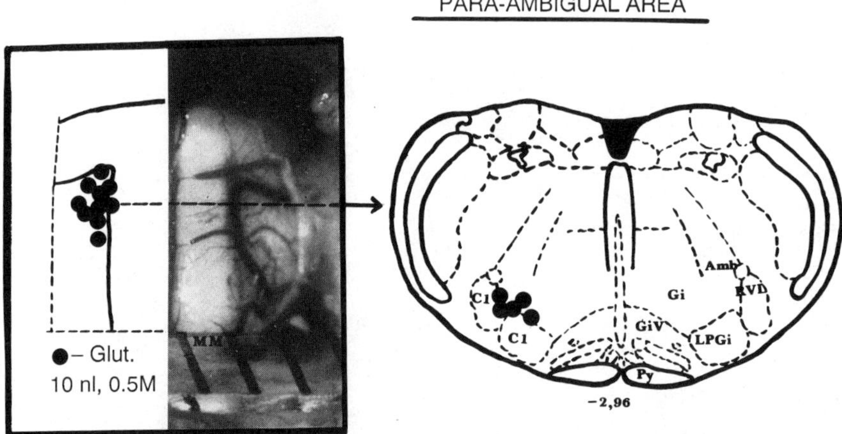



FIGURE 6.1. Photograph of the ventral surface of the brainstem (left) and schematic cross section of the rostral medulla (right). Sites of glutamate microinjections (10 nl, 0.5 M) are marked, by filled dots.

## Respiratory-Related Sympathetic Discharge Pattern is Species Dependent

Respiratory modulation of the spontaneous activity of sympathetic nerves has been well known since the original observation of Adrian et al. in 1932 (for references Koepchen et al., 1980). However, only more recently has it been recognized that the central modulation of sympathetic activity (SA) during the respiratory cycle shows species-dependent variation (Trzebski, 1989). In vagotomized and debuffered Wistar rats the pattern of SA is opposite to that seen in cats: a strong depression of sympathetic activity occurs in early inspiration and a peak sympathetic discharge is synchronized with early, phase I expiration (postinspiratory period) (Czyzyk et al., 1987). In the cat, the postinspiratory period corresponds to sympathoinhibtion (Bainton et al., 1985). Strain specific differences have also been observed, as in spontaneously hypertensive rats (SHR) the inspiratory-related sympathetic depression is lacking, which may contribute to the overall increase in sympathetic activity in hypertension (Czyzyk-Krzeska and Trzebski, 1990).

Fig. 6.2A shows the respiratory phase-related pattern of sympathetic discharge in the lumbar trunk of a normotensive Wistar rat anesthetized with pentobarbital, paralyzed, vagotomized with carotid sinus nerves cut, and artificially ventilated. Occasionally, a slight increase in spontaneous sympathetic activity (SA) occurred at the very onset of phrenic discharge, used

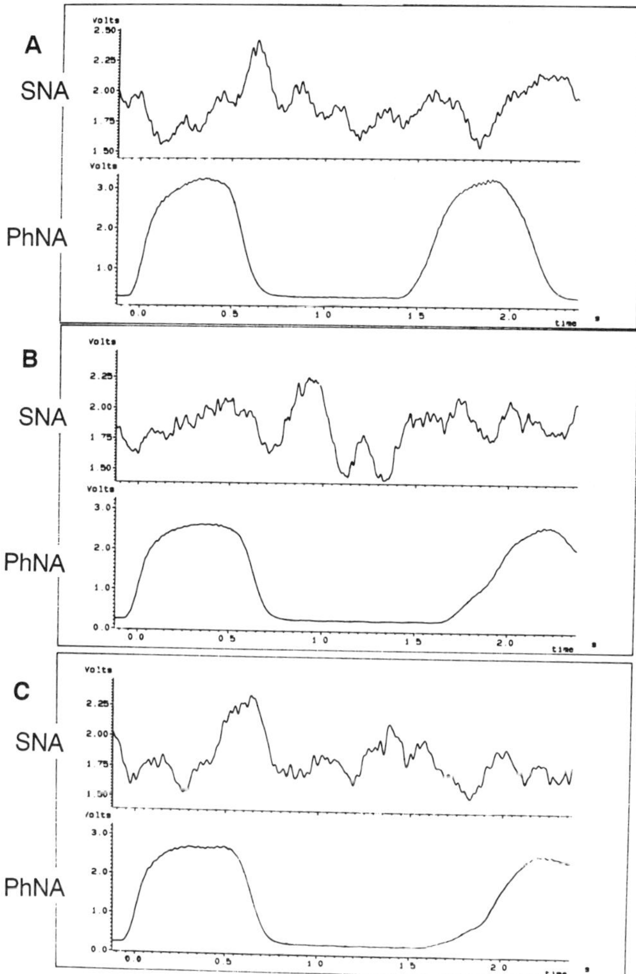

FIGURE 6.2. Averaged ($\times$16) integrated lumbar sympathetic activity (SNA) triggered by the onset of integrated phrenic nerve burst (PhNA). **A**: control; **B**: after 10 nl, 0.5 M, buffered glutamate microinjection into a site whithin the para-ambigual area; **C**: return to control.

as an index of central respiratory activity. This increase was followed by a deep, prolonged depression of SA reaching a nadir at mid-inspiration. The peak of the sympathetic discharge was synchronous with phase I expiration (postinspiratory phase), and SA remained elevated over phase II expiration. Sometimes the peak in SA activity appeared in phase II expiration or a bimodal expiratory-related discharge was observed (Czyzyk et al., 1987). This pattern is centrally generated as it is not influenced by baro- or chemoreceptor peripheral input or by frequency of breathing (Czyzyk et al. 1987).

## Para-Ambigual Area is Critical for the Timing of the Sympathetic Discharge Within the Respiratory Cycle

Ipsilateral, contralateral or bilateral microinjections of 10 nl 0.5 M buffered glutamate into a restricted area at the ventral and medial border of nucleus ambiguus (PA) 600–800 $\mu$m beneath the ventral surface (Fig. 6.1) change the timing of respiratory-sympathetic synchronization in a variable way depending on the site and volume of microinjection (Fig. 6.2B). Volumes of 10 nl, which caused reversible shifts of respiratory-sympathetic synchronization, did not change sympathetic or phrenic nerve activities or respiratory frequency. The responses lasted for 5 min after which the pattern of sympathetic synchronization returned to control. Among various

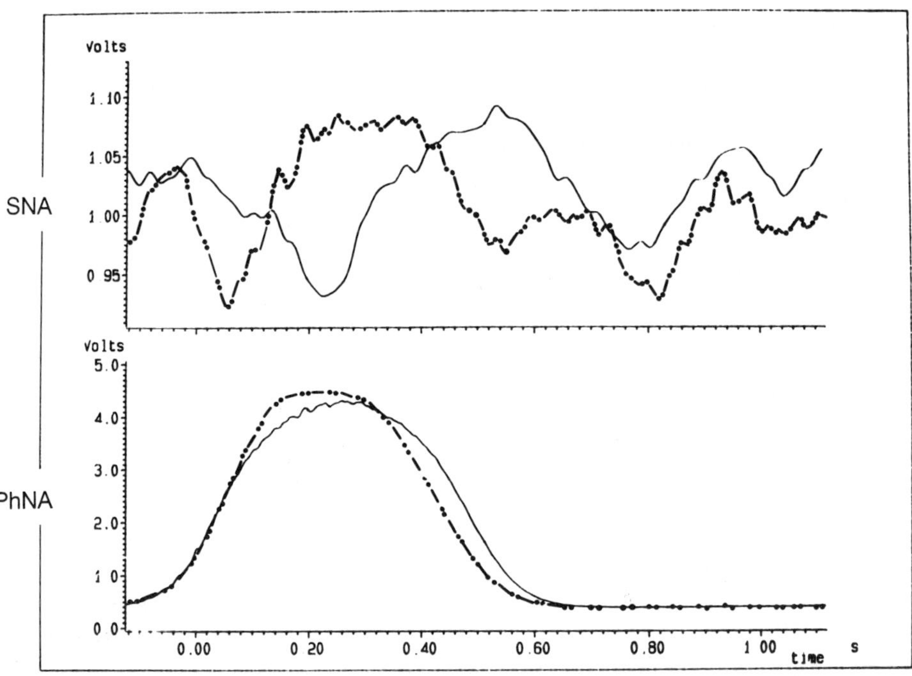


FIGURE 6.3. Averaged ($\times$16) integrated lumber trunk sympathetic activity (SNA) triggered by the onset of integrated phrenic nerve burst (PhNA). Solid line: control. Super-imposed dash-dotted line: after 10 nl, 0.5 M, glutamate microinjection into a site within the parambigual area.

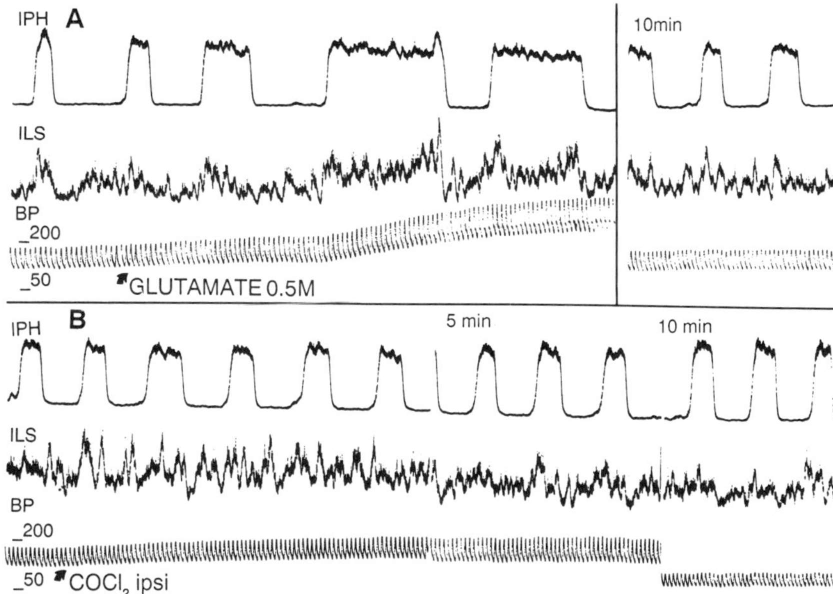



FIGURE 6.4. Effects of a glutamate (A) and CoCl$_2$ (B) micro-injected into the same area in the RVLM. **A**: Sympathoexcitatory response to glutamate (50 nl, 0.5 M). Traces from top to bottom: integrated phrenic nerve activity (IPh), integrated lumbar trunk sympathetic activity (ILS), arterial blood pressure (BP), immediately and 10 min after micro-injection. **B**: Sympathoexcitatory and pressor response to CoCl$_2$ (300 nl, 4 mM ipsilaterally). Records are the same as in A, immediately following microinjection, after 5 min and after 10 min.

induced patterns of respiratory-sympathetic synchronization a timing which characterizes spontaneously hypertensive rats (Czyzyk-Krzeska and Trzebski, 1990) was also produced by glutamate microinjections (Fig. 6.3). Larger volumes of glutamate (50 nl) applied in the same area produced significant pressor, sympathexcitatory and respiratory responses (Fig. 6.4A). Kainic acid (0.01 M, 20 nl) microinjections mimicked the effects of glutamate. 20–30 min following kainic acid microinjection phrenic nerve activity was depressed, then totally abolished, and respiratory modulation of SA disappeared. Kynurenic acid (0.5 M, 100 nl) microinjected into the PA reduced or abolished respiratory-sympathetic synchronization and altered the phrenic nerve activity pattern (Fig. 6.5C). 50 nl of 1 M GABA microinjected into the PA reduced sympathetic activity and the magnitude of respiratory-sympathetic synchronization. None of these substances were effective when microinjecteded outside of the PA. The para-ambigual area therefore has a critical role in the synchronization of the respiratory rhythm generator with the central sympathetic oscillator.

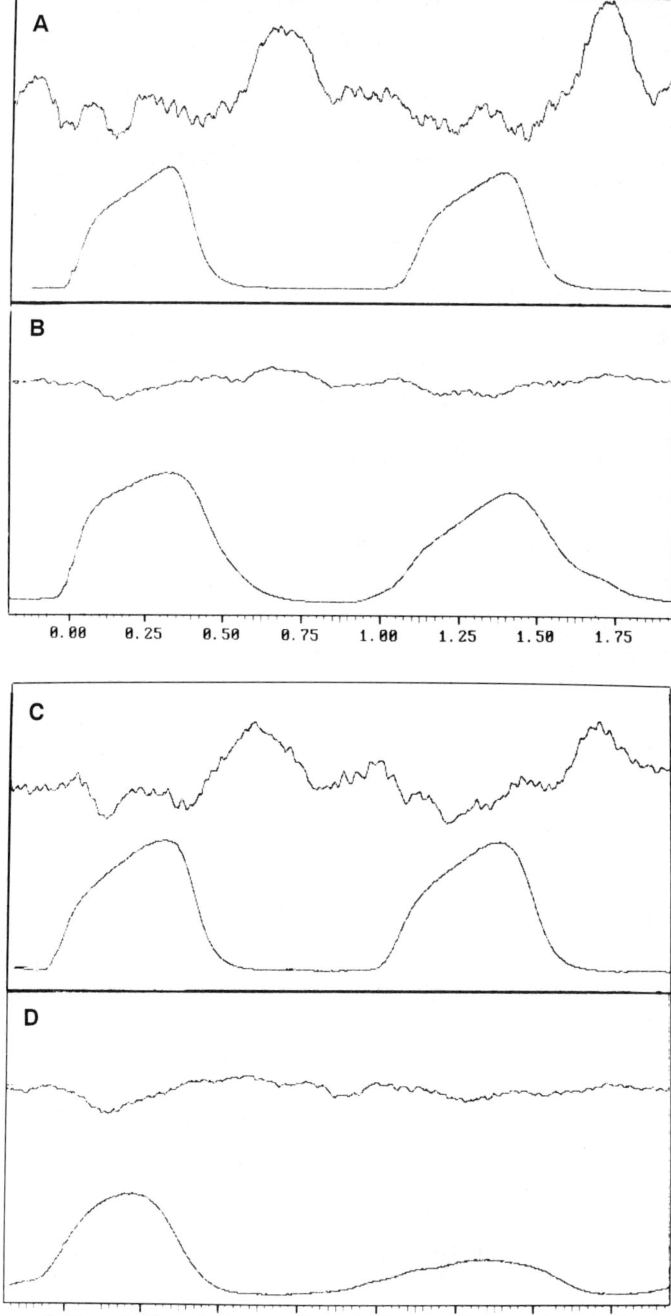

A
B
0.00  0.25  0.50  0.75  1.00  1.25  1.50  1.75
C
D
0.00  0.25  0.50  0.75  1.00  1.25  1.50  1.75

# Power Density Spectra (PDS) of Sympathetic Nerve Discharge Frequencies in Rat

In vagotomized, baro- and chemoreceptor denervated, paralyzed and artificially ventilated rats anesthetized with pentobarbital, power spectral analysis of cervical and lumbar sympathetic trunk activity was performed. Fast Fourier transform of time series of sympathetic activity was plotted as power of the signal against its frequency components. Whole nerve activity was band-pass filtered (0.2, 2000 Hz) and passed to an analog integrator with a time constant of 0.1 s, then it was fed to the amplifier with a gain of 5 to eliminate the DC component. The signal was sampled at 100 Hz by CED real-time computer. Power spectra were computed on 16 sequential time windows each being 10 s long and averaged. 1024 block size was used. Total power was contained between 0.4–1 Hz frequency, corresponding to the usual respiratory rhythm and 7–7.5 Hz frequency corresponding to the cardiac rhythm (Fig. 6.6A). Peaks of power corresponding to respiratory frequency were usually evident in the spectrum. If respiratory rate was fast enough, the respiratory peak overlapped with the main range of power in frequencies contained between 2 Hz and 6 Hz. Peaks within this band of frequency appeared often (Fig. 6.6A). Some of them represented harmonics of respiratory or cardiac frequencies. In animals with vagus nerves and baroreceptors intact a peak corresponding to respiratory pump frequency was evident if central respiratory rhythm was not entrained to lung inflation. Also, the amplitude of the 7 Hz-frequency peak, corresponding to cardiac frequency, was significantly greater in baroreceptor intact animals. This is in agreement with the data of Barman and Gebber (1989) in the rat, although the frequency range in their recordings from splanchnic nerve was extended to 10 Hz. Furthermore, in the cat the maximal power in PDS is contained within the 2–6 Hz-frequency band (Barman and Gebber, 1989). Peak frequencies at 10 Hz were reported in cat (Gootman and Cohen, 1981). Taking into account a lower resting heart rate in the cat as compared to rat, it appears that the overall pattern of PDS, relative to cardiac frequencies, is slightly shifted to higher frequencies in the cat. This may be a species difference or an effect of different experimental conditions and the

FIGURE 6.5. Averaged lumbar trunk sympathetic activity (top trace) triggered by the onset of the integrated phrenic nerve burst (bottom trace) at point 0.00 s. A: control, corresponds to PDS in Fig. 6.6A; **B**: after microinjection of, MgCl$_2$ (300 nl, 4 mM) into the ipsilateral RVLM inluding PA area, corresponds to PDS in Fig. 6.6C; **C**: return to control after 10 min, corresponds to PDS in Fig. 6.6D; **D**: after kynurenic acid (300 nl, 0.5M) microinjected into the ipsilateral RVLM, corresponds to PDS in Fig. 6.6E.

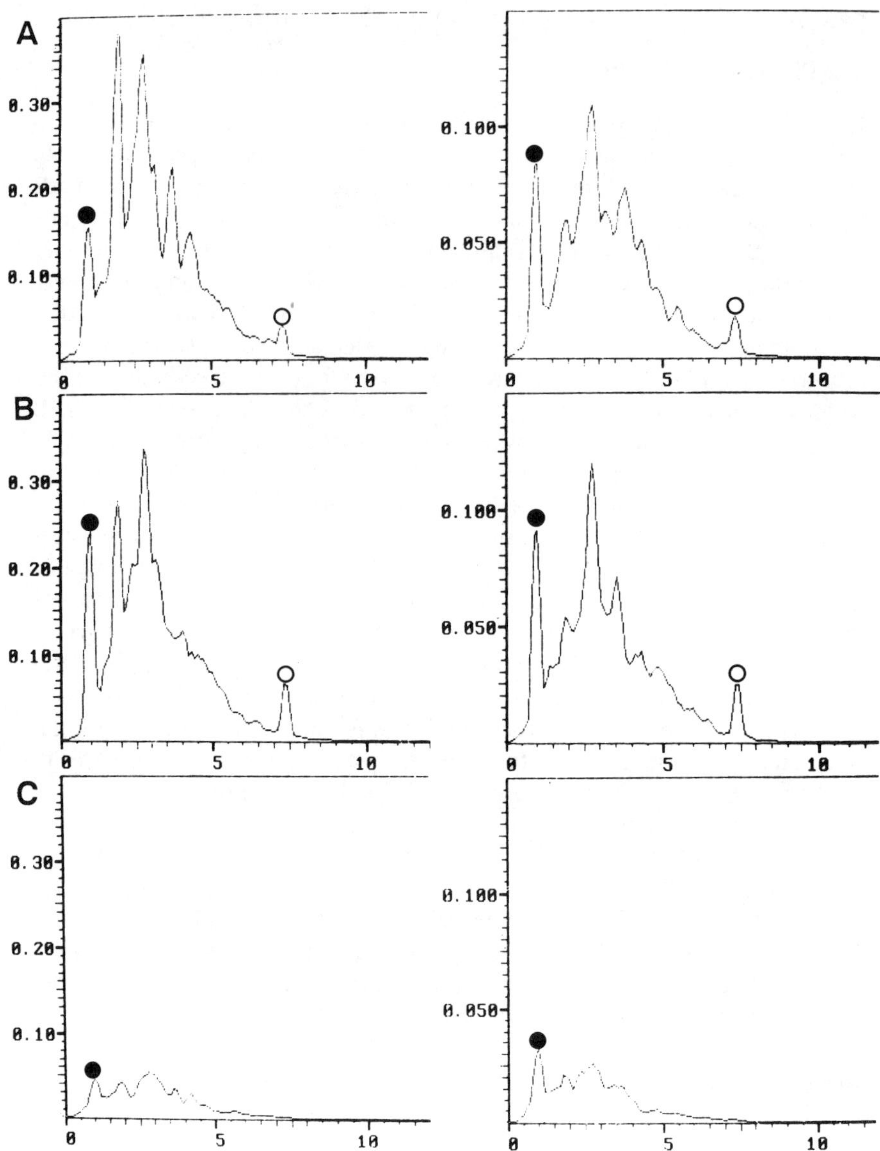

FIGURE 6.6. Power density spectra of the activities of two branches (left and right panels, respectively) separated from the lumbar sympathetic trunk (L4–L5) in a vagotomized and baroreceptor denervated rat. **A**: control, the PDS of both branches contained three components in the frequency range of 0.5–8 Hz. The first peak at 1 Hz corresponds to the rate of phrenic nerve activity (solid dot), the second diffuse component from 1 Hz to 6 Hz is related to the non-respiratory bulbar sympathetic tone generator, the thrid component peak at 7.5 Hz corresponds to cardiac frequency (open dot); **B**: sympathoexcitatory effect of glutamate (20 nl, 0.5 M) microinjected into the ipsilateral RVLM. **C**: Effects of $MgCl_2$ (300 nl, 4 mM)

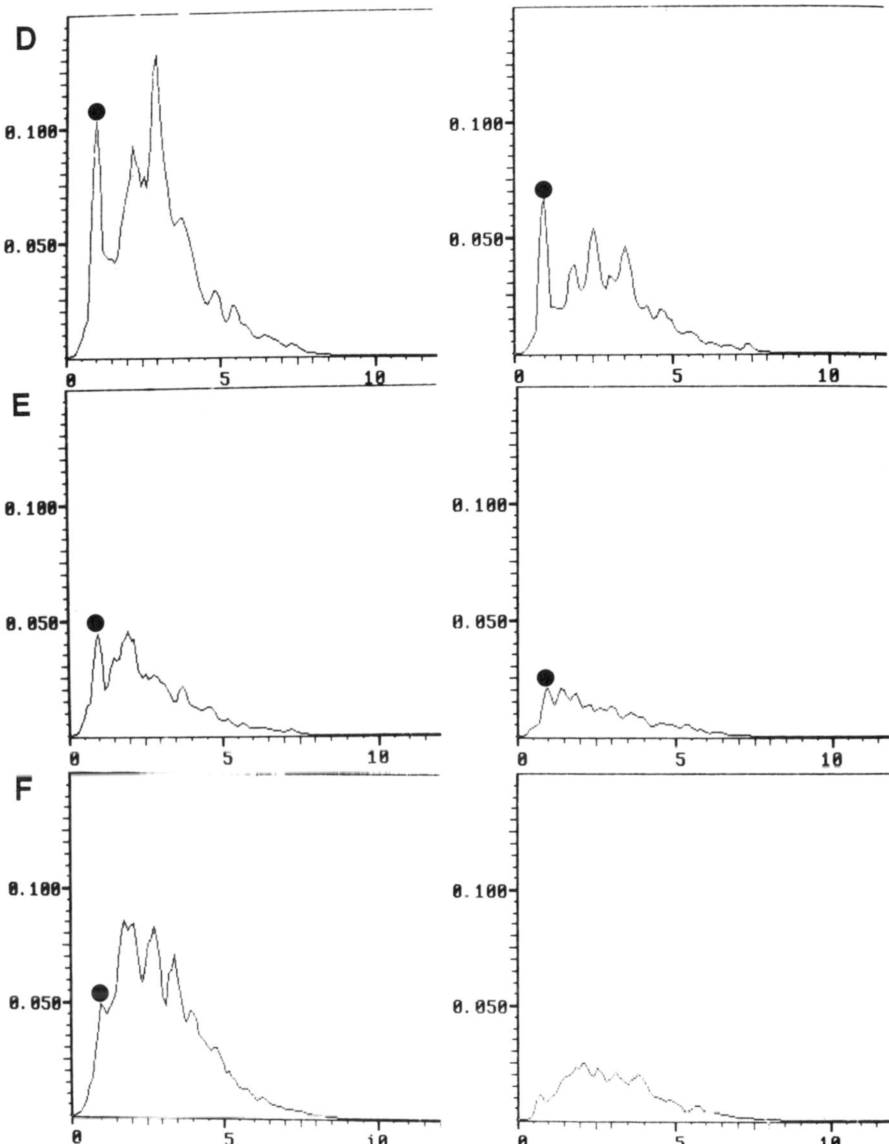

microinjected into the ipsilateral RVLM. sympathetic activity and blood pressure are slightly increased but respiratory activity is unchanged; **D**: return to control after 10 min; **E**: Effects of kynurenic acid (300 nl, 0.5 M) microinjected into the same area; **F**: PDS after 30 minutes. Phrenic nerve activity was decreased and periodicities in the right branch still reduced; **G**: Effects of CoCl₂ (300 nl, 12 mM) microinjected into the same area; **H**: PDS after high C1–C2 spinal cord section in the same rat.

x − axis: power (voltage$^2$); y − axis: frequency in Hz.

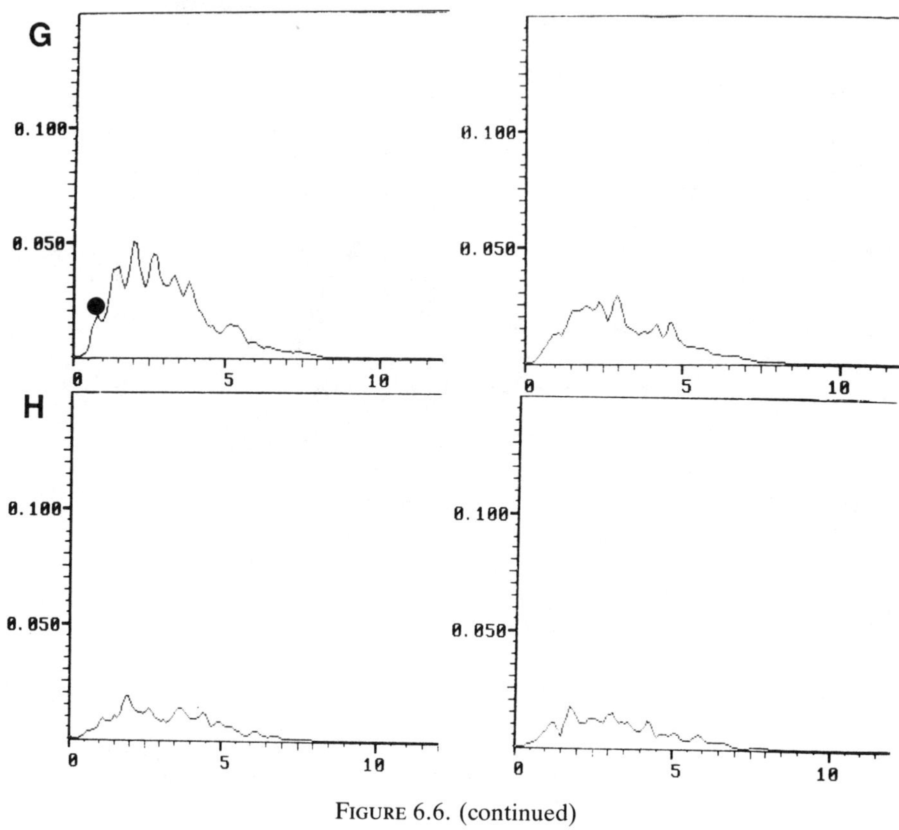

FIGURE 6.6. (continued)

type of anesthetic used. Some diffuse periodicities, although without distinct peaks, still remained in PDS after spinal cord section of rats (Fig 6.6H), an effect not significant in spinal cats unless in asphyxia or after strychnine administration (Gootman and Cohen, 1981).

## Effect of Synaptic Transmission Blockade in RVLM by Microinjections of $CoCL_{22}$ and $MgCL_2$ and Effect of Kynurenate Microinjections upon Sympathetic Rhythms

Microinjection of 150–300 nl of 4–12 mM $Mgcl_2$ or 4–12 mM $CoCl_2$ into RVLM reduced or abolished synaptic transmission in this region. This effect was verified by testing the sympathoinhibitory baroreflex. Norepinephrine administered i.v. in baroreceptor intact animals reduced SA and caused a pressor effect. After bilateral microinjections of $CoCl_2$ or $MgCl_2$ into the RVLM, the sympathoinhibitory baro-reflex was abolished

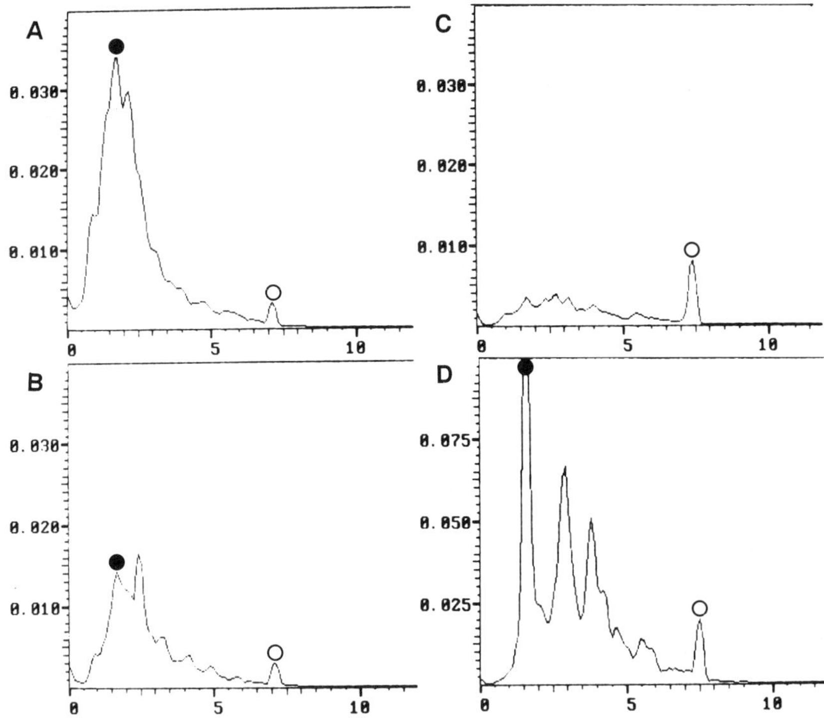

FIGURE 6.7. Power density spectra of lumbar sympathetic trunk activity in baroreceptor intact rat. **A**: control. PDS contains two sharp peaks at 1.9 Hz and 7.2 Hz. The first peak corresponds to the frequency of fast phrenic activity (solid dot), the second peak corresponds to the cardiac frequency (open dot); **B**: PDS after microinjection of $MgCl_2$ (150 nl, 4 mM) into the ipsilateral RVLM including the para-ambigual area. Blood pressure and overall sympathetic activity unchanged; **C**: PDS after microinjection of $MgCl_2$ (150 nl, 12 mM) into the symmetrical contra-lateral RVLM. Blood pressure and overall sympathetic activity increased; **D**: PDS after 20 min. Sympathetic activity and blood pressure continued to be elevated. x − axis: power (voltage$^2$); y − axis: frequency in Hz.

and, usually, blood pressure was slightly increased. $MgCl_2$ or $CoCl_2$ micro-injection into the RVLM reduced or totally abolished the PDS peak corresponding to respiratory rhythm (Fig. 6.6C, G, Fig. 6.7) and significantly depressed all other periodicities. In some experiments, presumably depending on the area of penetration, $Mg^{2+}$ or $Co^{2+}$ selectively suppressed respiratory frequency-related peaks and the 2–6 Hz band of frequencies, leaving the cardiac frequency-related component of PDS intact (Fig. 6.7). A desynchronizing effect was already evident in PDS after unilateral (ipsi- or contralateral) microinjection of $MgCl_2$ or $CoCl_2$. After bilateral micro-injections the desynchronization of PDS was more pronounced (Fig.

6.7). In some experiments, PDS appeared almost flat with only small power in the 2–6 Hz range. A similar significant desynchronization was observed after kynurenate microinjections into the RVLM (Fig. 6E). The desynchronization of PDS was associated with an almost total disappearance of the respiratory modulation of SA, as assessed by averaging SA triggered by the phrenic burst. Compare Fig. 6.5 and 6.6, in which recordings of PDS and averaged sympathetic discharge are taken from the same animal. Surprisingly, neither $Co^{2+}$ nor $Mg^{2+}$ microinjected into the RVLM or the para-ambigual area has any effect upon the pattern of central respiratory activity: the frequency and amplitude of phrenic bursts remained unchanged.

## Discussion and Conclusions

The present study provides further evidence that the para-ambigual area within the rostroventrolateral medulla contains populations of neurons of critical importance in the generation of respiratory-related periodicity and in the timing of rhythmical sympathetic discharge within the respiratory cycle, as reported before (Baradziej and Trzebski, 1989). In support of this conclusion is the specificity of pharmacological interventions which are effective only if applied within this restricted area. Microinjections of very small volumes of glutamate into PA caused a significant change in the timing of respiratory-sympathetic synchronization without affecting the central resporatory pattern, blood pressure, or overall sympathetic activity. Furthermore, microinjection of $Co^{2+}$ or $Mg^{2+}$ did not influence respiration, but completely abolished respiratory-related sympathetic periodicities. These results suggest that a population of interneurons in the RVLM acts as an interphase between the respiratory oscillator and sympathoexcitatory RVLM neurons. We hypothesize that in the rat, propriobulbar respiratory-related neurons in the proximity of the pars compacta of the rostral ambigual nucleus (Saether et al., 1987), relay excitatory and/or inhibitory inputs to sympathoexcitatory RVLM neurons from neurons involved in the generation of respiratory rhythm (Richter et al., 1986). Further research is needed, however, to test this possibility. So far our data indicate that the para-ambigual area within the RVLM is critical for the respiratory-coupled pattern of sympathetic discharge.

An even more interesting finding of this study is that the same area of the RVLM is involved in the expression of other, non-respiratory periodicities of sympathetic discharge. Desynchronization of PDS is evident after unilateral (ipsi- or contralateral) microinjections of $Co^{2+}$, $Mg^{2+}$ or kynurenate into the RVLM, which suggests that both symmetrical RVLM areas contribute to the generation of sympathetic rhythms. Our conclusion is consistent with findings that respiratory-related synchronization of the sympathetic discharge is reduced or abolished in split-medulla preparation in the cat (Kubin et al., 1985).

The present results do not conclusively prove that the RVLM and/or the para-ambigual area is the site of the origin of sympathetic rhythmicities, although this possibility has to be considered. The mechanism of the generation of sympathetic periodicities is still debated. It may be related to pacemaker-like neurons in the RVLM projecting to the spinal cord (Sun et al., 1988), it may originate in an antecendent probabilistic network oscillator (Barman and Gebber, 1989), or within a common diffuse oscillatory system of synaptically interconnected functional subsystems with sliding mutual coordination of rhythms between them (Koepchen et al., 1986; Bachoo and Polosa, 1986).

Whatever is the site of generation of sympathetic periodicities, they have to be projected to a very restricted area of the rostral ventrolateral medulla as defined in this study, as any intervention within this critical site disturbs or abolishes sympathetic oscillations including the respiratory-related rhythmicity of sympathetic discharge. It is tempting to suggest that the para-ambigual area of the RVLM, where synchronization of respiratory and sympathetic rhythmicities occurs, receives inputs from other neuronal oscillatory networks and represents a pivotal neuronal population which shapes these inputs into the final pattern of sympathetic periodicities.

*Acknowledgements.* Supported by the Wellcome Foundation and the Polish Academy of Sciences.

# References

Adrian ED, Bronk DW and Phillips G (1932): Discharges in mammalian sympathetic nerves. *J Physiol (Lond.)* 74:115–153.

Bachoo M and Polosa C (1986): Lack of evidence of coupled oscillator mechanisms in the generation of sympathetic Rhythm. In: *Organization of the Autonomic Nervous System. Central and Peripheral Mechanisms*, Ciriello J, Calaresu FR, Renaud LP, Polosa C, (eds.) New York, Alan R Liss, Inc., pp 189–202.

Bainton CR, Richter DW, Seller H, Ballantyne D and Klein JP (1985): Respiratory modulation of sympathetic activity. *J Auton Nerv Syst* 12:77–90.

Baradziej S and Trzebski A (1989): Specific areas of the ventral medulla controlling sympathetic and respiratory activities and their functional synchronization in the rat. In: *The Central Neural Organization of Cardiovascular Control*, Ciriello J, Caverson MM and Polosa C, (eds.) *Progress in Brain Res* 81:193–204.

Barman SM and Gebber GL (1989): Basis for the naturally occurring activity of rostral ventrolateral medullary sympathoexcitatory neurons. In: *The Central Neural Organization of Cardiovascular Control*, Ciriello J, Caverson MM and Polosa C, (eds.) *Progress in Brain Res*: Amsterdam-New York-Oxford, Elsevier 81:117–129.

Ciriello J, Caverson MM and Polosa C (eds). (1989): *Progress in Brain Research* 81: Amsterdam-New York-Oxford, Elsevier Czyzyk M, Fedorko L and Trzebski A (1987): Pattern of the respiratory modulation of the sympathetic activity is species dependent; synchronization of the sympathetic outflow over the respiratory cycle in the rat. In: *Organization of the Autonomic Nervous System. Central and*

*Peripheral Mechanisms*, Ciriello J, Calaresu FR, Renaud LP Polosa C, (eds.) New York, Alan R Liss, pp 143–152.

Czyzyk-Krzyska M and Trzebski A (1990): Respiratory related discharge pattern of sympathetic nerve activity in the spontaneously hypertensive rat. *J Physiol (London)*: 426, 355–368.

Gootman PM and Cohen MI (1981): Sympathetic rhythms in spinal cats. *J Auton Nerv Syst* 3:379–387.

Haselton JR and Guyenet PG (1989): Central respiratory modulation of medullary sympathoexcitatory neurons in rat. *Am J Physiol* 256:R739–R750

Koepchen HP, Hilton SM and Trzebski A (eds.) (1980): *Central Interaction between Respiratory and Cardiovascular Control Systems*, Berlin-Heidelberg-New York, Springer Verlag.

Koepchen HP, Abel HH and Klüssendorf D (1986): Brain stem generation of specific and non-specific rhythms. In: *Organization of the Autonomic Nervous System. Central and Peripheral Mechanisms*. Ciriello J, Calaresu FR, Renaud LP, Polosa C, (eds.) New York, Alan R. Liss, Inc., pp 179–188.

Kubin L, Trzebski A and Lipski J (1980): Split medulla preparation in the cat: arterial chemoreceptor reflex and respiratory modulation of the renal sympathetic nerve activity. *J Auton Nerv Syst* 12:211–225.

McAllen RM (1986): Action and specificity of ventral medullary vasopressor neurones in the cat. *Neuroscience* 18:51–59.

Morrison SF, Milner TA, Pickel BM and Reis DJ (1988): Reticulospinal vasomotor neurons of the rat rostral ventrolateral medulla (RVL): relationship to sympathetic nerve activity and the C1 adrenergic group. *J Neurosc* 8:1286–1301.

Richter DW, Ballantyne D and Remmers JE (1986): How is the respiratory rhythm generated? A model. *News Physiol Sci* 1:109–112.

Ross CA, Ruggiero DA and Reis DJ (1981): Projection to the spinal cord from neurons close to the ventral surface of the hindbrain of the rat. *Neurosci Lett* 21:143–148.

Ross CA, Ruggiero DA, Joh TH, Park DH and Reis DJ (1983): Rostral ventrolateral medulla: selective projection to the thoracic autonomic cell column from the region containing C1 adrenaline neurons. *J Comp Neurol* 228:168–185.

Ruggiero DA, Cravo SL, Arango V and Reis DJ (1989): Central control of the circulation by the rostral ventrolateral reticular nucleus: anatomical substrates. In: *The Central Neural Organization of Cardiovascular Control*, Ciriello J, Caverson MM and Polosa C, (eds.) *Progress in Brain Research*, Amsterdam-New York-Oxford, Elsevier 81:49–79.

Saether K, Hilaire G and Monteau R (1987): Dorsal and ventral respiratory groups of neurons in the medulla of the rat. *Brain Res* 419:87–96.

Sun MK, Hackett JT and Guyenet PG (1988): Sympathoexcitatory neurons of rostral ventrolateral medulla exhibit pacemaker properties in presence of glutamate-receptor antagonist. *Brain Res* 438:23–40.

Trzebski A (1990): Species differences in interaction between autonomic nervous system and respiratory system. In: *Cardiorespiratory and Motor Coordination*, Koepchen HP (ed.) Springer Verlag (in press).

# Section II
## Central Neurotransmitter Systems

# 7
# Interaction of Angiotensin II with Catecholamines in the Brain

Fatimunnisa Qadri, Emilio Badoer, Thilo Stadler,
Annette Veltmar, and Thomas Unger

Almost 30 years ago, the circulating effector hormone of the renin-angiotensin system (RAS), the octapeptide angiotensin II (ANG II), was first reported to act not only on peripheral vascular structures but also on the central nervous system (CNS) (Bickerton and Buckley, 1961). In the following years, evidence has accumulated that the brain, in addition to possessing ANG II-sensitive sites, contains the precursor molecule as well as the enzymatic apparatus to generate its own angiotensin peptides, suggesting a local synthesis of ANG II in the brain (Brosnihan et al., 1988; Ganten et al., 1971; Unger et al., 1988). In addition, the protein genes of the RAS are expressed in the CNS and mRNAs have been localized in specific brain areas (Hellmann et al., 1988; Jin et al., 1988), although not all components of the RAS were demonstrated within the same neuron. ANG II receptors were found in the rat brain mainly in the thalamus, hypothalamus, midbrain, septum, and medulla (Bennett and Snyder, 1976; Mendelsohn et al., 1984; Sirett et al., 1977), with higher concentrations in the lateral septum, superior colliculus, and area postrema and very high concentrations in the subfornical organ (SFO), median preoptic area (MnPO), organum vasculosum of the lamina terminalis (OVLT), medial preoptic area (MPO), paraventricular nucleus (PVN), supraoptic nucleus (SON), and nucleus tractus solitarii (NTS). In the PVN very high levels of ANG II binding sites were found in both the magnocellular and parvocellular regions (Felix et al., 1988; Imboden et al., 1989; Mendelsohn, 1988). Taken together, these data support the idea that ANG II acts in the brain as a neurotransmitter or neuromodulator (Moffet et al., 1987; Printz, 1988).

A comparison of the current findings on the distribution of ANG II immunoreactive neurons and fibers in the brain with the localization of catecholamine-containing neurons and catecholaminergic nerve endings reveals some striking associations. For example, angiotensin-containing neurons originating in the SFO have been shown to project nerve fibers to the MnPO, OVLT, PVN, and SON. Also, ANG II fibers from the PVN terminate in catecholamine-rich nuclei in the brainstem such as the locus coeruleus (LC) and the nucleus tractus solitarii (NTS) as well as in the spinal cord (Lind, 1988; Lind et al., 1985; McKinley et al., 1989; Simon et al., 1989). In addition, the NTS and LC in the brainstem contain high concentrations of both catecholamines (Saavedra et al., 1986) and ANG II receptors (Mendelsohn, 1988; Mendelsohn et al., 1984), as do many parts of the hypothalamus. Thus, components of the ANG II system and catecholamines are anatomically closely related in areas of the brain associated with ANG II-mediated blood pressure regulation (Fig. 7.1).

## Central Actions of ANG II

ANG II acts in the brain in a dual fashion: as a circulating hormone that can reach receptor sites in the brain, where the blood-brain barrier is not fully intact, and as a neuromodulator or neurotransmitter within a number

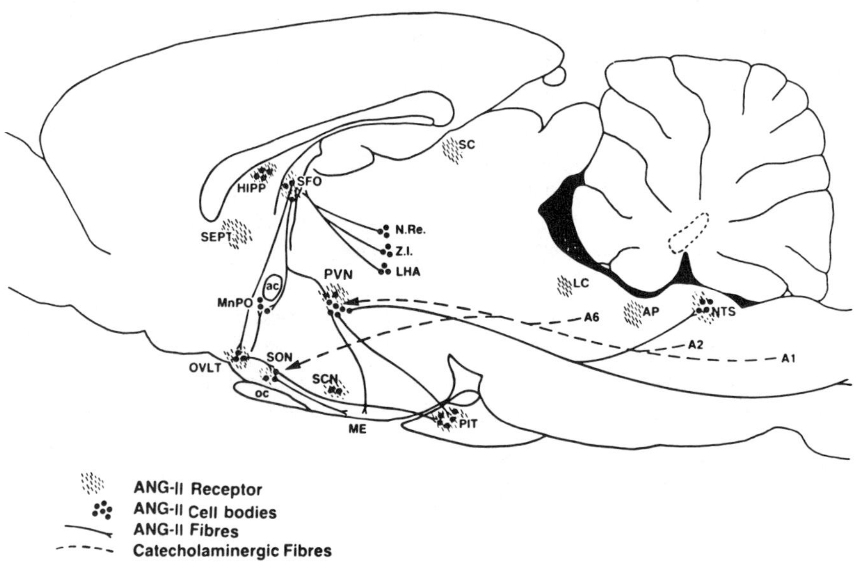


FIGURE 7.1. A schematic diagram representing main ANG II receptor sites (shaded areas) and ANG II containing cell bodies (dark circles) in the brain as well as neural angiotensinergic fibres and/or pathways (solid lines) and catecholaminergic projections (dashed lines). A1, A2, A6: catecholamine-containing nuclei in the brainstem; ANG II: angiotensin II; ac: anterior commisure; AP: area postrema; CC: corpus callosum; HIPP: hippocampus; LC: locus coeruleus; LHA: lateral hypothalamic area; ME: median eminence; MnPO: median preoptic nucleus; N. Re.: nucleus reuniens; NTS: nucleus tractus solitarii; OC: optic chiasm; OVLT: organum vasculosum of the lamina terminalis; PIT: pituitary gland; PVN: paraventricular nucleus; SC: superior colliculus; SCN: suprachiasmatic nucleus; SEPT: septum; SFO: subfornical organ; SON: supraoptic nucleus; Z.I.: zona incerta.

of anatomically discrete brain structures and pathways. Stimulation of ANG II receptors in the brain evokes a set of coordinated autonomic, endocrine, and behavioral responses including an increase in blood pressure and water intake as well as stimulation of natriuresis, salt appetite, and secretion of vasopressin, oxytocin, adrenocorticotropin (ACTH), and other pituitary hormones.

For more detailed information concerning the central ANG II-induced actions see reviews by Phillips (1987) and Unger et al. (1988).

## Interaction of Noradrenaline with ANG II in the Brain

The demonstration of an interaction between ANG II and noradrenaline (NA) in peripheral sympathetic nerve terminals (McCubbin and Page, 1963; Zimmermann, 1962) has stimulated research on whether a similar interaction would also take place in the brain.

In vitro studies suggested that ANG II may not release NA from brain tissues by itself but rather enhance electrically stimulated NA outflow (Meldrum et al., 1984). This finding was consistent with the previous observation that ANG II increased the $K^+$-induced release of NA in rabbit hypothalamic slices, an effect that was blocked by the ANG II-receptor antagonist saralasin (Garcia-Sevila et al., 1979).

On the other hand, a number of in vivo studies demonstrated that catecholamines were critical for the expression of ANG II's central actions. Smookler et al. (1966) showed that depletion of catecholamine stores in the brain by intracerebroventricular (i.c.v.) reserpine blunted the pressor response to i.c.v. ANG II. A subsequent study (Severs et al., 1971) showed that the pressor and dipsogenic actions of i.c.v. ANG II were associated with an activation of $\alpha$-adrenergic receptors in the brain, suggesting that NA was the catecholamine interacting with ANG II. Central pretreatment with 6-hydroxydopamine (6-OHDA) attenuated the pressor responses to i.c.v. ANG II in rats. In these animals the neurotoxin had significantly reduced the NA concentration in brain and spinal cord without having an influence on the dopamine (DA) concentration (Badoer et al., 1988; Bellin et al., 1987; Bellin et al., 1988).

Sumners and Phillips (1983), using $\alpha$-methyl-p-tyrosine ($\alpha$-MT), which blocks the neuronal synthesis of catecholamines, reported that i.c.v. ANG II injections increased the turnover of NA in specific brain regions associated with blood pressure control without changing the dopamine utilization. For example, an i.c.v. injection of a pressor dose of ANG II stimulated the NA utilization in the LC, the raphé magnus, and A1 regions of the brainstem and in the hypothalamus. This effect was not due to the rise in blood pressure caused by ANG II, since a similar pressor response induced by intravenous hypertonic saline did not alter NA utilization in any of the above regions. Areas such as the SFO and the OVLT that contain both catecholaminergic nerve terminals and ANG II receptors did not show a substantial change in catecholamine utilization after i.c.v. application of ANG II.

In an other in vivo study, ANG II given i.c.v. increased the concentration of NA in the cerebrospinal fluid (CSF) (Chevillard et al., 1979). However, these experiments did not answer the question as to whether ANG II stimulated the NA release into the CSF or inhibited NA reuptake. Further experiments, using primary neuronal cultures of neonatal rat brainstem cells, demonstrated that ANG II may increase NA uptake at concentrations as low as $10^{-10}$ M after a short incubation period (5 min). However, following a longer incubation period (15–30 min), an inhibition of NA uptake was observed (Sumners and Raizada, 1986; Sumners et al., 1990). Palaic and Khairallah (1967) demonstrated that large amounts of ANG II infused into the brain inhibited NA uptake from the cerebral ventricles. Subsequent in vitro experiments in brain slices (Khairallah, 1972) and brain synaptosomes (Janowsky et al. 1972) also indicated that ANG II inhibited NA uptake in the brain.

The above described studies provide evidence, although in most cases circumstantial, that ANG II may use NA to mediate its central (pressor) actions. To elucidate these interactions further, we investigated the effects of ANG II on central catecholamines in vivo by using the novel technique of brain microdialysis coupled with HPLC and electrochemical detection to measure the endogenous release of catecholamines in discrete brain nuclei (Badoer et al., 1989a; Ungerstedt, 1984; Westerink et al., 1987). With the help of this technique, monoamines and their metabolites can be measured in the same brain perfusate, including adrenaline (A), NA, DA, serotonin (5-HT), and their major intraneuronal metabolites, that is, 3,4-dihydroxyphenylethylene glycol (DOPEG), 3,4-dihydroxyphenylacetic acid (DOPAC), and 5-hydroxyindol acetic acid (5-HIAA).

We first studied the effects of ANG II on monoamine release from the anterior hypothalamus (AH), an area that was reported to play an important role in the central cardiovascular actions of ANG II (Benarroch et al., 1983; Hartle et al., 1982; Hartle and Brody, 1984). ANG II perfused directly into the AH of anesthetized normotensive rats via the microdialysis probe did not alter basal catecholamine release. However, after $K^+$-stimulation there was a striking increase of the main intraneuronal metabolite of DA, DOPAC, in the perfusate (Badoer et al., 1989b). Thus, in the anterior nucleus of the hypothalamus ANG II does not appear to interfere directly with NA release in vivo but has some previously unknown effects on the DA metabolism that need to be further investigated.

In further experiments we examined the effects of periventricular ANG II receptor stimulation on catecholamine release in discrete hypothalamic nuclei in vivo. In these experiments, ANG II was injected i.c.v. in conscious freely moving rats and the microdialysis probe was placed in the nucleus under investigation. In contrast to the previous experiments, where ANG II was directly perfused into the AH, ANG II injected i.c.v.

selectively increased the NA release from the AH without changing the release of other catecholamines or metabolites. This effect was abolished by i.c.v. pretreatment with the ANG II-receptor antagonist sarilesin (Qadri et al., 1990). We subsequently focused our experiments on the PVN and SON, since both areas are critically involved in the central actions of ANG II. Like in the AH, but even more impressively, ANG II increased NA outflow in both nuclei in a dose-dependent fashion at doses from 100 pg to 100 ng i.c.v. without altering the release of other monoamines or monoamine metabolites (unpublished data).

These data provide the first in vivo evidence that stimulation of periventricular ANG II receptors engenders a selective release of NA from anterior hypothalamic nuclei, especially the PVN and SON, which participate in the central actions of the peptide. Since this effect was observed only at pressor doses of ANG II, an indirect pathway including baroreceptor reflex activation and subsequent NA release from the brainstem to the PVN or SON cannot be excluded at present (Day et al., 1984a,b).

However, if NA release is instrumental in the well known ANG II-induced stimulation of vasopressin release from the PVN and SON—an important central pressor mechanism of ANG II (Unger et al., 1985)—such an indirect stimulation of NA release via the baroreceptor reflex does not appear to be likely, since it would tend to raise blood pressure even further instead of dampening the pressor response. Further studies, including baroreceptor reflex inactivation and blockade of central adrenergic receptors, will help to clarify the role of NA in the PVN and SON for the central actions of ANG II.

## Interaction of DA with ANG II in the Brain

Booth (1968) first demonstrated the involvement of DA in ANG II-induced dipsogenic actions. He could further demonstrate that the dipsogenic response induced by DA was slightly greater than the dipsogenic response to NA.

Shortly thereafter, Fitzsimons and Setler (1971) observed that low doses of phentolamine and propranolol injected locally into the preoptic region of the hypothalamus did not block the dipsogenic response to ANG II, suggesting that stimulation of $\alpha$- and $\beta$-adrenoceptors was not involved in the ANG II-induced drinking response. On the other hand, the dopaminergic receptor antagonists, haloperidol and spiroperidol, selectively inhibited ANG II-induced drinking. Moreover, i.c.v. administration of DA caused a dipsogenic response, if given at high doses (Fitzsimons and Setler, 1975). However, Camacho and Phillips (1981) could not reproduce these findings with either DA or with the dopaminergic receptor agonist apomorphine. These results indicate that DA is not a potent dipsogen by itself, but the possibility that DA may play a permissive role for ANG II-induced drinking still exists. Pharmacological studies revealed that DA may also be involved in the pressor responses to ANG II. For instance, pretreatment of rats with haloperidol reduced the pressor response to i.c.v. ANG II by nearly 50%, even though it did not reduce the vasopressin release to i.c.v. ANG II (Hoffman et al., 1977). Other studies also indicated an interaction between ANG II and DA in the brain. For example, ANG II caused an increased release of DA from the rat striatum measured in vitro and in vivo (Simmonet and Giorguieff-Chesselet, 1979; Simmonet et al., 1981).

A few reports suggest an involvement of DA in the ANG II-mediated release of pituitary hormones. Application of ANG II i.c.v. stimulated DA turnover in the nucleus accumbens and in the median eminence, where DA has been associated with a decrease in prolactin release from the anterior pituitary gland (Fuxe et al., 1980; Steele et al., 1982).

In vitro studies using neuronal cultures revealed a significant increase in neuronal DA levels in response to ANG II, but only at the highest concentrations of ANG II used in the culture medium (7.5 and 15 $\mu$m). This response was fully abolished by coincubation with the ANG II receptor antagonist, saralasin, implying that this action was ANG II-receptor mediated (Sumners et al., 1990).


## Interaction of A with ANG II in the Brain

Data in the literature regarding the effects of ANG II on A in the brain are scarce. This may be because of the low levels of A in the CNS implying methodological problems in the measurement of this amine. Nevertheless, an increased A turnover was observed in the caudal part of the dorsomedial medulla after i.c.v. injection of renin (Fuxe et al., 1980). Renin also increased A turnover in a block of brainstem tissue containing the NTS, the nucleus commissuralis, and the dorsal motor nucleus of the vagus. The effects were specifically mediated by ANG II (Schacht, 1984).


## Conclusion

There is ample evidence from in vitro and in vivo studies that catecholamines in the brain are involved in the various central actions of ANG II. It appears that release of NA in distinct brain nuclei contributes rather to the central pressor actions of the peptide, whereas DA might be instrumental in ANG II-induced drinking.

Critical issues for further investigation will be the elucidation of the exact sites of this peptide-neurotransmitter interaction as well as the description of the pathways involved. Further points of interest include the nature of the interaction, for example, catecholamine release versus uptake, and the effects of ANG II on catecholamine metabolism. Finally, the role of neurotransmitters other than catecholamines, such as serotonin or acetyl-choline, for the central actions of ANG II needs to be investigated in more detail.


# References


Badoer E, Würth H, Qadri F, Itoi K, Unger T (1988): Central noradrenergic pathways are not involved in the pressor response to intracerebroventricular substance P. *Eur J Pharmacol* 154:105–108.

Badoer E, Würth H, Türk D, et al. (1989a): The K$^+$-induced increases in noradrenaline and dopamine release are accompanied by reductions in the release of their intraneuronal metabolites from the rat anterior hypothalamus. An in vivo brain microdialysis study. *Naunyn-Schmiedeberg's Arch Pharmacol* 339:54–59.

Badoer E, Würth H, Türk D, et al. (1989b): Selective local action of angiotensin II on dopaminergic neurons in the rat hypothalamus in vivo. *Naunyn-Schmiedeberg's Arch Pharmacol* 340:3–35.

Bellin SI, Bhatnagar RK, Johnson AK (1987): Periventricular noradrenergic systems are critical for angiotensin-induced drinking and blood pressure responses. *Brain Res* 403:1105–112.

Bellin SI., Landas SK, Johnson AK (1988): Selective catecholamine depletion of structures along the ventral lamina terminalis: Effects on experimentally-induced drinking and pressor responses. *Brain Res* 456:9–16.

Bennarroch EE, Balada MS, Finkeilman S, Nahmod VE (1983): Neurogenic hypertension after depletion of norepinephrine in anterior hypothalamus induced by 6-hydroxydopamine administration into the ventral pons: Role of serotonin. *Neuropharmacology* 22:29–34.

Bennett JP, Snyder SH (1976): Angiotensin II binding to mammalian brain membranes. *J Biol Chem* 251:7423–7430.

Bickerton RK, Buckley JP (1961): Evidence for a central mechanism in angiotensin-induced hypertension. *Proc Soc Exp Biol Med* 1106:834–836

Booth DA (1968): Mechanism of action of norepinephrine in eliciting an eating response on injection into the rat hypothalamus. *J Pharmacol Exp Ther* 160:336–348.

Brosnihan KB, Schiavone MT, Sprunger AE, Chappell MC, Rio M, Ferrario AE (1988): In vivo release of angiotensin II from the rat hypothalamus. *Hypertension* 11(suppl I):I.1588–I.162.

Camacho A, Phillips MI (1981): separation of drinking and pressor responses to central angiotensin by monoamines. *Am J Physiol* 240:R106–R113.

Chevillard C, Duchene N, Pasquier R, Alexander JM (1979): Relation of the centrally evoked pressor effect of angiotensin II to central noradrenaline in the rabbit. *Eur J Pharmacol* 58:203.

Day TA, Ferguson AV, Renaud LP (1984a): Facilitatory influence of noradrenergic afferents on the excitability of rat paraventricular nucleus neurosecretory cells. *J Physiol (Lond)* 355:237–250.

Day TA, Renaud LP (1984b): Electrophysiological evidence that noradrenergic afferents selectively facilitate the activity of supraoptic vasopressin neurons. *Brain Res* 303:233–240.

Felix D, Harding JW, Imboden H (1988): The hypothalamic- angiotensin system: location and functional considerations. *Clin Exp Hypertens* A10 (suppl 1):45–62.

Fitzsimons JT, Setler PE (1971): Catecholaminergic mechanisms in angiotensin-induced drinking. *J Physiol* 218:43P–44P.

Fitzsimons JT, Setler PE (1975): The relative importance of central nervous catecholaminergic and cholinergic mechanisms in drinking in response to angiotensin and other thirst stimuli. *J Physiol* 250:63–631.

Fuxe K, Andersson K, Locatelli V, et al. (1980): Neuropeptides and central catecholamine systems: Interactions in neuroendocrine and central cardiovascular regulation. In: *Neural peptides and Neuronal Communication*, Costa E, Traabucchi M, eds. New York: Raven Press.

Ganten D, Minnich JL, Granger P, et al. (1971): Angiotensin forming enzyme in brain tissue. *Science* 173:64–65.

Garcia-Sevila JA, Dubocovich ML, Langer SZ (1979): Angiotensin II facilitates the potassium-evoked release of $^3$H-noradrenaline from the rabbit hypothalamus. *Eur J Pharmacol* 56:173–176.

Hartle DK, Brody M (1984): The angiotensin II pressor system of the rat forebrain. *Circ Res* 54:355–366.

Hartle DK, Lind W, Johnsohn AK, Brody M (1982): Localization of the anterior hypothalamic angiotensin II pressor system. *Hypertension* 4(suppl II):II.159–II.165.

Hellmann W, Suzuki F, Ohkubo H, Nakanishi S, Ludwig G, Ganten D (1988): Angiotensinogen gene expression in extrahepatic rat tissues: Application of a solution hybridization assay. *Naunyn-Schmiedeberg's Arch Pharmacol* 338: 327–331.

Hoffman WE, Phillips MI, and Schmid P (1977): The role of catecholamines in central antidiuretic and pressor mechanisms. *Neuropharmacology* 16:563–569.

Imboden H, Haarding JW, Felix D (1989): Hypothalamic angiotensinergic fibre systems terminate in the neurohypophysis. *Neurosci Lett* 96:42–46.

Janowsky DS, Davis JM, Fann WE, Freeman J, Nixon R, and Michelakis AA, (1972): Angiotensin effect on uptake of norepinephrine by synaptosomes, *Life Sci* 11, Pt 1:1–11

Jin M, Wilhelm M, Lang RE, et al. (1988): Endogenous tissue renin-angiotensin systems. From molecular biology to therapy. *Am J Med* 84(suppl 3A):28–36.

Khairallah PA (1972): Action of angiotensin on adrenergic nerve endings: inhibition of norepinephrine uptake. *Fed Proc* 31:1351–1357.

Lind WR (1988): Angiotensin and the lamina terminalis: illustration of a complex unity. *Clin Exp Hypertens* A10(suppl 1):79–105.

Lind RW, Sawson LW, Ganten D (1985): Organization of angiotensin II immunoreactive cells and fibres in the rat nervous system. *Neuroendocrinology* 40:2–24.

McCubbin JW, Page IH (1963): Renal pressor system and neurogenic control of arterial pressure. *Circ Res* 12:553–559.

McKinley MJ, Allen AM, Chai SY, Hards DK, Mendelsohn FAO, Oldfield BJ (1989): The lamina terminalis and its neural connections: neural circuitry involved in angiotensin action on fluid and electrolyte homeostasis. *Acta Physiol Scand* 136:113–118.

Meldrum MJ, Xne CS, Badino L, Westfall TC (1984): Angiotensin facilitation of noradrenergic neurotransmission in central tissues of the rat: Effects of sodium restriction. *J Cardiovasc Pharmacol* 6:989.

Mendelsohn FAO (1988): Localization of angiotensin II receptors in rat kidney and brain. In: *Angiotensin and Blood Pressure Regulation*, Harding JW, Wright JW, Speth RC, Barnes CD, eds. New York: Academic Press, pp 61–81.

Mendelsohn FAO, Quirion R, Saavedra JM, Aguilera G, Catt KJ (1984): Autoradiographic localization of angiotensin II receptors in rat brain. *Proc Natl Acad Sci USA* 81:1575–1579.

Moffet RB, Bumpus FM, Husain A (1987): Cellular organization of the brain renin-angiotensin system. *Life Sci* 41:1867–1897.

Palaic C, Khairallah PA (1967): Effects of angiotensin on uptake and release of norepinephrine by brain. *Biochem Pharmacol* 16:2291–2298.

Phillips MI (1987): Functions of angiotensin in the central nervous system. *Annu Rev Physiol* 49:413–435.

Printz MP (1988): Regulation of the brain angiotensin system: a thesis of multicellular involvement. *Clin Exp Hypertens* 10:17–35.

Qadri F, Badoer E, Stadler T, Unger T (1990): Stimulatory effect of angiotensin-II on noradrenaline release in anterior hypothalamus of conscious rats. An in vivo brain microdialysis study. *Eur J Pharmacol* 183(2):427–428.

Saavedra JM, Brownstein MJ, Kizer JS, Palkovits M (1976): Biogenic amines and related enzymes in the circumventricular organs of the rat. *Brain Res* 107:412–417.

Schacht U (1984): Effects of angiotensin II and ACE inhibitors on electrically stimulated noradrenaline release from superfused rat brain slices. *Clin Exp Hyperten* A6:1847.

Severs WB, Summy-Long J, Daniels-Severs A, Connor JD (1971): Influence of adrenergic blocking drugs on central angiotensin effects. *Phamacology* 5:205–214.

Simmonet G, Giorguieff-Chesselet MF (1979): Stimulating effect of angiotensin II on the spontaneous release of newly synthesized $^3$H-dopamine in rat striatal slices. *Neurosci Lett* 15:153–158.

Simmonet G, Giorguieff-Chesselet MF, Carayon A, Bioulac B, Chesselin F, Glowinski J, Vincent JD (1981): Angiotensin II and the nigrostriatal system. *J Physiol Paris* 77:71–79.

Simon E, Gerstberger R, Gray DA, Matsumura K (1989): Location and functional properties of angiotensin targets in the third ventricular region. *Acta Physiol Scand* 136(suppl 583):119–129.

Sirett NE, McLean AS, Bray JJ, Hubbard JI (1977): Distribution of angiotensin II receptors in rat brain. *Brain Res* 122:299–312.

Smookler HH, Severs WB, Kinnard WJ, Buckley JP (1966): Centrally mediated cardiovascular effects of angiotensin II. *J Pharmacol Exp Ther* 153(3):4885–494.

Steele MK, Negro-Vilar A, McCann SM (1982): Modulation by dopamine and estradiol of the central effects of angiotensin II on anterior pituitary hormone release. *Endocrinology* 111:722.

Sumners C, Myers LM, Kalberg CJ, Raizada MK (1990): Physiological and pharmacological comparisons of angiotensin II receptors in neuronal and astrocyte glial cultures. *Prog Neurobiol* 34:355–385.

Sumners C, Phillips MI (1983): Central injection of angiotensin II alters catecholamine activity in rat brain. *Am J Physiol* 244:R257–R263.

Sumners C, Raizada MK (1986): Angiotensin II stimulates norepinephrine uptake in hypothalamus/brainstem neuronal cultures. *Am J Physiol* 250:C236–C244.

Unger T, Badoer E, Ganten D, Lang RE, Rettig R (1988): Brain angiotensin:

Pathways and pharmacology. *Circulation* 77(suppl 1):1–40.

Unger T, Becker H, Petty M, et al. (1985): Differential effects of angiotensin II and substance P on sympathetic nerve activity in conscious rats. Implications for cardiovascular adaptation to behavioral responses. *Circ Res* 56:563–575.

Unger T, Itoi K, Badoer E, et al. (1989): Central catecholaminergic mechanisms of blood pressure control. *Curr Opin Cardiol* 4(suppl 4):S3–S11.

Ungerstedt U (1984): Measurement of neurotransmitter release by intracranial dialysis. In: *Measurement of Neurotransmitter Release in Vivo*, Marsden CA, ed. Chichester: John Wiley and Sons Ltd, pp 81–105.

Westerink BHC, Damsma G, Rollema H, De Vries JB, Horn AS (1987): Scope and limitation of in vivo brain dialysis: A comparison of its application to various neurotransmitter systems. *Life Sci* 41:1763–1776.

Zimmermann BG (1962): Effect of acute sympathectomy on responses to angiotensin and norepinephrine. *Circ Res* 11:780–786.

# 8
# Actions of Angiotensin II in the Ventrolateral Medulla Oblongata

ANDREW M. ALLEN, SHUICHI SASAKI, ROGER A.L. DAMPNEY, FREDERICK A.O. MENDELSOHN, AND WILLIAM W. BLESSING

Angiotensin II (ANG II) regulates numerous brain functions including drinking and salt appetite, release of both anterior and posterior pituitary hormones, and regulation of cardiovascular function through interactions with central control of efferent autonomic activity (see Phillips, 1987) as well as the well characterized actions on peripheral tissues (see Peach, 1977). The central actions are probably mediated by both systemic and endogenous neuronal angiotensin.

Receptor binding sites for ANG II, localized by in vitro autoradiography, occur in restricted sites in the mammalian central nervous system (Mendelsohn et al., 1984, 1988). The pharmacological specificity of the central ANG II binding site indicates that it may be a biologically relevant ANG II receptor, recognizing ANG II and ANG III with similar potency and having low affinity for the precursor ANG I. This contention is also supported by the very high correlation between the distribution of ANG II receptor binding sites, ANG II responsive neurons determined by electrophysiology, and ANG II-like immunoreactive nerve terminals (Lind, 1987).

A high density of ANG II receptor binding occurs in the rostral and caudal ventrolateral medulla (VLM), in the region of the C1 and A1 catecholamine-containing cell groups, respectively (Fig. 8.1) (Allen et al., 1988a; Mendelsohn et al., 1988). Both regions contain an ANG II-like immunoreactive terminal field (Lind et al., 1985), suggesting the possibility that ANG II may be released from nerve terminals in the VLM.

The rostral VLM contains bulbospinal neurons that project to the preganglionic sympathetic neurons in the intermediolateral cell column of the spinal cord (Dampney et al., 1987; Ross et al., 1984a). Stimulation of the rostral VLM results in widespread, sympathetically mediated vasoconstriction (Dampney et al., 1982; McAllen and Dampney, 1989). Conversely, inhibition or ablation of the rostral VLM reduces blood pressure to levels observed after cervical spinal cord section, suggesting that this region is the major source of tonic sympathetic efferent activity to the cardiovascular system (Dampney and Moon, 1980; Ross et al., 1984b). Several studies

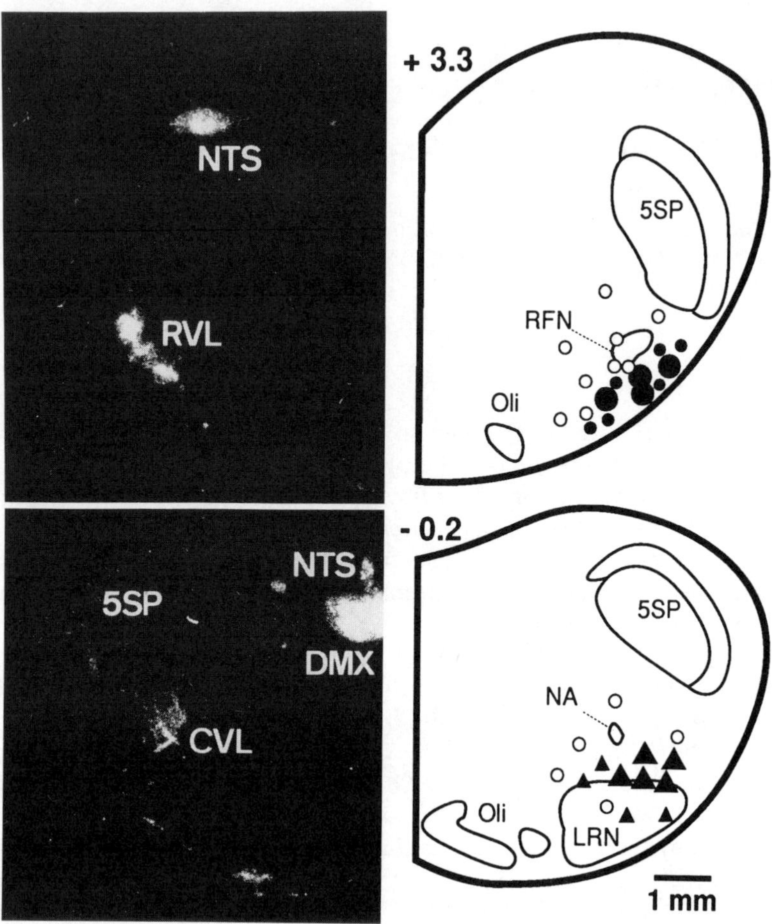


FIGURE 8.1. Comparison of the distributions of ANG II receptor binding sites, demonstrated by in vitro autoradiography (LHS), and sites where microinjections of ANG II alter mean arterial pressure (RHS), at two levels of the rabbit ventrolateral medulla (3.3 mm rostral and 0.2 mm caudal to the obex, respectively). ANG II receptor binding sites (white areas) occur in both the rostral (RVL) and caudal (CVL) ventrolateral medulla and also in the nucleus of the solitary tract (NTS), the dorsal motor nucleus of vagus (DMX), and the nucleus of the spinal trigeminal tract (5SP). The right hand side shows changes in mean arterial pressure elicited by microinjection of 20 pmol of ANG II (20 nl) into the ventrolateral medulla (small closed circles indicate a 6–20 mm Hg increase while large closed circles represent an increase of greater than 20 mm Hg; small closed triangles depict a 6- 1 5 mm Hg decrease and large closed triangles a decrease in mean arterial pressure of greater than 15 mm Hg). In both diagrams the open small circles indicate sites at which no response was observed. Oli: olivary nucleus; NA: nucleus ambiguus; RFN: retrofacial nucleus; LRN: lateral reticular nucleus. (The diagrams of changes in mean arterial pressure were adapted from Sasaki and Dampney, 1990, with permission.)

have also shown that the rostral VLM is involved in phasic regulation of blood pressure (Dampney and Moon, 1980; Granata et al., 1985; McAllen, 1986). Electrophysiological studies have demonstrated that there are neurons in the rostral VLM that have pacemaker properties indicative of sympathoexcitatory neurons (Barman and Gebber, 1985; Brown and Guyenet, 1984; Morrison et al., 1988). Some of these neurons exhibit a tonic pacemaker-like activity in the absence of external inputs (Sun et al., 1988a). The pacemaker cells do not contain catecholamines (Sun et al., 1988b), but at least some nonpacemaker sympathoexcitatory neurons are catecholaminergic (Haselton and Guyenet, 1989).

The A1 region, in the caudal VLM, exerts a tonic depressor action, probably through an inhibitory, gamma-aminobutyric acid (GABA)-ergic connection with the rostral VLM (Blessing, 1988). In addition to producing a depressor response, stimulation of neurons in the caudal VLM elicits release of vasopressin (Blessing and Reis, 1982; Blessing and Willoughby, 1985a; Kubo et al., 1985). Several lines of evidence indicate that stimulation of the catecholamine-containing A1 neurons within the caudal VLM, which project directly to the magnocellular neurosecretory neurons of the hypothalamic paraventricular and supraoptic nuclei, produces vasopressin release and that this pathway is involved in baroreflex control of vasopressin release (Blessing and Day et al., Day and Sibbald, 1988, 1989; Kannan et al., 1984; Sawchenko and Swanson, 1982; Willoughby, 1985b).

The striking localization of ANG II receptor binding sites in the region of the catecholamine-containing cells of the rostral and caudal VLM suggested that ANG II might be an important neuropeptide in this area, regulating cardiovascular and neuroendocrine function. We therefore examined this question by microinjecting ANG II into the rostral and caudal VLM to determine the effect on cardiovascular function and, in the caudal VLM, on vasopressin release.


## Rostral VLM

Unilateral microinjection of ANG II (10–50 pmol in 20 nl) into the rostral VLM of the chloralose-anesthetized cat produced a dose-dependent increase in mean arterial pressure and a secondary baroreflex-mediated bradycardia (Fig. 8.2) (Allen et al., 1988b). Ganglionic blockade by intravenous administration of hexamethonium abolished the pressor response to ANG II in the rostral VLM, demonstrating that the response was due to stimulation of sympathetic efferent activity. Histological verification of the injection sites revealed that responsive areas were confined to a highly localized region called the subretrofacial nucleus (McAllen and Dampney, 1989), which contains a very high density of ANG II receptor binding (Allen et al., 1988b).

In the rostral VLM of the pentobarbital-anesthetized rabbit, microinjec-

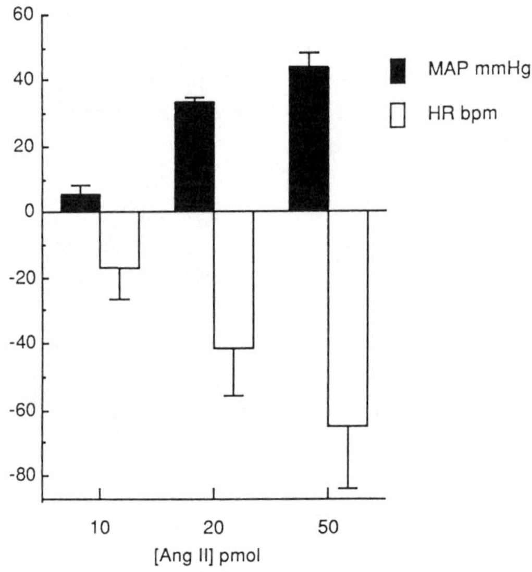


FIGURE 8.2. Histograms demonstrating the changes in mean arterial pressure (MAP, mm Hg) and heart rate (HR, bpm) produced by microinjections of ANG II into the rostral ventrolateral medulla of the anesthetized cat.

tion of ANG II (0.02–20 pmol in 20 nl) also increased blood pressure (Fig. 8.1)(Sasaki and Dampney, 1990). In contrast, microinjection of an ANG II receptor antagonist, [Sar$^1$, Thr$^8$] ANG II (sarthran) produced a long-lasting depressor effect (Sasaki and Dampney, 1990).

Similarly, Andreatta et al. (1988) found that application of ANG II or sarthran to the "glycine-sensitive area" on the ventral surface of the cat medulla, which is adjacent to the rostral VLM, also elicits an increase or decrease in blood pressure, respectively. Thus, the results of these experiments in both cats and rabbits indicate that ANG II, which may be tonically released in the rostral VLM, has an excitatory action on pressor neurons within this region.

It is not known whether ANG II exerts its excitatory effects by a presynaptic or postsynaptic action. In an electrophysiological study in the rat using an in vitro slice preparation, Sun and Guyenet (1989) found that direct application of ANG II to putative sympathoexcitatory pacemaker neurons did not alter their activity. This may indicate that ANG II normally acts only presynaptically, or, alternatively, that it acts only on non-pacemaker sympathoexcitatory neurons within the rostral VLM. As mentioned above, at least some of the latter group are catecholaminergic (Haselton and Guyenet, 1989). Another possibility is that, unlike its observed effects in the cat and rabbit, ANG II has little effect on any type of sympathoexcitatory neurons in the rat. Unlike other species (e.g., rabbit, cat, sheep, and human), the rat rostral VLM displays only a low density of ANG II receptor binding sites (Mendelsohn et al., 1984).

Intracisternal administration of very low doses of ANG II ($ED_{50}$—5 fmol) to the conscious rabbit elicits a dose-dependent pressor response (Head et al., 1988). The sensitivity of this response is increased 1000-old following sinoaortic denervation ($ED_{50}$—5 amol) (Head et al., 1988). Following sinoaortic denervation, intraspinal administration of 6-hydroxydopamine, which decreased spinal noradrenaline content without affecting serotonin levels, abolished the pressor response to intracerebroventricular ANG II (Elghozi and Head, 1990). In baroreceptor-intact anesthetized rabbits, the response to intracisternal administration of ANG II was significantly attenuated by the administration of [Sar[1], Ile[8]] ANG II, an ANG II receptor antagonist, into the rostral VLM (Head et al., 1990). These studies therefore suggest that the rostral VLM is exquisitely sensitive to ANG II in the conscious animal, lending support to the proposition that ANG II is physiologically important at this site.

Elghozi and Head (1990) also propose that the role of ANG II at the rostral VLM would be increased during inhibition of the baroreceptor reflex. It is interesting to note that microinjections of ANG II into the nucleus of the solitary tract suppress the baroreflex and that the spontaneously hypertensive rat also has inhibited baroreflex function (Casto and Phillips, 1986).

## Caudal VLM

Bilateral microinjections of ANG II (0.2–20 pmol in 20 nl or 0.1–100 pmol in 100 nl) into the caudal VLM of the anesthetized rabbit produced a depressor response and bradycardia (Figs. 8.1, 8.3) (Sasaki and Dampney, 1990; Allen et al., 1990). Microinjection of the ANG II receptor antagonist, sarthran, into the caudal VLM produced a small increase in blood pressure, suggesting that ANG II may also be tonically released in the caudal VLM, acting on the sympathoinhibitory neurons (Sasaki and Dampney, 1990).

Microinjection of ANG II into the caudal VLM of the urethane-anesthetized rabbit also stimulated vasopressin secretion (Fig. 8.3), presumably through activation of the A1 noradrenaline-containing neurons (Allen et al., 1990). This response was blocked by prior microinjection of sarthran into the caudal VLM. Sarthran alone did not affect vasopressin release and did not significantly alter the response to microinjections of the excitatory amino acid, N-methyl-D-aspartate (Allen et al., 1990). Stimulation of vasopressin release by ANG II in the caudal VLM was not dependent on the concomitant hypotension, but was due to a direct effect (Allen et al., 1990).

Bilateral microinjection of sarthran into the caudal VLM also significantly attenuated vasopressin release in response to hemorrhage (Allen et al., 1990). This dose of sarthran did not exert a general depressant effect, as the response to microinjections of N-methyl-D-aspartate was unaffected,

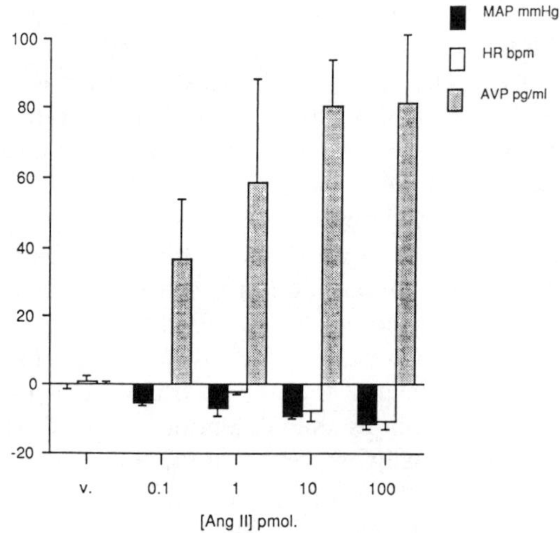


FIGURE 8.3. Histograms showing the changes in plasma vasopressin concentration (AVP, pg/ml), mean arterial pressure (MAP, mm Hg), and heart rate (HR, bpm) produced by ANG II microinjected into the caudal ventrolateral medulla of the anaesthetized rabbit. (Adapted from Allen et al., 1990.)

suggesting a specific role for ANG II in neural pathways mediating baroreflex control of vasopressin secretion.

Hemorrhage also stimulates production of systemic ANG II (Claybaugh and Share, 1973; Wang et al., 1983). However, blockade of the peripheral renin-angiotensin system does not alter hemorrhage-induced vasopressin release (Rose et al., 1987), indicating that the responses observed following microinjection of ANG II into the caudal VLM are not normally produced by systemic ANG II acting at this site. In addition, these observations strengthen the proposal that the blockade of hemorrhage-induced vasopressin secretion by sarthran in the caudal VLM is due to specific actions at this site and not to leakage of the antagonist into the circulation to block systemic ANG II acting at another site.

The results from our studies suggest that ANG II may be functionally important in the caudal VLM, mediating, or modulating, baroreceptor-initiated vasopressin release. At this site ANG II also tonically regulates cardiovascular function by excitation of the sympathoinhibitory neurones.

## Conclusion

ANG II receptor binding sites and ANG II-like immunoreactive nerve terminals occur in the VLM, where ANG II microinjections alter efferent sympathetic activity to the cardiovascular system and stimulate vasopressin release. As these sites are behind the blood-brain barrier, our observations strongly suggest a neurotransmitter or neuromodulatory role for ANG II in the VLM.

# References

Allen AM, Chai SY, Clevers, J, McKinley MJ, Paxinos G, Mendelsohn FAO (1988a): Localization and characterization of angiotensin II receptor binding and angiotensin converting enzyme in human medulla oblongata *J Comp Neurol* 269:249–264.

Allen AM, Dampney RAL, Mendelsohn FAO (1988b): Angiotensin receptor binding and pressor effects in cat subretrofacial nucleus *Am J Physiol* 255: H1011–H1017.

Allen AM, Mendelsohn FAO, Gieroba ZJ, Blessing WW (1990): Vasopressin release following microinjection of angiotensin II into the caudal ventrolateral medulla oblongata in the anaesthetized rabbit. *J Neuroendocrinol* 2:867–874.

Andreatta SH, Averill DB, Santos RAS, Ferrario CM (1988) The ventrolateral medulla: A new site of action of the renin-angiotensin system. *Hypertension* 11[S1]I-163–166.

Barman SM, Gebber GL (1985): Axonal projection patterns of ventrolateral medullospinal sympathoexcitatory neurons. *J Neurophysiol* 53:1551–1566.

Blessing WW (1988): Depressor neurons in rabbit caudal ventrolateral medulla act via GABA receptors in the rostral medulla. *Am J Physiol* 254:H686–H692.

Blessing WW, Reis DJ (1982): Inhibitory cardiovascular function of neurons in the caudal ventrolateral medulla of the rabbit: Relationship to the area containing A1 noradrenergic cells. *Brain Res* 253:161–171.

Blessing WW, Willoughby JO (1985a): Excitation of neuronal function in rabbit caudal ventrolateral medulla elevates plasma vasopressin. *Neurosci Lett* 58:189–194.

Blessing WW, Willoughby JO (1985b): Inhibiting the rabbit caudal ventrolateral medulla prevents baroreceptor-initiated secretion of vasopressin. *J Physiol (Lond)* 367:253–265.

Brown DL, Guyenet PG (1984): Cardiovascular neurons of brain stem with projections to spinal cord. *Am J Physiol* 247:R1009–R1016.

Casto R, Phillips MI (1986): Angiotensin II attenuates baroreflexes at nucleus tractus solitarius of rats. *Am J Physiol* 250:R193–R198.

Claybaugh JR, Share L (1973): Vasopressin, renin and cardiovascular responses to continuous slow hemorrhage. *Am J Physiol* 224:519–523.

Dampney RAL, Czachurski J, Dembowsky K, Goodchild AK, Seller H (1987): Afferent connections and spinal projections of the pressor region in the rostral ventrolateral medulla of the cat. *J Auton Nerv Sys* 20:73–86.

Dampney RAL, Goodchild AK, Robertson LG, Montgomery W (1982): Role of the ventrolateral medulla in vasomotor regulation: A correlative anatomical and physiological study. *Brain Res* 249:223–235.

Dampney RAL, Moon EA (1980): Role of the ventrolateral medulla in vasomotor response to cerebral ischemia. *Am J Physiol* 239:H349–H358.

Day TA, Ferguson AV, Renaud LP (1984): Facilitatory influence of noradrenergic afferents on the excitability of rat paraventricular nucleus neurosecretory cells. *J Physiol (Lond)* 355:237–249.

Day TA, Sibbald JR (1988): Solitary nucleus excitation of supraoptic vasopressin cells via adrenergic afferents. *Am J Physiol* 254:R711–R716.

Day TA, Sibbald JR (1989): A1 cell group mediates solitary nucleus excitation of supraoptic vasopressin cells. *Am J Physiol* 257:R1020–R1026.

Elghozi J-L, Head GA (1990): Spinal noradrenergic pathways and pressor responses to central angiotensin II. *Am J Physiol* 258:H240–H246.

Granata AR, Ruggerio DA, Park DH, Joh TH, Reis DJ (1985): Brain stem area with C1 epinephrine neurons mediates baroreflex vasodepressor responses. *Am J Physiol* 248:547–H567.

Haselton JR, Guyenet PG (1989): Electrophysiological characterization of putative C1 adrenergic neurons in the rat. *Neuroscience* 30:199–214.

Head GA, Elghozi J-L, Korner PI (1988): Baroreflex modulation of central angiotensin II pressor responses in conscious rabbits. *J Hypertens* 6[S4]:S505–S507.

Head GA, Williams NS, Goodwin SJ (1990): Evidence for central renin angiotensin system controlling sympathetic tone in the rabbit. *Proceedings of the Australian Physiological and Pharmacological Society*, 21:41P (abstract).

Kannan H, Yamashita H, Osaka T (1984): Paraventricular neurosecretory cells: Synaptic inputs from the ventrolateral medulla in rats. *Neurosci Lett* 51:183–188.

Kubo T, Amano H, Misu Y (1985): Caudal ventrolateral medulla. A region responsible for the mediation of vasopressin-induced pressor responses. *Naunyn-Schmiedberg's Arch Pharmacol* 328:368–372.

Lind RW (1987): Sites of action of angiotensin in the brain In: *Angiotensin and Blood Pressure Regulation*, Harding JW, Wright JW, Speth RC, Barnes CD, eds San Diego: Academic Press, pp 135–164.

Lind RW, Swanson LW, Ganten D (1985): Organization of angiotensin II immunoreactive cells and fibres in the rat central nervous system. *Neuroendocrinology* 40:2–24.

McAllen RM (1986) Identification and properties of subretrofacial bulbospinal neurones a descending cardiovascular pathway in the cat. *J Auton Nerv Syst* 17:151–164.

McAllen RM, Dampney RAL (1989) The selectivity of descending vasomotor control by subretrofacial neurons. In: *Progress in Brain Research Vol. 81. The Central Neural Organization of Cardiovascular Control*, Ciriello J, Caverson MM, Polosa C, eds Amsterdam: Elsevier, pp 233–242.

Mendelsohn FAO, Allen AM, Clevers J, Denton DA, Tarjan E, McKinley MJ (1988): Localization of angiotensin II receptor binding in rabbit brain by in vitro autoradiography. *J Comp Neurol* 270:372–384.

Mendelsohn FAO, Quirion R, Saavedra JM, Aguilera G, Catt KJ (1984): Autoradiographic localization of angiotensin receptor binding in rat brain. *Proc Natl Acad Sci USA* 81:1575–1579.

Morrison SF, Milner TA, Reis DJ (1988): Reticulospinal vasomotor neurons of the rat rostral ventrolateral medulla: Relationship to sympathetic nerve activity and the C1 adrenergic cell group. *J Neurosci* 8:1286–1301.

Peach MJ (1977): The renin angiotensin system: biochemistry and mechanism of action. *Physiol Rev* 55:313–369.

Phillips MI (1987): Functions of angiotensin in the central nervous system. *Annu Rev Physiol* 49:413–435.

Rose JC, Block SM, Flowe K, et al. (1987): Responses to converting-enzyme inhibition and hemorrhage in newborn lambs and adult sheep. *Am J Physiol* 252:R306–R313.

Ross CA, Ruggerio DA, Joh TH, Park DH, Reis DJ (1984a): Rostral ventrolateral medulla: selective projections to the thoracic autonomic cell column from the region containing C1 adrenaline neurons. *J Comp Neurol* 228:168–184.

Ross CA, Ruggiero GA, Park DH, et al. (1984b): Tonic vasomotor control by the rostral ventrolateral medulla: Effect of electrical or chemical stimulation of the area containing C1 adrenaline neurons on arterial pressure, heart rate, and plasma catecholamines and vasopressin. *J Neurosci* 4:479–494.

Sasaki S, Dampney RAL (1990): Tonic cardiovascular effects of angiotensin II in the ventrolateral medulla. *Hypertension* 15:274–283.

Sawchenko PE, Swanson LW (1982): The organisation of noradrenergic pathways from the brainstem to the paraventricular and supraoptic nuclei in the rat. *Brain Res Rev* 4:275–325.

Sun M-K, Guyenet PG (1989): Effects of vasopressin and other neuropeptides on rostral medullary sympathoexcitatory neurons "in vitro." *Brain Res* 492:261–270.

Sun M-K, Hackett JT, Guyenet PG (1988a): Sympathoexcitatory neurons of rostral ventrolateral medulla exhibit pacemaker properties in the presence of a glutamate-receptor antagonist. *Brain Res* 438:23–40.

Sun M- K, Young BS, Hackett JT, Guyenet PG (1988b): Reticulospinal pacemaker neurons of the rat rostral ventrolateral medulla with putative sympathoexcitatory function: an intracellular study in vitro. *Brain Res* 442:229–239.

Wang BC, Sundet WD, Hakumaki MOK, Goetz KL (1983): Vasopressin and renin responses to hemorrhage in concious, cardiac-denervated dogs. *Am J Physiol* 245:H399–H405.

# 9
# Cardiovascular Actions of Angiotensin II in the Ventrolateral Medulla

DAVID B. AVERILL, HIROMI MURATANI, KARLA J. MADALIN, AND CARLOS M. FERRARIO

Angiotensin II (ANG II) has received considerable attention as a humoral regulator of cardiovascular homeostasis because of its well known actions at resistance vessels, its stimulatory effects on neurohormonal systems and its role as a potent dipsogen via actions in the hypothalamus. Furthermore, evidence obtained over the last 25 years has shown that circulating Ang II acts at restricted sites in the central nervous system lacking an intact blood-brain barrier to influence the regulation of the autonomic nervous system. ANG II enhances the activity of the sympathetic nervous system by an action of the peptide at the area postrema. Many aspects of ANG II involvement in circulatory homeostasis are directly related to the plasma concentration of this peptide. However, local tissue renin-angiotensin systems (RAS) have been recognized as contributing to the regulation of arterial pressure. Evidence shows that the brain contains a functional RAS. Angiotensinogen is a major protein component of cerebrospinal fluid (Brosnihan et al., 1987) and glial cells contain abundant mRNA necessary for the synthesis of the renin substrate (Deschepper et al., 1986). Immuno-histochemical and anatomical studies have shown that ANG II and binding sites for this peptide are found in brain regions important in the regulation of hydromineral balance and cardiovascular function (Aguirre et al., 1989; Diz et al., 1986; Lind et al., 1985a,b; Speth et al., 1985). In the hypothalamus, circumventricular organs that respond to blood-borne ANG II by eliciting dipsogenic and pressor responses may utilize neural pathways exhibiting ANG II immunoreactivity. (Hartle and Brody, 1984; Hartle et al., 1982; Mogenson and Kucharczyk, 1978). At the level of the lower brain stem ANG II acts at a number of sites in the vagal-solitarii complex to influence cardiovascular function (Averill et al., 1987; Campagnole-Santos et al., 1988; Casto and Phillips, 1984a,b, 1985; Diz et al., 1984). Additional studies have provided evidence that actions of ANG II in the brain contribute to the pathogenesis of hypertension (for review see Unger et al., 1988). As a circumventricular organ permeable to blood-borne ANG II, the area postrema may play an important pathogenic role in certain models

104

of ANG II-dependent hypertension (Fink et al., 1987a,b; Mangiapane et al., 1989). Furthermore, it has been suggested that the elevated blood pressure of spontaneously hypertensive rats (SHR) may be related to an overactivity of the brain RAS. In part, this is based on the demonstration that central administration of ANG II antagonists or angiotensin-converting enzyme (ACE) inhibitors ameliorate this form of hypertension (Mann et al., 1978; McDonald et al., 1980; Okuno et al., 1983; Unger et al., 1981).

Recent studies have demonstrated ANG II binding sites as well as ANG II-containing cells and fibers in the ventrolateral medulla at sites that participate in cardiovascular regulation (Allen et al., 1987; Allen et al., 1988; Mendelsohn et al., 1988; Speth et al., 1985). Therefore, we undertook studies to determine the role that ANG II plays in cardiovascular regulation by actions of this peptide at discrete regions of the ventrolateral medulla. Furthermore, we investigated whether vasomotor regions of the ventrolateral medulla could represent sites where ANG II participates in the pathogenesis of hypertension.

In this chapter we review recent findings that implicate the vasomotor regions of the ventrolateral medulla as an important site at which intrinsic ANG II contributes to the regulation of sympathetic nervous system function and possibly the expression of hypertension. To understand how ANG II influences cardiovascular regulation via actions in the medulla oblongata, a number of aspects of peptide function should be appreciated. These include the demonstration that the cardiovascular effects of the peptide are mediated by functionally specific cell groups of the ventrolateral medulla, knowledge about the location and density of ANG II receptors in the lower brain stem, and elucidation of the biochemical cascade that leads to the formation of peptide at sites appropriate for cardiovascular responses. In reviewing the cardiovascular actions of ANG II in the medulla, two terms require some clarification. First, endogenous denotes the presence of the peptide in the vicinity of neurons that participate in the regulation of circulatory function. The use of this term does not necessarily imply the source of the peptide. Second, exogenous denotes administration of the peptide from an external source. In most cases this will be either by microinjection into the brain parenchyma or by topical application of the peptide to the surface of the medulla oblongata.

## Cardiovascular Functions of the Ventrolateral Medulla

The importance of the ventral medulla in circulatory control was first indicated by observations made in the 1870's (Dittmar, 1873; Owsjannikow, 1871). However, Guertzenstein and colleagues (Feldberg and Guertzenstein, 1972; Guertzenstein, 1973; Guertzenstein and Lopes, 1984; Guertzenstein and Silver, 1974) demonstrated that the ventrolateral medulla is composed of functionally distinct regions involved in cardiovascular regulation. Recent studies have shown that neurons of the rostral and caudal ventrolateral medulla participate in baroreceptor reflex control of sympathetic outflow (for reviews see Calaresu and Yardley, 1988; Ciriello et al., 1986). Neurons restricted to the subretrofacial nucleus of the rostral ventrolateral medulla (RVLM) are crucial to the maintenance of sympathetic nerve activity compatible with normal cardiovascular function. Stimulation of this region augments sympathetic nerve activity, whereas inhibition or lesion of these neurons suppresses sympathetic discharge and reduces blood pressure to spinal levels. Anatomical (Amendt et al., 1979; Caverson et al., 1983) and electrophysiologic (Barman and Gebber, 1985; Brown and Guyenet, 1984, 1985; Caverson et al., 1983) studies have shown that RVLM neurons have bulbospinal axons projecting to sympathetic preganglionic neurons of the thoracic and lumbar spinal cord. These bulbospinal neurons provide the predominant facilitatory drive to sympathetic preganglionic neurons. They also act as a major integrating site for baroreceptor-related and nonbaroreceptor input for sympathofacilitatory drive from the brain stem.

Neurons of the caudal ventrolateral medulla (CVLM) are an important source of GABAergic input to RVLM neurons (Blessing, 1988; Dampney et al., 1988; Sun and Guyenet, 1985; Willette et al., 1984). Stimulation of CVLM neurons produces a large decrease in blood pressure and sympathetic nerve activity (Gordon, 1987; Minson et al., 1987; Willette et al., 1983). Conversely, inhibition or lesion of CVLM neurons in normotensive animals substantially augments sympathetic nerve activity and results in significant elevations of blood pressure (Granata et al., 1985; Granata et al., 1986). A number of recent studies provide convincing evidence that CVLM neurons participate in baroreflex inhibition of RVLM pressor neurons and sympathetic outflow (Agarwal et al., 1989; Agarwal et al., 1990; Gordon, 1987; Urbanski and Sapru, 1988a,b). The results of these studies are consistent with the view that CVLM neurons are indirectly excited by baroreceptor input impinging upon second order neurons of the nucleus tractus solitarius (nTS). Excitation of these CVLM neurons then augments GABAergic inhibitory drive to RVLM neurons. As such, these neurons constitute the inhibitory link in the negative feedback loop that characterizes baroreflex control of sympathetic nerve activity. What is particularly interesting is the apparent multiplicity of roles that the CVLM plays in circulatory control. CVLM neurons also participate in chemoreflex control of vasopressin release from the neurohypophysis. Renaud et al. (1988) and colleagues suggest that noradrenergic CVLM neurons augment vasopressin release via a stimulatory effect on hypothalamic paraventricular neurons.

# Tissue Concentration of ANG II Peptide and Location of ANG II Receptors in the Medulla Oblongata

The demonstration of high affinity binding sites for ANG II in brain stem nuclei that participate in cardiovascular regulation has often been an important step in determining a central neurogenic role for ANG II in circulatory function. Thus, the observation of high affinity binding sites for ANG II in the RVLM of the dog (personal communication from D. Diz; Speth et al., 1985) and rat (Gehlert et al., 1986) initially provided us with the impetus to determine if this peptide acted at vasomotor neurons to produce cardiovascular responses. Allen and coworkers (Allen et al., 1987; Allen et al., 1988) and Mendelsohn et al. (1988) also used in vitro receptor autoradiography to identify high affinity binding sites for ANG II in both the RVLM and CVLM of rabbits and humans. Since the ventrolateral medulla contains neurons that subserve respiratory function as well as cardiovascular regulation, we determined whether the ANG II binding sites revealed in autoradiograms were receptors linked to cardiovascular regulation.

Other anatomical information that supports a role for the brain RAS in cardiovascular regulation is the demonstration by immunocytochemical techniques that the RVLM and CVLM contain cells and fibers immunoreactive to ANG II. Lind et al., (1985b) revealed a sparse distribution of ANG II-immunoreactive fibers residing in the dorsolateral aspect of the nucleus ambiguus. On the other hand, Aguirre et al. (1989) found neural elements immunoreactive to ANG II in the Bötzinger complex, nucleus ambiguus, and nucleus retroambiguus of the cat. The ability of Aguirre et al. (1989) to identify ANG II immunoreactive perikarya and fibers restricted to ventrolateral medullary structures involved in respiration may have been related to the intraparenchymal injection of colchicine used by these investigators. The possibility that ANG II participates in cardiovascular regulation by acting as a neurotransmitter is suggested by the recent observation that a significant proportion of A1 and C1 neurons contain both ANG II-like and tyrosine hydroxylase-like immunoreactivities (Covenas et al., 1990). In addition, the use of ANG II antagonists has permitted us and other investigators (Sasaki and Dampney, 1990) to uncover cardiovascular functions of ANG II endogenous to the ventrolateral medulla.

# Cardiovascular Actions of Exogenously Applied Ang II to the Ventrolateral Medulla

The seminal paper of Guertzenstein and Silver (1974) showed that neurons of the RVLM contribute significantly to the maintenance of tonic sympathetic outflow. One of the techniques that these investigators used to reach this conclusion was bilateral topical application of glycine to the ventral surface of the RVLM, which profoundly decreased blood pressure. Hence, this region was labeled as the glycine-sensitive area (GSA). In our first demonstration that ANG II acted in the ventrolateral medulla to affect cardiovascular function, we applied the peptide to the GSA of cats (Andreatta et al., 1988). We showed that topical application of the peptide to the GSA produced dose-dependent increases in blood pressure over a dose range of 12.5 to 100 pmol of ANG II. At the largest dose (100 pmol), blood pressure increased by $31.3 \pm 34.5$ (SEM) mm Hg. More recently, we found that unilateral microinjection of ANG II in the RVLM of normotensive rats evoked dose-dependent increases in blood pressure and heart rate (Muratani et al., 1991) (Fig. 9.1). In the rat experiments, we established that the microinjection pipette was located in the pressor neurons of the RVLM by evoking an increase in blood pressure of at least 30 mm Hg in response to a 2-nmol injection of L-glutamate (L-Glu). Furthermore, marking of injection sites with dye and histological examination of the brain stems revealed that pressor responses mediated by both ANG II and L-Glu were restricted to a region immediately caudal to the facial nu-

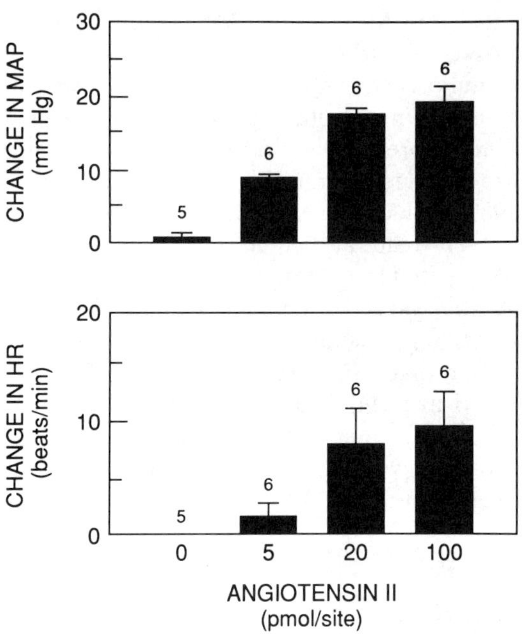



FIGURE 9.1. Changes in mean arterial pressure (MAP) and heart rate (HR) produced by graded doses of ANG II injected in the RVLM of 14 to 16-week-old WKY rats. At all doses used, ANG II evoked significant increases in blood pressure ($p < 0.01$) and heart rate ($p < 0.01$). The effect of vehicle (artificial cerebrospinal fluid) is indicated by the 0 dose of ANG II. Numbers above bars denote the number of rats studied at each dose of peptide.

cleus that corresponded to the dorsolateral aspect of the lateral paragigan-tocellular nucleus (LPGi) and dorsolateral to the LPGi. Our observations in the cat and rat agree with the findings of Allen et al. (1988) and Sasaki and Dampney (1990) that peptide injection in the RVLM of the cat and rabbit, respectively, elicit pressor responses. However, variable changes in heart rate have been observed when the peptide has been applied to the RVLM. In cats, topical application of ANG II did not consistently increase heart rate (Andreatta et al., 1988; Averill et al., 1991) whereas Allen et al. (1988) observed that injection of ANG II in the RVLM of cats elicited a pressor response accompanied by a decrease in heart rate. Allen et al. (1988) have interpreted that the bradycardia was mediated by the baroreflex in response to the increase in blood pressure. However, one might consider that injection of the peptide directly activated cardiac vagal motoneurons of the nucleus ambiguus. In contrast, microinjection of ANG II in the RVLM of the rabbits (Sasaki and Dampney, 1990) and Wistar Kyoto rats (WKY) (Muratani et al., 1991) evoked increases in heart rate in concert with the pressor response. Although these studies provide evidence that activation of ANG II receptors in the RVLM elicits cardiovascular responses, it is equally important to establish that the peptide did not have nonspecific excitatory effects on brain stem neurons. Sasaki and Dampney (1990) have shown that ANG II did not evoke pressor responses when injected in the lateral tegmental field of the rabbit at a site where L-Glu injection produced significant increases in blood pressure. Furthermore, in vitro receptor autoradiography has shown that dense collections of high affinity binding sites for the peptide are not found in the lateral tegmental field.

One of the distinguishing characteristics of the response produced by ANG II administration to the RVLM is the slow time course of the increase in blood pressure and the prolonged elevation of blood pressure that follows application of the peptide. This is a consistent feature of the pressor response produced by either topical application of ANG II to the GSA of cats (Andreatta et al., 1988) or by microinjection of the peptide in the RVLM of rats (Muratani et al., 1991). Sasaki and Dampney (1990) also observed that microinjection of the peptide in the RVLM of rabbits was characterized by this slow time course. By injecting L-Glu at the same site as ANG II we showed in rats that the time course for the pressor response to L-Glu is significantly faster than that for ANG II ($p < 0.01$) (Muratani et al., 1991). This difference in time course suggests that ANG II and L-Glu excite neurons through different mechanisms. The reuptake processes for the two agents probably differ. Furthermore, ANG II may suppress the M-current that affects $K^+$ flux across the cell membrane (Brown et al., 1980). A consequence of this proposed alteration in M-current is a change in neuronal excitability that occurs over a period of minutes (Jones, 1987). This matches the time course for responses evoked by microinjection of ANG II in both dorsomedial medulla (Averill et al., 1987; Diz et al., 1984) and ventrolateral medulla (Allen et al. 1988; Andreatta et al., 1988; Muratani et al., 1991; Sasaki and Dampney, 1990).

Since application of ANG II to the RVLM elicits a pressor response, we hypothesized that ANG II acts in the RVLM to excite neurons that contribute sympathofacilitatory drive to sympathetic preganglionic neurons. Several observations support this hypothesis. The pressor response elicited either by topical application of ANG II to the GSA of cats (Averill et al., 1991) or by microinjection of the peptide in the RVLM of rats (Muratani et al., 1991) was completely eliminated by blockade of ganglionic neurotransmission. Allen et al. (1988) also observed that microinjection of ANG II in the subretrofacial nucleus of the cat was abolished by ganglionic blockade. However, blockade of ganglionic neurotransmission often produces a substantial hypotension that could alter the responsiveness of brain stem neurons to ANG II. Therefore, additional support for this hypothesis was provided by the demonstration that topical application of ANG II to the GSA of cats (Averill et al., 1991) and microinjection of ANG II in the RVLM of rabbits (Sasaki and Dampney, 1990) significantly increased renal sympathetic nerve activity. Sasaki and Dampney (1990) have also shown that an increase in sympathetic nerve activity is accompanied by an increase in hindlimb vascular resistance.

In vitro receptor autoradiography has revealed ANG II binding sites in the CVLM as well as in the RVLM (Allen et al., 1987; Allen et al., 1988; Mendelsohn et al., 1988). These binding sites appear coincident with a region from which stimulation elicits depressor responses. In rats and rabbits, this corresponds to a region ventral to the nucleus ambiguus and dorsal to the lateral reticular nucleus. When ANG II was injected in the CVLM of rats (Fig. 9.2) (Muratani et al., 1991) and rabbits (Sasaki and Dampney, 1990), dose-dependent decreases in blood pressure were obtained. In both species, ANG II produced significant decreases in heart rate (Muratani et al., 1991; Sasaki and Dampney, 1990). Since recent studies indicate that CVLM neurons exert their depressor action through inhibition of sympathofacilitatory neurons of the RVLM (Agarwal et al., 1989; Blessing, 1988; Urbanski and Sapru, 1988a), we hypothesized that ANG II injected in the CVLM achieved its depressor response through reduction of central sympathetic outflow. Figure 9.3A shows that unilateral injection of ANG II in the CVLM of a Sprague-Dawley rat reduced blood pressure by 12 mm Hg. This depressor response was associated with an 18% decrease in splanchnic sympathetic nerve activity (SpSNA). The work of Sasaki and Dampney (1990), in rabbits, suggests that the reduction in sympathetic outflow evoked by ANG II injection in the CVLM may apply to other vascular beds as well. These investigators observed a sustained decrease in renal sympathetic nerve activity coincident with the ANG II-induced depressor response. Furthermore, the ANG II-induced depressor responses observed by Sasaki and Dampney were obtained in rabbits in which parasympathetic control of heart rate had been eliminated by bi-

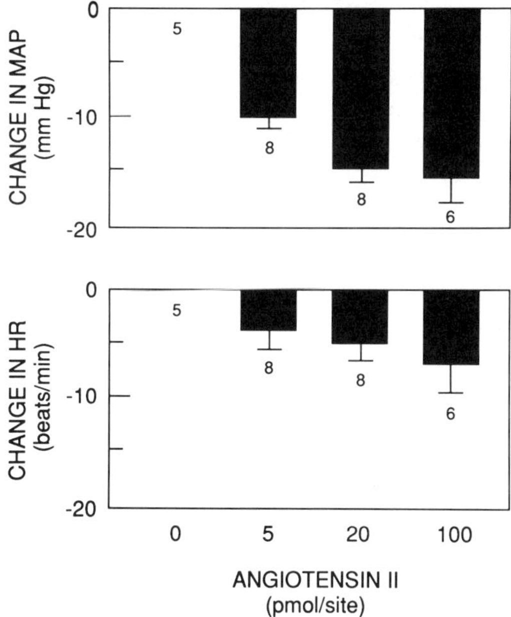



FIGURE 9.2. Changes in mean arterial pressure (MAP) and heart rate (HR) produced by graded doses of ANG II injected in the caudal ventrolateral medulla of 14 to 16-week-old WKY rats. ANG II evoked significant decreases in blood pressure ($p < 0.01$). The effect of vehicle (artificial cerebrospinal fluid) is indicated by the 0 dose of ANG II. Numbers above bars denote the number of rats studied at each dose of peptide.

lateral vagotomy. Thus, it appears that ANG II acts in the CVLM to enhance the activity of CVLM neurons that inhibit sympatho-facilitatory neurons of the RVLM. The most likely candidate for this ANG II-mediated inhibition is through a GABAergic pathway to RVLM neurons. These findings in rabbits and rats also indicate that the ANG II-induced depressor response in the CVLM is mediated by a reduction of cardiac and vasoconstrictor sympathetic outflow.

In rats, the caudal depressor region was identified routinely by the injection of L-Glu (2 nmol) (Muratani et al., 1991). The results of this strategy yielded interesting information about the probable organization of inhibitory pathways from the CVLM to pressor neurons of the RVLM. In WKY rats, unilateral injection of L-Glu decreased blood pressure from a control value of $90 \pm 2$ mm Hg to $54 \pm 1$ mm Hg. In some of these rats, hexamethonium bromide (40 mg/kg) was given intravenously to estimate the contribution of the sympathetic nervous system to the level of resting blood pressure. Ganglionic blockade reduced blood pressure to $48 \pm 2$ mm Hg, which was only 6 mm Hg lower than the level of blood pressure achieved by the

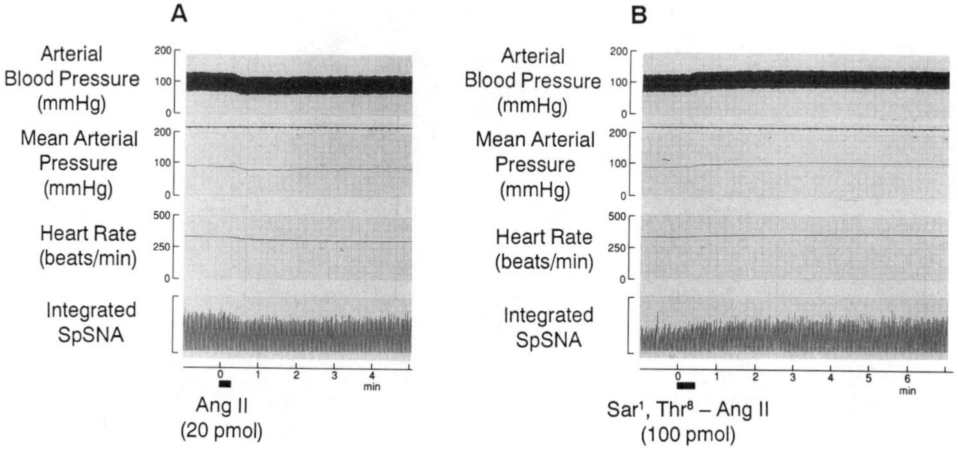



FIGURE 9.3. Hemodynamic and sympathetic effects produced by unilateral injection of ANG II or [Sar$^1$, Thr$^8$]-ANG II into the caudal ventrolateral medulla (CVLM) of a Sprague-Dawley rat. **A**: A single 50 nl injection of ANG II (20 pmol) in the CVLM reduced mean arterial pressure (MAP) by 12 mm Hg, heart rate (HR) by 23 bpm, and SpSNA by 18%. **B**: Injection of an ANG II antagonist (50 nl, 100 pmol) at the same site had an effect opposite to that of the agonist. MAP and HR increased by 16 mm Hg and 25 beats per minute, respectively, and SpSNA increased by 50%. Injection of peptide is indicated by the solid bar at the bottom traces in each panel.

unilateral injection of L-Glu in rats with an intact baroreflex. Because blood pressure is controlled by neurohormonal factors in addition to changes in autonomic outflow, we recorded SpSNA to obtain a more direct estimate of the role of the CVLM in the regulation of sympathetic outflow. Figure 9.4 shows that unilateral injection of L-Glu (2 nmol) in the CVLM of a Sprague-Dawley rat produced a greater than 80% reduction in SpSNA. This suppression of SpSNA significantly preceded the depressor (−47 mm Hg) and bradycardic (−50 bpm) responses evoked by L-Glu. In this particular animal, the L-Glu-induced reduction of SpSNA was very close to the total suppression of SpSNA that could be achieved through the baroreceptor reflex. These findings suggest that caudal inhibitory neurons (GABAergic) have a substantial bilateral projection to rostral pressor neurons. In contrast, unilateral excitation of RVLM neurons by L-Glu has the effect of partially activating (or augmenting) sympathetic outflow. Furthermore, the magnitude of the pressor response produced by unilateral RVLM stimulation may be compensated by the baroreflex operating through the contralateral pool of rostral pressor neurons. This view is supported by the observation of Sasaki and Dampney (1990) that the pressor responses to injection of ANG II in the RVLM of the rabbit were twice as large in baroreceptor denervated animals as in rabbits with carotid baroreceptor afferents intact.

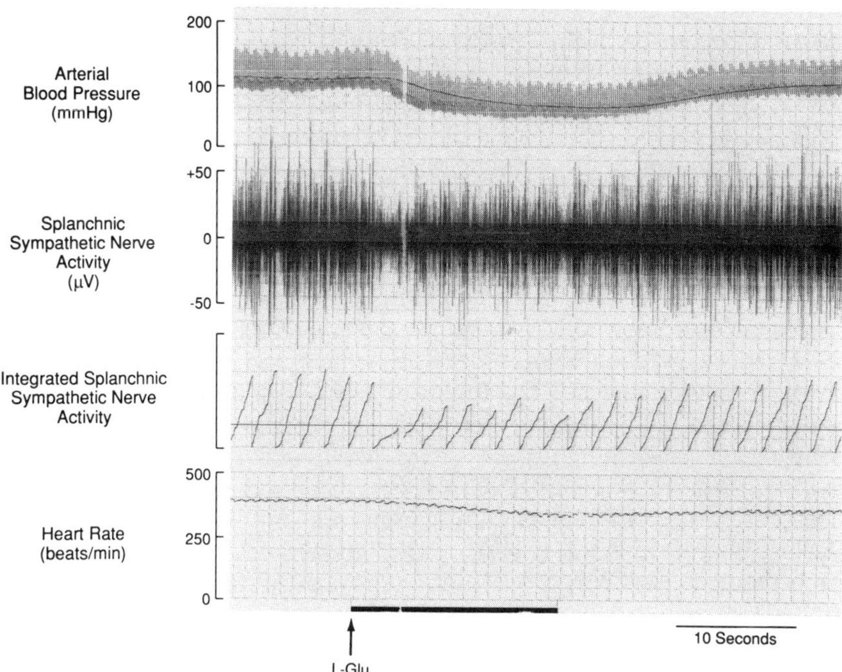


FIGURE 9.4. Profound inhibition of SpSNA and mean arterial pressure (MAP) produced by unilateral injection of L-Glu (2 nmol) in the caudal ventrolateral medulla of a Sprague-Dawley rat. The largest reduction in SpSNA was observed approximately $2\frac{1}{2}$ sec after initiation of L-Glu injection whereas the nadir in MAP and heart rate (HR) occurred 20 sec after initiation of L-Glu injection. The largest response in MAP and HR occurred at a time when SpSNA had recovered by about 50%. The solid bar at the bottom of the traces denotes the time of L-Glu injection.

# Role of Endogenous ANG II in Cardiovascular Regulation

With the demonstration that exogenously applied ANG II acted in the ventrolateral medulla to produce cardiovascular responses, we pursued the hypothesis that ANG II endogenous to the ventrolateral medulla contributes to the tonic activity of ventrolateral medullary neurons involved in circulatory regulation. We first demonstrated in the cat (Andreatta et al., 1988) that topical application of [Sar[1], Thr[8]]-ANG II to the GSA produced a significant reduction ($-8$ mm Hg, $p < 0.05$) in blood pressure. This observation has now been confirmed and expanded by studying the response to microinjection of [Sar[1], Thr[8]]-ANG II in the RVLM and CVLM of normotensive rats. Figure 9.3B shows that injection of the antagonist

(100 pmol) into the CVLM of a Sprague-Dawley rat increased blood pressure by 16 mm Hg and produced a 50% increase in SpSNA. Injection of this ANG II antagonist in the RVLM of normotensive rats decreased blood pressure. These data obtained in the rat agree with the observations of Sasaki and Dampney (1990) that this peptide antagonist injected in the RVLM and CVLM of the rabbit produced changes in blood pressure that are opposite to those produced by the agonist. Furthermore those investigators showed that the changes in blood pressure produced by the antagonist in either region were mediated by changes in sympathetic nerve activity.

At present we can appreciate that the activity of CVLM and RVLM vasomotor neurons is significantly influenced by baroreceptor-related afferent input (Agarwal et al., 1990; Brown and Guyenet, 1984, 1985; Gordon, 1987). However, other inputs or local tissue factors may set the tonic activity of vasomotor neurons. The results obtained with injections of ANG II antagonists in the ventrolateral medulla suggest that endogenous ANG II contributes significantly to the tonic activity of RVLM and CVLM neurons. But, the extent of ANG II involvement in the regulation of baseline activity of CVLM and RVLM neurons remains to be studied. Nevertheless, the role of ANG II in the ventrolateral medulla appears to differ from the action of the peptide in the dorsomedial medulla. Injection of ANG II antagonists in the nTS had no effect on the baseline blood pressure (Campagnole-Santos et al., 1988; Casto and Phillips, 1985). However, injection of [Sar$^1$, Thr$^8$]-ANG II in the nTS enhanced the baroreflex control of heart rate (Campagnole- Santos et al., 1988). These seemingly different modes of action for ANG II at either the dorsomedial medulla or the ventrolateral medulla await studies that will define the precise mechanisms by which the peptide affects neurotransmission.

Clearly, a pertinent issue related to the action of ANG II in the ventrolateral medulla is the source of the peptide. We have shown that topical application of ANG I to the GSA of the cat evokes pressor responses equal in magnitude to that produced by ANG II (Andreatta et al., 1988). Further, the Ang I-induced pressor response was eliminated by prior treatment of the GSA with an ACE inhibitor. Although all the components of the RAS cascade have not been examined in the ventrolateral medulla, the possibility of in situ generation of ANG II is supported by observations in the rat (Chevillard and Saavedra, 1982) and dog (Santos et al., 1988) that higher levels of ACE activity are found in the Al and C1 regions of the ventrolateral medulla. The area postrema and nTS also contain high levels of ACE activity (Santos et al., 1988). Moreover, ACE activity in the nTS was inhibited 6 hr after intravenous injection of a single dose of an ACE inhibitor (Santos et al., 1988). Thus, these data reinforce the view that ACE inhibitors have important sites of action in regions of the medulla oblongata where ANG II modulates the baroreflex and influences the regulation of sympathetic drive. These regions include the CVLM and RVLM as well as the nTS.

# Do Vasomotor Actions of ANG II in the Ventrolateral Medulla Contribute to Hypertension?

The SHR has been employed as a genetic model of essential hypertension. SHRs have augmented sympathetic drive directed to the peripheral vasculature during the development and maintenance of hypertension (Judy and Farrell, 1979). Furthermore, the accentuated sympathetic outflow is accompanied by a diminution in baroreflex control of sympathetic nerve activity (Hayashi et al., 1988). Additional evidence suggests that the elevation of sympathetic nerve activity in SHR may be the result of accentuated central drive for sympathetic outflow rather than altered central baroreflex control of sympathetic nerve activity (Judy and Farrell, 1979). Other studies suggest that the central neurogenic actions of ANG II may be intimately involved in the progression of hypertension in SHR (Unger et al., 1988). The involvement of the brain RAS in the disturbed circulatory regulation of SHR is further supported by the antihypertensive effects of intracerebroventricularly administered ANG II antagonists (McDonald et al., 1980) and ACE inhibitors (Okuno et al., 1983; Unger et al., 1981). Since our initial data in the cat implicated the RVLM as a site where ANG II could influence the tonic level of sympathetic outflow, we hypothesized that SHR would be characterized by an accentuated responsiveness to ANG II in the RVLM. The action of ANG II in the CVLM of SHR was also investigated since the work of Granata et al., (1985, 1986) indicated that CVLM neurons had a significant tonic inhibitory influence on rostral pressor neurons.

Injection of L-Glu and ANG II in the RVLM of SHR produced comparable pressor responses to those obtained in WKY (Fig. 9.5). Thus, SHR did not exhibit any greater sensitivity to ANG II acting at RVLM neurons. This result differs from the preliminary findings of Punnen et al. (1984) that SHR had a potentiated pressor response to ANG II injected in the RVLM. On the other hand, both L-Glu and ANG II injected in the CVLM produced significantly greater decreases in blood pressure in SHRs than in WKY rats (Fig. 9.5). We suspect that the greater depressor responses observed in SHRs for injections of either agent in the CVLM were not the result of accentuated vascular responsiveness (Folkow, 1982). This interpretation is based on the observation that similar increases in blood pressure were obtained in both strains when these two agents were injected in the RVLM. However, the definitive evidence for the comparison of the vasomotor actions of ANG II in the CVLM and RVLM of SHRs to the effects of the peptide on vasomotor neurons of WKY rats will require recording of sympathetic nerve activity in both strains. Our observations of similar pressor responses to L-Glu injection in the RVLM of each strain and a larger depressor response for L-Glu injection of the CVLM of the SHRs agree with the recent findings of Smith and Barron (1990a). These

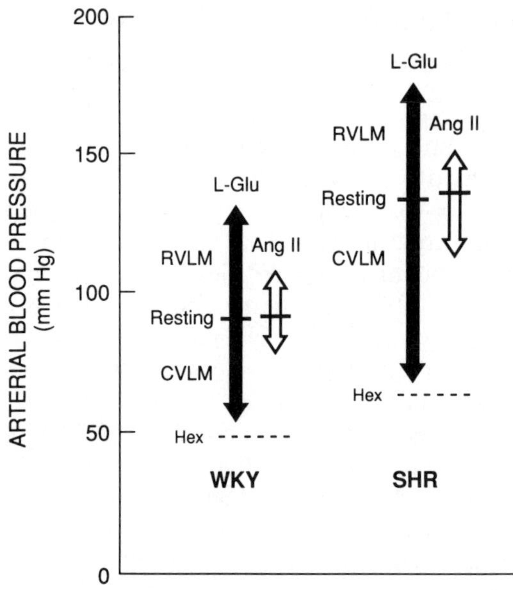



FIGURE 9.5. Blood pressures achieved by injection of L-Glu and ANG II in the rostral (RVLM) and caudal ventrolateral medulla (CVLM) of Wistar-Kyoto rats (WKY) and spontaneously hypertensive rats (SHR). WKY rats that received L-Glu injections had resting blood pressures ($90 \pm 2$ mm Hg, n = 25) that did not differ from WKY rats that received ANG II injections ($91 \pm 2$ mm Hg, n = 18). In contrast, SHR had significantly higher resting blood pressures: $133 \pm 2$ mm Hg (n = 27) before L-Glu injection and $135 \pm 2$ mm Hg (n = 21) before ANG II injection. L-Glu injection in the RVLM produced similar increases in blood pressure in WKY and SHR rats. Although ANG II injected in the RVLM evoked pressor responses that were smaller than those elicited by L-Glu, the pressor responses to the peptide were of the same magnitude in WKY and SHR. ANG II produced a larger fall in blood pressure in SHR compared to WKY ($p < 0.001$). However, the depressor response to ANG II was smaller than that evoked by L-Glu. L-Glu injected in the CVLM produced larger depressor responses in SHR compared to WKY ($p < 0.001$). In both the WKY and SHR the blood pressure achieved by L-Glu injection in the CVLM was 6 mm Hg above the blood pressure measured subsequent to ganglionic blockade (hexamethonium bromide, 40 mg/kg; indicated by the dotted line) in either strain.

investigators showed that inhibition of CVLM neurons by tetrodotoxin (TTX) injection produced negligible increases in blood pressure in SHR whereas TTX injection in the CVLM of WKY rats significantly elevated blood pressure. They hypothesized that RVLM neurons of SHRs received substantially less inhibitory GABAergic input from the CVLM; consequently, sympathetic outflow was enhanced. This view is supported by their more recent finding that injection of bicuculline in the RVLM had little effect on the prevailing level of blood pressure of SHRs whereas blockade of GABAergic synapses in the RVLM of WKY rats elevated the baseline blood pressure of the normotensive strain (Smith and Barron, 1990b). However, the plausibility of this hypothesis may be questioned, since data obtained recently in our laboratory showed that [Sar[1], Thr[8]]-ANG II injected in the CVLM of SHRs increased blood pressure. Alternatively, these data may suggest that the action of ANG II in the CVLM is not mediated by a direct GABAergic pathway to pressor neurons of the RVLM.

## Summary

Recent findings are reviewed that implicate the ventrolateral medulla as an additional site in the central nervous system where ANG II participates in the central regulation of cardiovascular function. Evidence shows that ANG II applied to rostral pressor or caudal depressor neurons of the ventrolateral medulla produces cardiovascular responses and changes in sympathetic nerve activity that are consistent with the peptide acting as an excitatory neurotransmitter at these locations. In addition, injection of ANG II antagonists at these same locations demonstrates that ANG II endogenous to the ventrolateral medulla participates in setting the tonic activity of neurons integral to the regulation of the sympathetic nervous system. This may be a unique property of ANG II actions in the central nervous system. That is, the ventrolateral medulla is one of the few sites in the central nervous system where brain ANG II can influence directly the tonic activity of sympathetic motoneurons.

## References

Agarwal SK, Gelsema AJ, Calaresu FR (1989): Neurons in rostral VLM are inhibited by chemical stimulation of caudal VLM in rats. *Am J Physiol* 257:R265–R270.

Agarwal SK, Gelsema AJ, Calaresu FR (1990): Inhibition of rostral VLM by baroreceptor activation is relayed through caudal VLM. *Am J Physiol* 258:R1271– R1278.

Aguirre JA, Covenas R. Croix D, et al. (1989): Immunocytochemical study of angiotensin-II fibres and cell bodies in the brainstem respiratory areas of the cat. *Brain Res* 489:311–317.

Allen AM, Chai SY, Clevers J, McKinley MJ, Paxinos G, Mendelsohn FAO (1988): Localization and characterization of angiotensin II receptor binding and angiotensin converting enzyme in the human medulla oblongata. *J Comp Neurol* 269:249–264.

Allen AM, Chai SY, Sexton PM, et al. (1987): Angiotensin II receptors and angiotensin converting enzyme in the medulla oblongata. *Hypertension* 9:III-198-III-205.

Allen AM, Dampney RAL, Mendelsohn FAO (1988): Angiotensin receptor bind-

118    D.B. Averill et al.

ing and pressor effects in cat subretrofacial nucleus. *Am J Physiol* 255:H1011–H1017.

Amendt K, Czachurski J, Dembowsky K, Seller H (1979): Bulbospinal projections to the intermediolateral cell column: a neuroanatomical study. *J Auton Nerv Syst* 1:103–117.

Andreatta SH, Averill DB, Santos RAS, Ferrario CM (1988): The ventrolateral medulla: a new site of the action of the renin-angiotensin system. *Hypertension* 11 (suppl I):I-163–I-166.

Averill DB, Andreatta- Van Leyen S, Ferrario CM (1991): Angiotensin II acts at the rostral ventrolateral medulla to augment sympathetic activity. *Peptides* (Submitted).

Averill DB, Diz Dl, Barnes KL, Ferrario CM (1987): Pressor responses of angiotensin II microinjected into the dorsomedial medulla of the dog. *Brain Res* 414:294–300.

Barman SM, Gebber GL ( 1985): Axonal projection patterns of ventrolateral medullospinal sympathoexcitatory neurons. *J Neurophysiol* 53:1551–1566.

Blessing WW (1988): Depressor neurons in rabbit caudal medulla act via GABA receptors in rostral medulla. *Am J Physiol* 254:H686–H692.

Brosnihan KB, Diz DI, Schiavone MT, Averill DB, Ferrario CM (1987): Approaches to establishing angiotensin II as a neurotransmitter. In: *Brain Peptides and Catecholamines in Cardiovascular Regulation*, Buckley JP, Ferrario CM, eds. New York: Raven Press, pp 313–328.

Brown DA, Constanti A, Marsh S (1980): Angiotensin mimics the action of muscarinic agonists on rat sympathetic neurones. *Brain Res* 193:614–619.

Brown DL, Guyenet PG (1984): Cardiovascular neurons of brain stem with projections to spinal cord. *Am J Physiol* 247:R1009–R1016.

Brown DL, Guyenet PG (1985): Electrophysiological study of cardiovascular neurons in the rostral ventrolateral medulla in rats. *Circ Res* 56:359–369.

Calaresu FR, Yardley CP (1988): Medullary basal sympathetic tone. *Annu Rev Physiol* 50:511–524.

Campagnole-Santos MJ, Diz DI, Ferrario CM (1988): Baroreceptor reflex modulation by angiotensin II at the nucleus tractus solitarii. *Hypertension* 11 (suppl I):I-167–I-171.

Casto R, Phillips MI (1984a): Cardiovascular actions of microinjections of angiotensin II in the brain stem of rats. *Am J Physiol* 247:R811–R816.

Casto R, Phillips MI (1984b): Mechanism of pressor effects by angiotensin in the nucleus tractus solitarius of rats. *Am J Physiol* 247:R575–R581.

Casto R, Phillips MI (1985): Neuropeptide action in nucleus tractus solitarius: angiotensin specificity and hypertensive rats. *Am J Physiol* 249:R341–R347.

Caverson MM, Ciriello J, Calaresu FR (1983): Direct pathway from cardiovascular neurons in the ventrolateral medulla to the region of the intermediolateral nucleus of the upper thoracic cord: an anatomical and electrophysiological investigation in the cat. *J Auton Nerv Syst* 9:451–475.

Chevillard C, Saavedra JM (1982): Distribution of angiotensin-converting enzyme activity in specific areas of the rat brain stem. *J Neurochem* 38:281–284.

Ciriello J, Caverson MM, Polosa C (1986): Function of the ventrolateral medulla in the control of the circulation. *Brain Res Rev* 11:359 – 391.

Covenas R, Fuxe K, Cintra A, Aguirre JA, Goldstein M, Ganten D (1990): Evidence for the existence of angiotensin II-like immunoreactivity in subpopulations of tyrosine hydroxylase immunoreactive neurons in the A1 and C1 area of the ventral medulla of the male rat. *Neurosci Lett* 114:160–166.

Dampney RAL, Blessing WW, Tan E (1988): Origin of tonic GABAergic inputs to vasopressor neurons in the subretrofacial nucleus of the rabbit. *J Auton Nerv Syst* 24:227–239.

Deschepper CF, Bouhnik J, Ganong WF (1986): Colocalization of angiotensinogen and glial fibrillary acidic protein in astrocytes in rat brain. *Brain Res* 355:195–198.

Dittmar C, (1873): Uber die lage des sogenannten gefasscentrums der medulla oblongata. *Ber Verh Saechs Wiss Leipzig Phys Kl* 25:449–479.

Diz DI, Barnes KL, Ferrario CM ( 1984): Hypotensive action of angiotensin II microinjected into the dorsal motor nucleus of the vagus. *J Hypertens* 2(suppl 3):53–56.

Diz Dl, Barnes KL, Ferrario CM (1986): Contribution of the vagus nerve to angiotensin Il binding sites in the canine medulla. *Brain Res Bull* 17:497–505.

Feldberg W, Guertzenstein PG (1972): A vasodepressor effect of pentobarbital sodium. *J Physiol (Lond)* 224:83–103.

Fink GD, Bruner CA, Mangiapane ML (1987a): Area postrema is critical for angiotensin-induced hypertension in rats. *Hypertension* 9:355–361.

Fink GD, Pawloski CM, Blair ML, Mangiapane ML (1987b): The area postrema in deoxycorticosterone-salt hypertension in rats. *Hypertension* 9:III-206–III-209.

Folkow B (1982): Physiological aspects of primary hypertension. *Physiol Rev* 62:347–504.

Gehlert DR, Speth RC, Wamsley JK (1986): Distribution of [$^{125}$I]angiotensin II binding sites in the rat brain: a quantitative autoradiographic study. *Neuroscience* 18:837–856.

Gordon FJ (1987): Aortic baroreceptor reflexes are mediated by NMDA receptors in caudal ventrolateral medulla. *Am J Physiol* 252:R628–R633.

Granata AR, Kumada M, Reis DJ (1985): Sympathoinhibition by A1-noradrenergic neurons is mediated by neurons in the C1 area of the rostral medulla. *J Auton Nerv Syst* 14:387–395.

Granata AR, Numao Y, Kumada M, Reis DJ (1986): Al noradrenergic neurons tonically inhibit sympathoexcitatory neurons of C1 area in rat brainstem. *Brain Res* 377:127–146.

Guertzenstein PG (1973): Blood pressure effects obtained by drugs applied to the ventral surface of the brain stem. *J Physiol (Lond)* 229:395–408.

Guertzenstein PG, Lopes OU (1984): Cardiovascular responses evoked from the nicotine-sensitive area on the ventral surface of the medulla oblongata in the cat. *J Physiol (Lond)* 347:345–360.

Guertzenstein PG, Silver A (1974): Fall in blood pressure produced from discrete regions of the ventral surface of the medulla by glycine and lesions. *J Physiol (Lond)* 242:489–503.

Hartle DK, Brody MJ (1984): The angiotensin II pressor system of the rat forebrain. *Circ Res* 54:355–366.

Hartle DK, Lind RW, Johnson AK, Brody MJ (1982): Localization of the anterior hypothalamic angiotensin II pressor system. *Hypertension* 4 (suppl II):II-159–II-165.

Hayashi J, Takeda K, Kawasaki S, et al. (1988): Central attentuation of baroreflex by angiotensin II in normotensive and spontaneously hypertensive rats. *Am J*

*Hypertens* 1:15S–22S.

Jones SW (1987): Luteinizing hormone-releasing hormone as a neurotransmitter in bullfrog sympathetic ganglia. *Ann NY Acad Sci* 519:310–322.

Judy WV, Farrell SK (1979): Arterial baroreceptor reflex control of sympathetic nerve activity in the spontaneously hypertensive rat. *Hypertension* 1:604–614.

Lind RW, Swanson LW, Bruhn TO, Ganten D (1985a): The distribution of angiotensin II-immunoreactive cells and fibers in the paraventriculo-hypophysial system of the rat. *Brain Res* 338:81–89.

Lind RW, Swanson LW, Ganten D ( 1985b): Organization of angiotensin II immunoreactive cells and fibers in the rat central nervous system. *Neuroendocrinology* 40:2–24.

Mangiapane ML, Skoog KM, Rittenhouse P, Blair ML, Sladek CD (1989): Lesion of the area postrema region attenuates hypertension in spontaneously hypertensive rats. *Circ Res* 64:129–135.

Mann JFE, Phillips MI, Dietz R, Haebara H, Ganten D (1978): Effects of central and peripheral angiotensin blockade in hypertensive rats. *Am J Physiol* 234:H629–H637.

McDonald W, Wickre C, Aumann S, Ban S, Moffitt B (1980): The sustained antihypertensive effect of chronic cerebroventricular infusion of angiotensin antagonist in spontaneously hypertensive rats. *Endocrinology* 107:1305 – 1308.

Mendelsohn FAO, Allen AM, Clevers J, Denton DA, Tarjan E, McKinley MJ (1988): Localization of angiotensin II receptor binding in rabbit brain by in vitro autoradiography. *J Comp Neurol* 270:372–384.

Minson JB, Chalmers JP, Caon AC, Renaud B (1987): Separate areas of rat medulla oblongata with populations of serotonin- and adrenaline-containing neurons alter blood pressure after L-glutamate stimulation. *J Auton Nerv Syst* 19:39–50.

Mogenson GJ, Kucharczyk J (1978): Central neural pathways for angiotensin-induced thirst. *Fed Proc* 37:2683–2688.

Muratani H, Averill DB, Ferrario CM (1991): Effect of angiotensin II in the caudal ventrolateral medulla of spontaneously hypertensive rats. (In press) *Am J Physiol*.

Okuno T, Nagahama S, Lindheimer MD, Oparil S (1983): Attenuation of the development of spontaneous hypertension in rats by chronic central administration of captopril. *Hypertension* 5:653–662.

Owsjannikow P, (1871): Die tonischen und reflectorischen centren der gefassnerven. *Ber Verh Saechs Wiss Leipzig Math Phys Kl* 23:135–143.

Punnen S, Krieger AJ, Sapru HN (1984): Exaggerated blood pressure responses to microinjections of angiotensin-II into the medullary pressor area of spontaneously hypertensive rats. *Fed Proc* 43:443 (abstract).

Renaud LP, Jhamandas JH, Buijis R, Raby W, Randle JCR (1988): Cardiovascular input to hypothalamic neurosecretory neurons. *Brain Res Bull* 20:771–777.

Santos RAS, Brosnihan KB, Chappell MC, et al. (1988): Converting enzyme activity and angiotensin metabolism in the dog brain stem. *Hypertension* 11 (suppl I):I-153–I-157.

Sasaki S, Dampney RAL (1990): Tonic cardiovascular effects of angiotensin II in the ventrolateral medulla. *Hypertension* 15:274–283.

Smith JK, Barron KW (1990a): Cardiovascular effects of L-glutamate and tetrodotoxin microinjected into the rostral and caudal ventrolateral medulla in normotensive and spontaneously hypertensive rats. *Brain Res* 506:1–8.

Smith JK, Barron KW (1990b): GABAergic responses in ventrolateral medulla in spontaneously hypertensive rats. *Am J Physiol* 258:R450 – R456.

Speth RC, Wamsley JK, Gehlert DR, Chernicky CL, Barnes KL, Ferrario CM (1985): Angiotensin II receptor localization in the canine CNS. *Brain Res* 326:137–143.

Sun MK, Guyenet PG (1985): GABA-mediated baroreceptor inhibition of reticulospinal neurons. *Am J Physiol* 249:R672–R680.

Unger T, Badoer E, Ganten D, Lang RE, Rettig R (1988): Brain angiotensin: pathways and pharmacology. *Circulation* 77 (suppl I):I-40–I-54.

Unger T, Kaufmann-Buhler I, Scholkens B, Ganten D (1981): Brain converting enzyme inhibition: a possible mechanism for the antihypertensive action of captopril in spontaneously hypertensive rats. *Eur J Pharmacol* 70:467–478,

Urbanski RW, Sapru HN (1988a): Evidence for a sympathoexcitatory pathway from the nucleus tractus solitarii to the ventrolateral medullary pressor area. *J Auton Nerv Syst* 23:161–174.

Urbanski RW, Sapru HN (1988b): Putative neurotransmitters involved in medullary cardiovascular regulation. *J Auton Nerv Syst* 25:181–193.

Willette RN, Barcas PP, Krieger AJ, Sapru HN (1983): Vasopressor and depressor areas in the rat medulla. Identification by microinjection of l-glutamate. *Neuropharmacology* 22:1071–1079.

Willette RN, Barcas PP Krieger AJ, Sapru HN (1984): Endogenous GABAergic mechanisms in the medulla and the regulation of blood pressure. *J Pharmacol Exp Ther* 230:34–39.

# 10
# Endorphinergic Neurons in the Brainstem: Role in Cardiovascular Regulation

GEORGE KUNOS, JAMES A. MASTRIANNI,
ROGELIO MOSQUEDA-GARCIA, AND KAROLY VARGA

The dorsal vagal complex (DVC) in the lower brainstem, a structure that comprises the nucleus of the solitary tract (NTS) and the adjacent dorsal vagal nucleus, has a key role in the reflex regulation of blood pressure and heart rate. The DVC contains the first synapse of the baroreflex, activation of which lowers blood pressure and heart rate. Although the nature of the primary chemical transmitter of the baroreflex synapse is still debated, a number of endogenous substances as well as drugs have been shown to modulate baroreflex sensitivity in the DVC, or produce cardiovascular effects by direct activation of effector baroreflex pathways.

Two of these endogenous transmitter systems have been of particular interest to us and are the focus of this chapter. The DVC is rich in catecholamines (Dahlstrom and Fuxe, 1964) as well as adrenergic receptors, particularly the $\alpha_2$-subtype (Unnerstall et al., 1984; Dashwood et al., 1985). Stimulation of $\alpha_2$-receptors in the DVC by catecholamines or certain antihypertensive agents such as clonidine or $\alpha$-methyldopa reduces blood pressure and heart rate through inhibition of sympathetic outflow to the heart and peripheral vasculature and an increase in vagal outflow to the myocardium (Laubie and Schmitt, 1977). Stimulation of $\alpha_2$-receptors in the NTS has also been shown to facilitate baroreflex bradycardia (Kobinger & Walland, 1972).

The DVC is also rich in all three classes of endogenous opioid peptides (Khachaturian et al., 1985), and it has a high concentration of opiate receptors (Dashwood et al., 1985). Stimulation of these receptors by morphine and some endogenous opioids can elicit responses similar to the effects of $\alpha_2$-receptor stimulation: hypotension and bradycardia (Feldberg and Wei, 1986) as well as facilitation of the depressor baroreflex response (Laubie & Schmitt, 1981), although pressor effects can also be elicited by opiates in the DVC, as discussed later in this chapter. Catecholamine and opioid-containing neurons in the DVC overlap and may impinge upon common targets (Pickel et al., 1989). In view of these functional and morphological similarities, it is not surprising to find interactions between the $\alpha_2$-adrenergic and opioid systems of the brainstem.

# Adrenergic-Opioid Interaction in the Dorsal Vagal Complex

Observations from several laboratories indicate that the centrally mediated cardiovascular effects of agents that activate $\alpha_2$-receptors (clonidine, some clonidine analogs, $\alpha$-methyldopa) are inhibited by naloxone or naltrexone (Farsang and Kunos, 1979; Farsang et al., 1980; Baum and Becker, 1982; Petty and de Jong, 1982a, 1984; Marmo et al., 1984; Naranjo et al., 1985; Medvedev, 1986; Mastrianni and Ingenito, 1987; Tackett and Laskey, 1987; Kunos et al., 1987; Williams et al., 1987; Van Giersbergen and de Jong, 1988; Van Giersbergen et al., 1989a, 1989b; Chang et al., 1989). Failure to observe such an interaction in some studies (Conway et al., 1984; Head and de Jong, 1985) appears to be related to the use of supramaximal doses of the $\alpha_2$-adrenergic agonists (Mastrianni & Ingenito. 1987; Van Giersbergen et al., 1989b). Intra-DVC microinjections of low doses (10–100 ng) of 1-naloxone but not d-naloxone inhibit the effects of clonidine or $\alpha$-methyldopa (Mosqueda-Garcia et al., 1986; Mosqueda-Garcia & Kunos, 1987, 1988; Van Giersbergen et al., 1989a), which suggests that the site of the adrenergic-opioid interaction is in the DVC and involves the activation of stereoselective opiate receptors.

Since clonidine and naloxone do not interact with each other's specific binding sites (Farsang & Kunos, 1979), activation of opiate receptors in the DVC is most likely caused by the release of an endogenous opioid peptide. We suspected $\beta$-endorphin because centrally administered $\beta$-endorphin had been reported to cause hypotension and bradycardia (Laubie et al., 1977) whereas similarly administered enkephalins elicited pressor effects (Schaz et al., 1980). Indeed, we reported that clonidine and $\alpha$-methylnoradrenaline release $\beta$-endorphinlike immunoreactivity from rat brain stem slices in vitro (Kunos et al., 1981), and others found that the same drugs reduce hypothalamic levels of $\beta$-endorphin in vivo (Mastrianni & Ingenito, 1987). Furthermore, microinjection of antisera against $\beta$-endorphin into the fourth cerebral ventricle or into the NTS were subsequently reported to inhibit the effects of clonidine and $\alpha$-methylnorepinephrine (Petty & de Jong, 1982a, 1984; Ramirez-Gonzalez et al., 1983; Naranjo et al., 1985; Van Giersbergen et al., 1989a,b). This supported our hypothesis (Kunos et al., 1981) that activation of central $\alpha_2$-adrenergic receptors leads to the release of $\beta$-endorphin or a $\beta$-endorphinlike substance in the DVC, which contributes to the cardiovascular depressor response.

The main source of $\beta$-endorphin in the brain is neurons in the hypothalamic arcuate nucleus, which project into many areas including the DVC in the lower brainstem. In addition to endorphinergic terminals, endorphin-containing perikarya have also been detected in the DVC (Joseph et al., 1983). Studies in rats have demonstrated that selective destruction of the endorphinergic neuronal system of the arcuate by neonatal treatment with monosodium glutamate (Krieger et al., 1979) eliminates the naloxone-sensitive component in the effects of clonidine (Mosqueda-Garcia et al., 1986). Similar results were obtained after electrolytic lesioning of the arcuate nucleus (Mastrianni and Ingenito, 1987). These findings indicate that the likely source of the $\beta$-endorphin released by clonidine-like agents is an endorphinergic neuronal pathway originating in the arcuate nucleus and projecting to structures in the DVC. Activation of these neurons by physiological or pharmacological stimuli would sensitize depressor baroreflex responses and elicit hypotension and bradycardia through stimulation of opiate receptors in the DVC.

## Cardiovascular Effects of Stimulation of the Arcuate Nucleus

To test the above hypothesis, we studied the cardiovascular effects of electrical stimulation of the arcuate nucleus in urethane-anesthetized rats (Mastrianni et al., 1989). In the first set of experiments the tip of the bipolar stainless steel microelectrode was inserted into the midanterior portion of the arcuate nucleus between 2.4 to 3.0 mm posterior from the bregma, as verified by postmortem microscopic examination and illustrated by the asterisks in Figure 10.1. Stimulation at these sites with currents of 40 to 200 $\mu$A, 80 Hz, 0.8 msec, typically caused a biphasic, depressor/pressor response and moderate bradycardia (Fig. 10.2A, solid lines). The pressor response could be inhibited by the intravenous (i.v.) administration of a vasopressin $V_1$-receptor antagonist, which unmasked a pure depressor response (Fig. 10.2A, dashed lines). This depressor response, in turn, was significantly reduced by pretreatment with naltrexone, 2 mg/kg i.v., or by intra-NTS administration of an antiserum against $\beta$-endorphin (Fig. 10.3).

The vasopressin-mediated pressor component of the response to arcuate stimulation is similar to observations by Brody et al. (1986), who found that the effect could be inhibited not only by systemic administration of a $V_1$-receptor antagonist but also by lidocaine infiltration of the magnocellular region of the paraventricular nucleus (PVN). Hence, they proposed that the mechanism of this effect involved activation of the magnocellular region of the PVN, with subsequent release of pressor amounts of vasopressin from the posterior pituitary (Brody et al., 1986). The mechanism of the pressor response observed in our experiments may be the same.

The sensitivity of the depressor response to inhibition by naltrexone or by intra-NTS injection of $\beta$-endorphin antiserum suggests that it is mediated by an endorphinlike opioid released in the DVC. To test further whether this endorphinergic pathway projects to the DVC region, we deafferentated the DVC by an ipsilateral, dorsolateral knife-cut. The cardiovascular response to arcuate stimulation was then tested following the

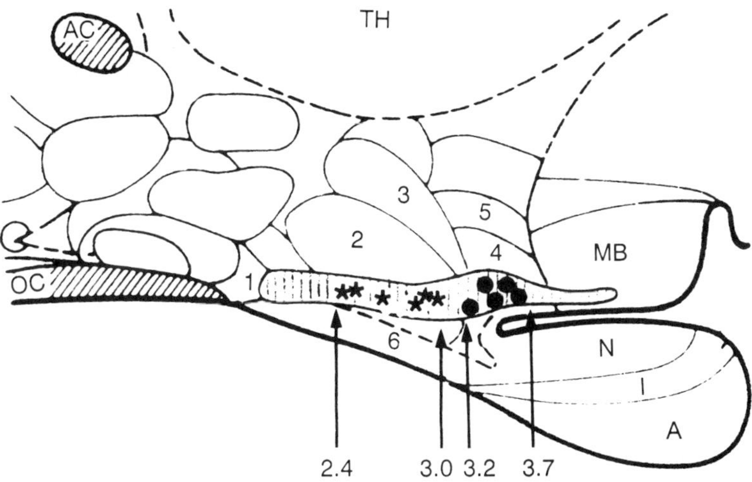



FIGURE 10.1. Anatomical localization of the sites of electrical stimulation of the arcuate nucleus. Stimulation sites, as verified by postmortem microscopic examination, are marked by * in the midanterior segment (see responses in Fig. 10.2A) and by filled dots in the postinfundibular segment of the arcuate nucleus (see responses in Fig. 10.2B) on the sagittal section of the rat brain. Numbers under the arrows represent the A-P distance in mm from the bregma; AC: anterior commissure; TH: thalamus; MB: mamillary bodies; OC: optic chiasm; N: neural; I: intermediate; A: anterior pituitary; 1: retrochiasmatic area; 2: ventromedial nucleus; 3: dorsomedial nucleus; 4: ventral premamillary nucleus; 5: dorsal premamillary nucleus; 6: median eminence and pituitary stalk.

i.v. administration of a $V_1$-antagonist. The results indicate that electrical stimulation of the arcuate ipsilateral to the knife-cut produced no change in blood pressure and heart rate, while stimulation of the contralateral side produced hypotension and bradycardia similar to that seen in sham-operated controls (Mastrianni et al., 1989). These findings strongly suggest that the depressor response to arcuate stimulation is mediated through an endorphinergic neuronal pathway projecting from the arcuate nucleus to the DVC.

In the experiments of Brody et al. (1986), no depressor response to arcuate stimulation was noted, although the pressor response was potentiated after sinoaortic denervation. The arcuate nucleus is a narrow and long structure, extending over more than 3 mm in the anteroposterior direction. It is possible that neurons projecting to the PVN and those projecting to the DVC are located at distinct, albeit overlapping, areas of the nucleus. We examined this possibility by stimulating the arcuate nucleus at sites posterior to those stimulated in the first series of experiments. The coordinates for these sites, similarly verified by postmortem examination, were 3.3 to 4.0 mm posterior from the bregma (see filled dots in Fig. 10.1).

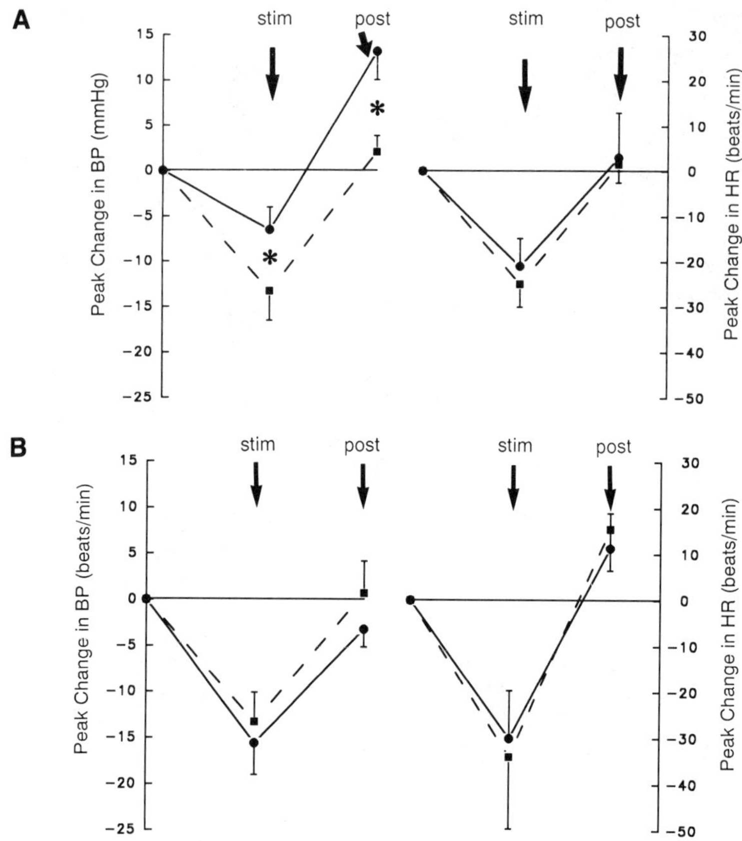

FIGURE 10.2. The effects on blood pressure (BP) and heart rate (HR) of the electrical stimulation of the midanterior (**A**) or postinfundibular segment (**B**) of the arcuate nucleus in urethane-anesthetized rats. The location of the bipolar, concentric, stainless steel microelectrode was as indicated in Fig. 10.1. Stimulation parameters were 60–200 $\mu$A, 0.8 msec, 80 Hz over 10 sec. Peak changes during (stim.) and after stimulation (post.) were established before (solid lines) and after (dashed lines) the i.v. administration of a $V_1$-vasopressin receptor antagonist (Mastrianni et al., 1989). Means and SE from 6 to 8 experiments are shown. Note the absence of the post-stimulatory pressor response when postinfundibular sites were stimulated (**B**). *indicates significant difference between corresponding control and post-$V_1$ antagonist values.

Electrical stimulation at these sites caused hypotension and bradycardia without a secondary rise in blood pressure. (Fig. 10.2B, solid lines). The absence of a significant pressor component was also indicated by the inability of the vasopressin $V_1$-antagonist to modify the blood pressure response to electrical stimulation (Fig. 10.2B, dashed lines). These experiments therefore indicate that arcuate neurons projecting to the paraventricular

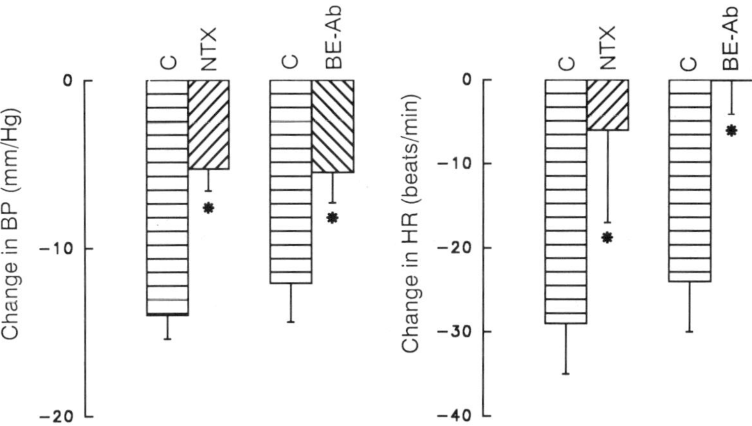

FIGURE 10.3. Inhibition of the hypotensive and bradycardic response to arcuate stimulation by naltrexone (NTX, 2 mg/kg i.v.) or by $\beta$-endorphin antiserum (BE-Ab, 100 nl intra-NTS). Means and SE from 5 to 7 experiments are shown. *indicates significant difference from corresponding control value ($p < 0.05$).

nucleus and those projecting to the DVC are located at distinct, albeit partially overlapping, regions of the narrow and long arcuate nucleus: although endorphinergic neurons projecting to the DVC are present in both segments of the arcuate tested, only the more rostral of the two appears to have neurons that initiate the vasopressin-mediated pressor response.

The depressor response triggered by $\beta$-endorphin in the DVC is mediated by opiate receptors of the $\mu$ subtype (Mosqueda-Garcia and Kunos, 1987). These receptors may be localized postsynaptically to baroreflex afferents, and their stimulation may inhibit or activate neurons that form an integral part of the efferent sympathetic or vagal pathways, respectively. However, there is evidence that most of the $\mu$ receptors in the DVC are localized presynaptically on vagal afferents (Dashwood et al., 1987). Therefore, the endorphin-induced depressor response may be due to a presynaptic effect, such as facilitation of release of the baroreflex transmitter. Indeed, the finding by Brody et al. (1986) that sinoaortic denervation potentiated the pressor response to arcuate stimulation could be due to climination of a depressor influence dependent on intact baroreflex afferents. To verify such a possibility, we examined the effect of arcuate stimulation on baroreflex bradycardia elicited by i.v. injection of graded doses of phenylephrine. When phenylephrine injections were repeated during stimulation of the arcuate nucleus with currents too low to alter baseline blood pressure and heart rate, the phenylephrine-induced rise in blood pressure was the same as without arcuate stimulation, while the corresponding bradycardia was significantly enhanced. This stimulation-induced potentiation of baroreflex bradycardia was completely eliminated by naltrexone, 2 mg/kg, administered intravenously prior to stimulation of the arcuate nucleus (Mastrianni et al., 1989).

The above observations indicate that endogenous opioids, most likely $\beta$-endorphin released from neurons that project from the arcuate nucleus to the DVC, can facilitate baroreflex bradycardia. It is likely that the same neuronal pool of $\beta$-endorphin is involved in facilitation of baroreflex bradycardia and in the depressor and bradycardic response observed during stimulation of the arcuate at higher current intensity. However, the finding that a relatively high dose of naltrexone completely blocked facilitation of baroreflex bradycardia (see Mastrianni et al., 1989), but only partially inhibited the direct depressor response (Fig. 10.3) could suggest the involvement of additional nonopioid factors in the latter response.

## Is the Arcuate Nucleus a Site of the Cardiovascular Actions of Clonidine?

The role of the arcuate-DVC endorphinergic pathway in depressor cardiovascular regulation (Mastrianni et al., 1989) and in the effects of clonidine (Mosqueda-Garcia et al., 1986) raises the possibility that the arcuate nucleus may be a site of action for the cardiovascular actions of clonidine. The mediobasal hypothalamus is rich in $\alpha_2$-receptors, stimulation of which

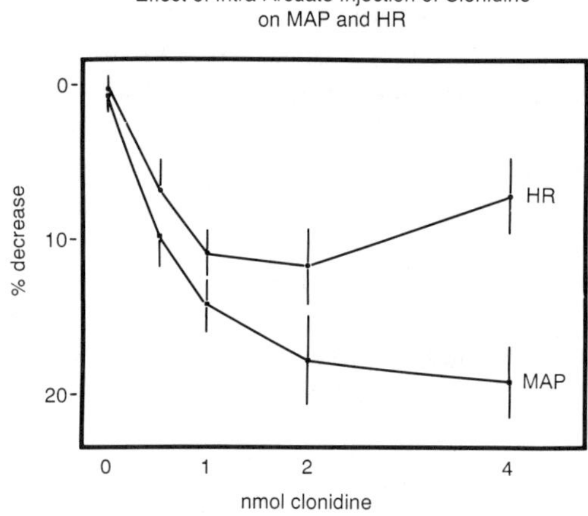


FIGURE 10.4. Hypotensive and bradycardic responses to unilateral intraarcuate microinjections of clonidine. Clonidine was microinjected in volumes of 50–100 nl through a glass microcannula stereotaxically inserted into the arcuate nucleus of urethane-anesthetized Sprague-Dawley rats. The coordinates used were as described in Mastrianni et al. (1989). Means and SE from 8 experiments are shown.

by catecholamines or clonidine leads to the release of growth hormone (Krulich et al., 1982) and prolactin (Lawson & Gala, 1975; Negro-Vilar et al., 1979). Recent reports indicate that, similar to the cardiovascular effects, these effects of clonidine are also mediated through the release of an endogenous opiate, most likely $\beta$-endorphin (Bramnert & Hokfelt, 1984; Koshiyama et al., 1989; Bruhn et al., 1989). We tested whether microinjection of clonidine into the arcuate nucleus is also able to elicit cardiovascular effects. As seen in Figure 10.4, unilateral microinjection of clonidine into the arcuate nucleus of urethane-anesthetized rats caused dose-dependent hypotension and bradycardia. It is noteworthy that significant effects are seen with as little as 0.5 nmol of clonidine, which is lower than the threshold dose required to produce similar effects in the DVC (1–5 nmol). These findings therefore indicate that the arcuate nucleus is a hitherto unrecognized site for the centrally mediated cardiovascular effects of clonidine.

## Opioid Peptides and Baroreflex Regulation

The potential role of endogenous opioid peptides in the regulation of the baroreflex has been studied extensively. Central administration of opiates and opioid peptides can elicit both depressor responses (Farsang et al., 1980; Petty and de Jong, 1982b; Ramirez-Gonzalez et al., 1983; Feldberg and Wei, 1986) and facilitation of the depressor baroreflex response (Laubie & Schmitt, 1981) as well as pressor responses (Schaz et al., 1980; Petty and de Jong, 1983; Hassen and Feuerstein, 1987) and inhibition of the baroreflex (Yukimura et al., 1981; Gordon, 1986; Wang and Li, 1988). The effects of naloxone on baroreflex sensitivity are similarly variable. Naloxone has been reported to inhibit (Miura and Takayama, 1983; Szilagyi, 1987), not to change (Gordon, 1986), or potentiate the depressor baroreflex response (Schaz et al., 1980; Ramirez-Gonzalez et al., 1983; Koyama et al., 1983; Szilagyi, 1988). The cardiovascular effects of centrally administered opioid peptides are known to be influenced by species, dose, type, and level of anesthesia and the opiate receptor subtype involved in the effect (Sitsen et al., 1982; Feuerstein, 1985), and some of the variability in responses can be attributed to such factors. It is possible, however, that neurons in the DVC containing different types of opioid peptides impinge on different but overlapping populations of target cells to trigger depressor or pressor responses, respectively. The involvement of different opiate receptor subtypes is not relevant in this respect, as $\mu$ receptors appear to be involved in both pressor (Hassen and Feuerstein, 1987) and depressor responses in the DVC (Mosqueda-Garcia and Kunos, 1987). For this reason, subtype-specific opiate receptor antagonists will not be useful for distinguishing between these mechanisms. Microinjection of the different peptides is also of limited use because the distribution of the injected peptide and of the receptors it activates is unlikely to match the unique distribution of receptors stimulated by endogenous peptides released from discrete nerve terminals. Nevertheless, most studies to date indicate that enkephalins cause pressor effects when injected intracerebroventricularly (i.c.v.) or into the DVC (Schaz et al., 1980; Petty and de Jong, 1983; Hassen and Feuerstein, 1987). In contrast, similar injections of low physiological amounts of $\beta$-endorphin cause hypotension and bradycardia (Petty and de Jong, 1983; Ramirez-Gonzalez et al., 1983; Mosqueda-Garcia and Kunos, 1987). The pressor response and sympathetic activation observed with much higher doses of $\beta$-endorphin (Petty and de Jong, 1982b; Appel & Van Loon, 1986) may be mediated indirectly through the release of enkephalins (Tseng et al., 1986). Antisera against opioid peptides are highly specific for individual peptides, and the localized release of the peptides they neutralize also provides topographical selectivity. Petty and de Jong (1983) found that intra-DVC injection of a $\beta$-endorphin antiserum caused a pressor response whereas similar injection of a met-enkephalin antiserum elicited a depressor response, suggesting the existence of tonically active endorphinergic depressor and enkephalinergic pressor systems in the

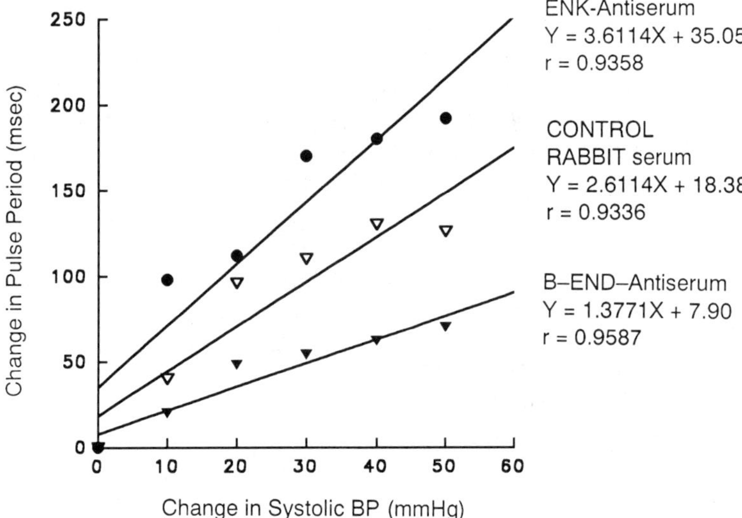


FIGURE 10.5. The effects of antisera against $\beta$-endorphin or leu-enkephalin on baroreflex sensitivity in urethane-anesthetized rats. The undiluted antisera were microinjected slowly in volumes of 200 nl into the bilateral DVC. Controls received normal rabbit serum intra-DVC. Baroreflex sensitivity was determined by regression analysis of the pulse period/blood pressure relationship during the response to a single i.v. dose of phenylephrine. The points represent the means from 3 to 4 experiments. The $\beta$-endorphin and leu-enkephalin antisera were kindly provided by Dr. Robert Eskay (NIAAA, Bethesda, MD) and Dr. Lee Eiden (NIMH, Betheda, MD), respectively.

DVC. We tested the effects of intra-DVC microinjections of antisera against $\beta$-endorphin and leu-enkephalin on baroreflex bradycardia elicited by phenylephrine. As illustrated in Figure 10.5, the antiserum against $\beta$-endorphin reduced the slope of the baroreflex curve, indicating reduced baroreflex sensitivity, whereas the antiserum against leu-enkephalin had the opposite effect. These findings suggest that baroreflex sensitivity is under the opposing control of facilitatory endorphinergic and inhibitory enkephalinergic influences at the level of the DVC. These mechanisms in the dorsomedial medulla represent only part of the net effect of opioids on the central segment of the baroreflex, as additional sites of interaction in the caudal and rostral ventrolateral medulla have also been documented (Punnen and Sapru, 1986; Morilak et al., 1990).

## Opioid Peptides and Central Cardiovascular Drug Action

The evidence presented above indicates that endorphinergic neurons in the brainstem are involved in the regulation of the baroreflex as well as in the centrally mediated cardiovascular depressor effects of $\alpha_2$-adrenergic agonists. Recent observations indicate that the centrally mediated hypotensive and bradycardic effects of a number of drugs or endogenous substances other than clonidine are similarly inhibited by naloxone. The list includes $\beta$-adrenergic blockers (Ramirez-Gonzalez et al., 1982; Jones and Tackett, 1989), atrial natriuretic peptide (Levin et al., 1989), the amino acid taurine (Fujita and Sato, 1988), Hageman factor (Goldstein et al., 1982), and the calcium antagonist dihydropyridine (Champeroux et al., 1988). Based on such findings it has been proposed that endogenous opioid release represents a common mechanism in the central sympathoinhibitory effect induced by various antihypertensive agents (Champeroux et al., 1988).

Recently, immunohistochemical evidence has been presented to suggest that the immunomodulator cytokine, interleukin-1$\beta$ (IL-1$\beta$), is widely distributed in the central nervous system including the arcuate nucleus and other brain stem structures involved in cardiovascular regulation (Breder et al., 1988). There is also evidence that lymphocytes express proopiomelanocortin-derived peptides including $\beta$-endorphin, and IL-1 can increase the secretion of $\beta$-endorphin in lymphocytes (Kavelaars et al., 1989). We therefore tested whether microinjection of IL-1$\beta$ into the DVC has any effect on blood pressure and heart rate and if it does, whether such effect involves endogenous opioids. Microinjection of 1 pmol of recombinant human IL-1$\beta$ unilaterally into the DVC of urethane-anesthetized rats caused a slight reduction in blood pressure and a marked decrease in heart rate. When the injection was repeated after the i.v. administration of naltrexone, 2 mg/kg, the bradycardic response was reduced by more than 50% (Fig. 10.6). These preliminary findings suggest that low physiological

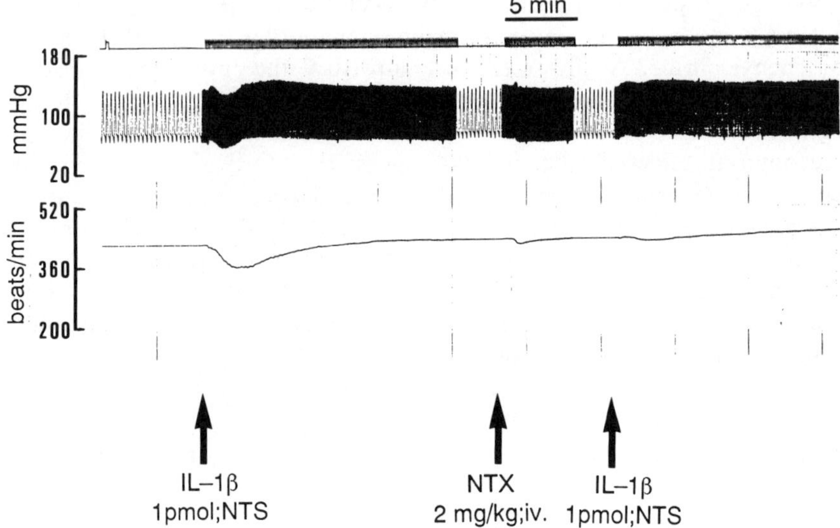



FIGURE 10.6. Centrally mediated bradycardic response to recombinant human IL-1β is inhibited by naltrexone. One pmol of IL-1β was microinjected into the left DVC of a urethane-anesthetized rat before and after the i.v. injection of 2 mg/kg naltrexone. Similar effects were observed in 6 additional experiments.

amounts of IL-1β can potently affect cardiovascular function at a central site of action, and the effect appears to have an opioid-mediated component.

## Summary

The observations reviewed in this chapter indicate that activation of an endorphinergic pathway projecting from the hypothalamic arcuate nucleus to the dorsal medullary vagal complex facilitates baroreflex bradycardia, and is also involved in the cardiovascular depressor action of various drugs and hormonelike substances.

## References

Appel NM, Van Loon GR (1986): β-Endorphin-induced stimulation of central sympathetic outflow: Inhibitory modulation by central noradrenergic neurons. *J Pharmacol Exp Ther* 237:697–701.

Baum T, Becker FT (1982): Alpha-adrenergic and 5-hydroxytryptaminergic receptor stimulants as new antihypertensive drugs, with observations on involvement of opiate receptors. *Clin Exp Hypertens* A4:235–248.

Bramnert M, Hokfelt B (1984): Partial blockade by naloxone of clonidine-induced increase in plasma growth hormone in hypertensive patients. *J Clin Endocrin Metab* 58:374–377.

Breder CD, Dinarello CA, Saper CB (1988): Interleukin-1 immunoreactive innervation of the human hypothalamus. *Science* 240:321–324.

Brody MJ, O'Neill TP, Porter JP (1986): Role of paraventricular and arcuate nuclei in cardiovascular regulation. In: *Central and Peripheral Mechanisms of Cardiovascular Regulation*, Magro A, Osswald W, Reis D, eds. New York: Plenum.

Bruhn TO, Tresco PA, Mueller GP, Jackson IMD (1989): Beta-endorphin mediates clonidine-stimulated growth hormone release. *Neuroendocrinology* 50:460–463.

Champeroux P, Brisac A-M, Laurent S, Schmitt H (1988): Endogenous opiate system and dihydropyridine-induced central regulation of sympathetic tone in rats. *Eur J Pharmacol* 158:157–160.

Chang APL, Dillard M, Dixon WR (1989): Effect of naloxone on blood pressure responses and plasma catecholamine levels following clonidine injection in conscious, unrestrained rats. *J Cardiovasc Pharmacol* 13:277–282.

Conway EL, Brown MJ, Dollery CT (1984): The evidence for involvement of endogenous opioid peptides in effects of clonidine on blood pressure, heart rate and plasma norepinephrine in anesthetized rats. *J Pharmacol Exp Ther* 229:803–809.

Dahlstrom A, Fuxe K (1964): Evidence for the existence of monoamine-containing neurons in the central nervous system. I. Demonstration of monoamines in the cell bodies of brainstem neurons. *Acta Physiol Scand* 232(suppl 62):1–55.

Dashwood MR, Gilbey MP, Spyer KM (1985): The localization of adrenoceptors and opiate receptors in regions of the cat central nervous system involved in cardiovascular control. *Neuroscience* 15:537–551.

Dashwood MR, Muddle JR, Spyer KM (1987): Opiate receptor subtypes in the nucleus tractus solitarii of the cat: The effect of vagal section. *Eur J Pharmacol* 155:85–92.

Farsang C, Kunos G (1979): Naloxone reverses the antihypertensive effect of clonidine. *Br J Pharmacol* 67:161–164.

Farsang C, Ramirez-Gonzalez MD, Mucci L, Kunos G (1980): Possible role of an endogenous opiate in the cardiovascular effects of central $\alpha$-adrenoceptor stimulation in spontaneously hypertensive rats. *J Pharmacol Exp Ther* 211:203–208.

Feldberg W, Wei E (1986): Analysis of cardiovascular effects of morphine in the cat. *Neuroscience* 17:495–506.

Feuerstein G (1985): The opioid system and central cardiovascular control: Analysis of controversies. *Peptides* 2(suppl 2):51–56.

Fujita T, Sato Y (1988): Hypotensive effect of taurine: Possible involvement of the sympathetic nervous system and endogenous opiates. *J Clin Invest* 82:993–997.

Goldstein DJ, Pitterman AB, Frech M, Kelly G, Pisano JJ, Keiser HR (1982): Naloxone attenuates the hypotension induced by Hageman factor. *Life Sci* 31:341–345.

Gordon FJ (1986): Central opioid receptors and baroreflex control of sympathetic and cardiovascular function. *J Pharmacol Exp Ther* 237:428–436.

Hassen AH, Feuerstein G (1987): $\mu$-Opioid receptors in NTS elicit pressor responses via sympathetic pathways. *Am J Physiol* 252:H156–H162.

Head GA, de Jong W (1985): Cardiovascular responses to central clonidine, $\alpha$-

134    G. Kunos et al.

methyldopa, and 6-hydroxydopamine in conscious normotensive and spontaneously hypertensive rats following naloxone. *J Cardiovasc Pharmacol* 7:321–326.

Jones LF, Tackett RL (1989): Catecholaminergic and opioidergic mechanisms involved in the hypotensive response of pindolol. *Eur J Pharmacol* 165:123–128.

Joseph SA, Pilcher WH, Bennett-Clarke C (1983): Immunocytochemical localization of ACTH perikarya in nucleus tractus solitarius: Evidence for a second opiocortin neuronal system. *Neurosci Lett* 38:221–228.

Kavelaars A, Ballieux RE, Heijnen CJ (1989): The role of IL-1 in the corticotropin-releasing factor and arginine-vasopressin-induced secretion of immunoreactive $\beta$-endorphin by human peripheral blood mononuclear cells. *J Immunol* 142:2338–2342.

Khachaturian H, Lewis ME, Schafer MKH, Watson SJ (1985): Anatomy of the CNS opioid systems. *Trends Neurosci* 8:111–119.

Kobinger W, Walland A (1972): Facilitation of vagal reflex bradycardia by an action of clonidine on central $\alpha$-receptors. *Eur J Pharmacol* 19:210–217.

Koshiyama H, Kato Y, Shimatsu A, et al. (1989): Possible involvement of endogenous opioid peptides in prolactin secretion induced by $\alpha_2$-adrenergic stimulation in rats. *Proc Soc Exp Biol Med* 192:105–108.

Koyama S, Manugian V, Ammons WS, Santiesteban HL, Manning JW (1983): Effect of naloxone on baroreflex, sympathetic tone and blood pressure in the cat. *Eur J Pharmacol* 90:367–376.

Krieger D, Liotta A, Nicholsen G, Kizer JS (1979): Brain ACTH and endorphin reduced in rats with monosodium glutamate-induced arcuate nuclear lesions. *Nature* 278:562–564.

Krulich L, Mayfield MA, Steele MK, McMillen BA, McCann SM, Koenig JI (1982): Differential effects of pharmacological manipulations of central $\alpha$-1 and $\alpha$-2 adrenergic receptors on the secretion of thyrotropin and growth hormone in male rats. *Endocrinology* 11:796–804.

Kunos G, Farsang C, Ramirez-Gonzalez MD (1981): $\beta$-Endorphin: Possible involvement in the antihypertensive effect of central $\alpha$-receptor activation. *Science* 211:82–84.

Kunos G, Mosqueda-Garcia R, Mastrianni JA (1987): Endorphinergic mechanism in the central cardiovascular and analgesic effects of clonidine. *Can J Physiol Pharmacol* 65:1624–1632.

Laubie M, Schmitt H (1977): Sites of action of clonidine: Centrally mediated increase in vagal tone and sympathoinhibitory effects. *Prog Brain Res* 47:337–348.

Laubie M, Schmitt H (1981): Sites of vagally mediated bradycardia induced by morphine-like agents and opioid peptides. In: *Central Nervous System Mechanisms in Hypertension*, Buckley JP, Ferrario CM, eds. New York: Raven Press.

Laubie M, Schmitt H, Vincent M, Remond G (1977): Central cardiovascular effects of morphinomimetic peptides in dogs. *Eur J Pharmcol* 47:67–71.

Lawson DM, Gala RR (1975): The influence of adrenergic, dopaminergic, cholinergic and serotoninergic drugs on plasma prolactin levels in ovariectomized, estrogen–treated rats. *Endocrinology* 96:313–318.

Levin ER, Mills S, Weber MA (1989): Central nervous system mediated vasodepressor action of atrial natriuretic factor. *Life Sci* 44:1617–1624.

Marmo E, Rossi F, Lampa E, et al. (1984): Participation of opiate peptidergic central mechanism in the hypotension and bradycardia of $\alpha_2$-adrenergic stimulating drugs: An experimental study in dogs with clonidine, flutonidine, guanabenz and guanfacine. *Curr Therapent Res* 36:1145–1151.

Mastrianni JA, Ingenito AJ (1987): On the relationship between clonidine hypotension and brain β-endorphin in the spontaneously hypertensive rat: Studies with alpha adrenergic and opiate blockers. *J Pharmacol Exp Ther* 242:378–387.

Mastrianni JA, Palkovits M, Kunos G (1989): Activation of brainstem endorphinergic neurons causes cardiovascular depression and facilitates baroreflex bradycardia. *Neuroscience* 33:559–566.

Medvedev OS (1986): Vascular effect of clonidine mediated via endogenous opiate receptors. *Bull Exp Biol Med* 1:52–55.

Miura M, Takayama K (1983): Naloxone inhibition of the carotid sinus nerve reflex in the nucleus of the solitary tract of the cat. *Brain Res* 288:389–392.

Morilak DA, Drolet G, Chalmers J (1990): Cardiovascular effects of the opioid antagonist naloxone in the rostral ventrolateral medulla of rabbits. *Am J Physiol* 258:R325–R333.

Mosqueda-Garcia R, Eskay R, Zamir N, Palkovits M, Kunos G (1986): Opioid-mediated effects of clonidine in spontaneously hypertensive rats: Elimination by neonatal treatment with monosodium glutamate. *Endocrinology* 118:1814–1822.

Mosqueda-Garcia R, Kunos G (1987): Opiate receptors and the endorphin-mediated cardiovascular effects of clonidine: Evidence for hypertension- induced μ-subtype to δ-subtype changes. *Proc Natl Acad Sci USA* 84:8637–8641.

Mosqueda-Garcia R, Kunos G (1988): Peripheral opiate receptors are not involved in the naloxone-sensitive cardiovascular effects of clonidine in rats. *Brain Res* 442:119–123.

Naranjo JR, Fernandez-Roman M, Urdin MDC, Fuentes JA (1985): β-Endorphin: A common factor in the antihypertensive action of clonidine-type imidazolines in spontaneously hypertensive rats. *Gen Pharmacol* 16:3–8.

Negro-Vilar A, Ojeda SR, Advis JP, McCann SM (1979): Evidence for noradrenergic involvement in episodic prolactin and growth hormone release in ovariectomized rats. *Endocrinology* 105:86–91.

Petty MA, de Jong W (1982a): Does β-endorphin contribute to the central antihypertensive action of α-methyldopa in rats? *Clin Sci* 63:293s–296s.

Petty MA, de Jong W (1982b): Cardiovascular effects of β-endorphin after microinjection into the nucleus tractus solitarii of the anesthetised rat. *Eur J Pharmacol* 81:449–457.

Petty MA, de Jong W (1983): Enkephalins induce a centrally mediated rise in blood pressure in rats. *Brain Res* 260:322–325.

Petty MA, de Jong W (1984): Endorphins and the hypotensive response to stimulation of alpha-receptors in the brainstem by alpha-methylnoradrenaline. *Neuropharmacology* 23:643–648.

Pickel VM, Chan J, Milner TA (1989): Ultrastructural basis for interactions between central opioids and catecholamines II. Nuclei of the solitary tracts. *J Neurosci* 9:2519–2535.

Punnen S, Sapru HN (1986): Cardiovascular responses to medullary microinjections of opiate agonists in urethane-anesthetized rats. *J Cardiovasc Pharmacol* 8:950–956.

Ramirez-Gonzalez MD, Farsang C, Tchakarov L, Kunos G (1982): Opiate antagonists reverse the centrally mediated antihypertensive action of propranolol in spontaneously hypertensive rats. *Eur J Pharmacol* 81:167–171.

Ramirez-Gonzalez MD, Tchakarov L, Mosqueda-Garcia R, Kunos G (1983): $\beta$-endorphin acting on the brainstem is involved in the antihypertensive action of clonidine and $\alpha$-methyldopa in rats. *Circ Res* 53:153–157.

Schaz K, Stock G, Simon W, et al. (1980): Enkephalin effects on blood pressure, heart rate, and baroreceptor reflex. *Hypertension* 2:395–407.

Sitsen JMA, Van Ree JM, de Jong W (1982): Cardiovascular and respiratory effects of $\beta$-endorphin in anesthetized and conscious rats. *J Cardiovasc Pharmacol* 4:883–889.

Szilagyi JE (1987): Opioid modulation of baroreceptor reflex sensitivity in dogs. *Am J Physiol* 252:H733–H737.

Szilagyi JE (1988): Endogenous opioid modulation of baroreflexes in normotensive and hypertensive rats. *Am J Physiol* 255:H987–H991.

Tackett RL, Laskey R (1987): Naloxone inhibits the centrally mediated hypotensive actions of BHT-933 (Azapexole). *Life Sci* 41:2063–2067.

Tseng LF, King RC, Fujimoto JM (1986): Release of immunoreactive met-enkephalin by intraventricular beta-endorphin in anesthetized rats. *Reg* Peptides 14:181–192.

Unnerstall JR, Kopajtic TA, Kuhar MJ (1984): Distribution of $\alpha_2$ agonist binding sites in the rat and human central nervous system: analysis of some functional, anatomic correlates of the pharmacologic effects of clonidine and related adrenergic agents. *Brain Res Rev* 7:69–101.

Van Giersbergen PLM, de Jong W (1988): Antagonism by naltrexone of the hypotension and bradycardia induced by $\alpha$-methyldopa in conscious normotensive rats. *J Pharmacol Exp Ther* 244:341 –347.

Van Giersbergen, PLM, Roording P, de Lang H, de Jong W (1989a): Participation of opiate receptors located in the nucleus tractus solitarii in the hypotension induced by $\alpha$-methyldopa. *Brain Res* 498:154–158.

Van Giersbergen PLM, Tierney SAV, Wiegant VM, de Jong W (1989b): Possible role of brain opioid peptides in clonidine-induced hypotension in spontaneously hypertensive rats. *Hypertension* 13:83–90.

Wang Q, Li P (1988): Inhibition of the baroreflex following microinjection of GABA or morphine into the nucleus tractus solitarii in rabbits. *J Auton Nerv Syst* 25:165–172.

Williams CA, Blevins LS, Paul DJ (1987): Possible catecholaminergic-opioidergic control of blood pressure during muscular contraction. *Cardiovasc Res* 21:471–480.

Yukimura T, Stock G, Stumpf H, Unger T, Ganten D (1981): Effects of [D-Ala$^2$]-methionine enkephalin on blood pressure, heart rate, and baroreceptor reflex sensitivity in conscious cats. *Hypertension* 3:528–533.

# 11
# Endogenous Opioid Peptides, Glucocorticoids, and Shock: Specificity, Site, and Mechanism of Action

PAUL L.M. VAN GIERSBERGEN, MARIA H. VAN DEN BERG, MARCEL H.J. EIJGELSHOVEN, JOKE COX-VAN PUT, DESIRÉE T.W.M. VAN DEN BERG, E. RONALD DE KLOET, AND WYBREN DE JONG

In 1973, when the presence of brain binding sites for compounds with opiate activity was demonstrated (Pert and Snyder, 1973; Simon et al., 1973; Terenius, 1973), the search for endogenous ligands for these putative opiate receptors was initiated. Two years later, Hughes et al. (1975) isolated two related pentapeptides from the brain of pigs that were called [Leu$^5$]- and [Met$^5$]enkephalin. Subsequently, $\beta$-endorphin (Li and Chung, 1976) and dynorphin B (Goldstein et al., 1979) were isolated. Interestingly, although opioid peptides are derived from different precursor molecules (for review see Höllt, 1986), they share at their N-terminal a [Met$^5$]- or [Leu$^5$]enkephalin sequence. The opioid peptides exert their biological effects via stimulation of specific receptors. Four major categories of opiate receptors have been identified, $\mu$, $\delta$, $\kappa$, and $\sigma$ receptors. Since the "classic" opiate receptor antagonist naloxone has no affinity for the $\sigma$ receptor (Schmidt et al., 1985), this receptor is considered by some investigators not to be an opioid receptor. At present, evidence is accumulating for the existence of subtypes of the $\mu$ and $\kappa$ receptor.

Endogenous opioid peptides have been implicated to play a role in many (patho)physiological processes (for review see Olson et al., 1987). Cardiovascular control was among the first putative functions of these peptides. The hypotensive and bradycardic effects of morphine had long been known (Evans et al., 1952; Feldberg and Paton, 1951) and similar cardiovascular responses were soon observed after i.v. administration of $\beta$-endorphin (Lemaire et al., 1978). The fact that administration of opioid peptides could reduce blood pressure together with the observation that $\beta$-endorphin is coreleased with adenosine corticotropic hormone (ACTH) during stress (Guillemin et al., 1977) prompted Holaday and Faden (1978) to study a possible involvement of endogenous opioid peptides in the pathogenesis of shock. They found that naloxone, injected in rats after the induction of endotoxic shock, reversed endotoxin-induced hypotension and increased survival rate (Holaday and Faden, 1978). The beneficial effects of naloxone on the cardiovascular system have been confirmed in other forms of shock such as hemorrhagic, spinal, and anaphylactic (for review see Holaday, 1983). Since then, numerous studies have been reported concerning the site of action of naloxone, its mechanism of action, the type of opiate receptor involved, and so forth. Little is still known regarding the precise location within the central nervous system and in the periphery of the opiate receptors that are blocked by naloxone and what the endogenous ligands are for these receptors. In this chapter we review the information in the literature on the role of endogenous opioid peptides in the pathophysiology of shock as well as report our recent findings on the location of the opiate receptors involved and their endogenous ligands in the central nervous system and on a possible interaction between brain endogenous opioid peptides and glucocorticosteroids.

## Methods

A method developed by Sandor et al. (1987) was used with which the blood pressure–blood volume relationship can be assessed. Briefly, urethane-anesthetized, artificially ventilated male Wistar rats, weighing between 220 and 300 gm, were used. Both femoral arteries were catheterized for continuous measurement of blood pressure and for standardized bleeding. Substances were administered either intracerebroventricularly (i.c.v.), according to Brakkee et al. (1979), or subcutaneously (s.c.). After determination of basal blood pressure and heart rate, the rats were treated with the test substance and 15 min later bleeding was started. Blood pressure was reduced stepwise to 80, 60, and 40 mm Hg by withdrawing blood. At the end of each 8-min bleeding period, the bleeding volume was determined. An increase, as compared to vehicle injected animals, in the bleeding volumes required to reduce blood pressure to the predetermined levels indicates a better capability of maintaining blood pressure whereas a decrease in the bleeding volumes indicates a worsened cardiovascular regulation.

## Are Central and/or Peripheral Opiate Receptors Activated During Shock?

Several studies show an effect of low, peripherally inactive doses of naloxone on cardiovascular function of animals in shock, indicating involvement of central opiate receptors. Administration of peripherally inactive doses of naloxone into the brain ventricular system resulted in an improvement of cardiovascular function in endotoxemic rats (Faden and Holaday, 1980) and dogs (Jansen, 1983), in rats with hemorrhagic shock (Holaday et al., 1981), in mice with experimental anaphylaxis (Amir, 1984a), and in rats with spinal shock (Holaday and Faden, 1980). In contrast, Lechner et al. (1985) were unable to demonstrate a hypertensive response after central injection of naloxone in a dog model of hemorrhagic shock, but beneficial effects of naloxone were observed after peripheral administration, thus suggesting a peripheral site of action for naloxone. Although demonstration of an effect of naloxone after central administration, but not after peripheral injection of the same dose, strongly suggests involvement of brain opiate receptors, a role for peripheral receptors cannot be excluded.

The use of quaternary analogs of naloxone or naltrexone may help resolve this problem, since such compounds do not readily cross the blood-brain barrier. It was previously, shown that the iodomethylate of naloxone could reverse endotoxic hypotension in rats after central, but not after peripheral, administration (Rios and Jacob, 1981). A similar observation was reported by Amir (1984) using naltrexone methyl bromide to reverse the hypotension induced by the histamine-releasing compound 48/80. Recently, we have shown that a dose of 1 mg/kg s.c. of naloxone methobromide (a generous gift from Boehringer, Ingelheim, FRG) increased the bleeding volume to reduce blood pressure whereas a dose of 10 mg/kg s.c. was ineffective (Van Giersbergen et al., 1989a) (Table 1). Our results indicate that activation of both peripheral and central opiate receptors play a role in the control of blood pressure during hemorrhage in rats. In other forms of shock, central opiate receptors appear to be more important (Amir, 1984a; Rios and Jacob, 1981). The lack of an effect of the higher dose of naloxone methobromide in our experiments might be explained by a mixed opiate agonistic and antagonistic action.

Little is known about the precise location of the opiate receptors that are activated during shock. Lechner et al. (1985) reported evidence that naloxone might act on cardiac opiate receptors. Naloxone had beneficial effects after both intracoronary and intravenous administration in dogs in a hemorrhagic shock state, but intracoronary naloxone was 10 times more potent. Opiate receptors in liver and pancreas have also been implicated as

TABLE 11.1. Effect of naloxone and naloxone methobromide on bleeding volumes during standardized, stepwise hemorrhagic hypotension in anesthetized rats.

| Treatment | Dose (mg/kg s.c.) | Blood pressure level | | |
| --- | --- | --- | --- | --- |
| | | 80 mm Hg | 60 mm Hg | 40 mm Hg |
| Saline | | $0.31 \pm 0.08$ | $0.56 \pm 0.09$ | $1.11 \pm 0.10$ |
| Naloxone | 1.0 | $0.50 \pm 0.12$ | $0.90 \pm 0.16$ | $1.72 \pm 0.13$[a] |
| Naloxone Methobromide | 1.0 | $0.40 \pm 0.09$ | $0.78 \pm 0.11$ | $1.53 \pm 0.07$[a] |
| Naloxone Methobromide | 10 | $0.38 \pm 0.12$ | $0.64 \pm 0.15$ | $1.15 \pm 0.16$ |

Values are expressed as ml blood/100gm body weight as mean $\pm$ SEM (n = 5–10).
[a]$p < 0.05$ as compared to saline-treated control rats.

sites of action of naloxone in the periphery (Curtis and Lefer, 1980). Few attempts have been made to localize the opiate receptors in the central nervous system. The nucleus tractus solitarii (NTS) is an important center for the regulation of autonomic nervous activity and could be a possible site of action. Furthermore, the NTS has been shown to contain opiate receptors (Atweh and Kuhar, 1977), and microinjection of opioid peptides into the NTS can result in hypotension (Hassen et al., 1982; Petty and De Jong, 1982). Therefore, we examined if opiate receptors in the NTS are involved in the regulation of blood pressure during controlled stepwise hemorrhagic hypotension in rats. Preliminary data indicate that bilateral microinjection of 10 ng of naloxone into the NTS of anesthetized rats tends to increase the bleeding volume required for a specific level of hypotension. Thus, opiate receptors in the NTS, or a closely located region, might be activated during blood loss. Recently, it was shown that naloxone microinjected into the rostral ventrolateral medulla produced a gradual increase in blood pressure of rabbits subjected to hemorrhage (Morilak et al., 1990) indicating that other sites in the medulla might also mediate the cardiovascular effects of naloxone (see also Chalmers et al., Chapter 1 in this volume) The anteroventral hypothalamus (AV3V) might be yet another site in the brain where opioid peptides can influence blood pressure regulation during blood loss. It was shown that injection of [D-Ala$^2$-MePhe$^4$- Gly-ol]-enkephalin (DAGO), a $\mu$ receptor agonist, into the AV3V region produced an enhanced recovery of blood pressure of rats in a hypovolemic shock state (Feuerstein et al., 1985). Lesioning of the AV3V exacerbated the effects of hypovolemia (Feuerstein et al., 1985). These results suggest that $\mu$ receptor stimulation in the AV3V activates/ facilitates compensatory systems in hemorrhagic shock. However, the opioid peptide-mediated depression of cardiovascular function seems to override the opioid peptide-dependent compensatory mechanisms, since the overall effect of naloxone is an improvement of cardiovascular function.

## What are the Endogenous Ligands?

Increased levels of circulating $\beta$-endorphin have been demonstrated in humans with septic shock (Hinds et al., 1985), in hypovolemic dogs (Vargish and Beamer, 1985), hypovolemic pigs (O'Benar et al., 1987), hypovolemic sheep (Hamilton et al., 1986 Smith et al., 1986), and in endotoxic sheep (Hamilton et al., 1986). An increased release of plasma enkephalins also has been reported (Gaumann et al., 1987; Inoue et al., 1987). Furthermore, Daly et al. (1987) reported a significant correlation between the decrease in blood pressure during shock and the increase in the plasma concentration of $\beta$-endorphin. Thus, both the enkephalins and $\beta$-endorphin might be endogenous ligands in the periphery. Naloxone blocks

$\mu$, $\delta$, and $\kappa$ opiate receptors (Schmidt et al., 1985) and inhibits most of the biological effects of both endorphins and of enkephalins; these endogenous opioids are not very selective for any one type of opiate receptor. Therefore, it is not possible to review the contribution of the individual peripheral opioid peptides to the pathophysiology of shock. Selective inhibition of one opioid system by an antiserum could shed light on this matter. The removal of a major source of circulating $\beta$-endorphin and enkephalins (i.e., pituitary and adrenal medulla, respectively) resulted in marked sensitization of animals to shock rather than a protective effect (Holaday et al., 1981; Holaday et al., 1983). These results do not necessarily argue against a possible role for the peripheral opioid peptides, but they do suggest that these peptides appear not to be essential for the development of shock. Moreover, they demonstrate that the pituitary–adrenal axis contains components that protect the animal from the consequences of shock.

In a series of experiments using antisera raised against different opioid peptides, we have attempted to elucidate the nature of the opioid peptides in the brain involved in the regulation of blood pressure during stepwise hemorrhagic hypotension. Previously, Sandor et al. (1987) have demonstrated that i.c.v. administration of a $\beta$-endorphin antiserum resulted in an increase in the bleeding volumes required to reduce blood pressure, whereas antisera against [Met$^5$]enkephalin and dynorphin A(1–13) were not effective. In addition, decreased bleeding volumes were observed after central administration of $\beta$-endorphin and dynorphin A(1–13), but not after [Met$^5$]enkephalin (Sandor et al., 1987). It was concluded that in the central nervous system $\beta$-endorphin might be the endogenous ligand whereas enkephalins and dynorphins appear not to be important. We have extended these earlier observations. Since the $\beta$-endorphin antiserum B4 that was used by Sandor et al. (1987) recognizes the 9–16 segment of the $\beta$-endorphin molecule and, therefore, also cross-reacts with $\alpha$-endorphin and $\gamma$-endorphin, more specific antisera against these endorphins were tested for their ability to influence the blood pressure–blood volume relationship. Furthermore, various dilutions of the same [Met$^5$]enkephalin and dynorphin A(1–13) antisera as used by Sandor et al. (1987) were tested to evaluate the negative findings of these investigators. We confirmed that, at least in the rat brains, enkephalin-like peptides are not important in the control of blood pressure during blood loss (Van den Berg et al., unpublished data). The use of the specific endorphin antisera revealed that both the $\beta$-endorphin antiserum X5 and the $\alpha$-endorphin antiserum A2 significantly elevated the required bleeding volumes whereas the $\gamma$-endorphin antiserum L10 tended to decrease bleeding volume at all blood pressure levels (Van den Berg et al., unpublished data). At the level of the NTS $\beta$-endorphin (Petty and De Jong, 1982) and $\alpha$-endorphin (De Jong et al., 1982) decrease blood pressure whereas microinjection of $\gamma$-endorphin at this site causes an increase in blood pressure (Petty et al., 1983). Together these results suggest that $\beta$-, $\alpha$- and perhaps $\gamma$-endorphin play a role in central cardiovascular control during hemorrhage in such a way that $\gamma$-endorphin might exert a blood pressure increasing action whereas $\beta$-endorphin and $\alpha$-endorphin exert a hypotensive influence. The tendency of the $\gamma$-endorphin antiserum to decrease the required bleeding volume correlates with the observation of Amir and Van Ree (1985), who reported a beneficial effect of $\gamma$-type endorphins in mice subjected to anaphylactic shock. In contrast to the study of Sandor et al. (1987), we found that i.c.v. administered dynorphin A(1–13) antiserum could mimic the effect of naloxone and of the $\beta$-endorphin antiserum under identical experimental conditions. The discrepancy regarding the dynorphin A(1–13) antiserum between the present results and the study by Sandor et al. (1987) cannot now be explained. However, our observation that the dynorphin antiserum increased the required bleeding volume is in agreement with the observation that administration of dynorphin A(1–13) itself decreased bleeding volume (Sandor et al., 1987). Thus, $\beta$-endorphin and $\alpha$-endorphin, dynorphin A(1–13) and possibly $\gamma$-endorphin, or closely related peptides, but not the enkephalins, appear to be the endogenous ligands of the brain opiate receptors that are activated during hemorrhagic hypotension. It remains to be established which opioid peptides play a role in other forms of shock.

## Possible Mechanisms of Action

The attention on the mechanism of action of naloxone in the treatment of shock has been focused on the sympathoadrenal medulla and pituitary–adrenal cortex axes. Both hypophysectomy (HYPOX) (Davis et al., 1984; Holaday et al., 1981) and adrenalectomy (ADX) (Holaday et al., 1983; Patton et al., 1983) sensitized animals to shock. This sensitization can be explained by an impaired cardiovascular regulation due to the disturbance of hormonal homeostasis. Both ADX and HYPOX result in a significant decrease in blood pressure. The effect of ADX on arterial pressure in anesthetized rats is illustrated in Figure 11.1.

The observation in hemorrhagic shock models that less blood removal from HYPOX (Holaday et al., 1981) and ADX (Patton et al., 1983) animals was required to induce shock compared to sham-operated (SHAM) controls does not necessarily mean that these animals are sensitized to blood loss because they already have a lower blood pressure. Recently, we have shown that the bleeding volume required to reduce blood pressure from 60 to 40 mm Hg is decreased in ADX rats in which surgery was performed 2 to 14 days before the experiment (Fig. 11.1). In addition, this bleeding volume in ADX rats was constant and did not change in time although blood pressure and total bleeding volume gradually decreased in time (Fig. 11.1). Thus, we have shown that ADX rats have, as expected, a disturbed blood pressure regulation that is not dependent on the time point of adrenalectomy.

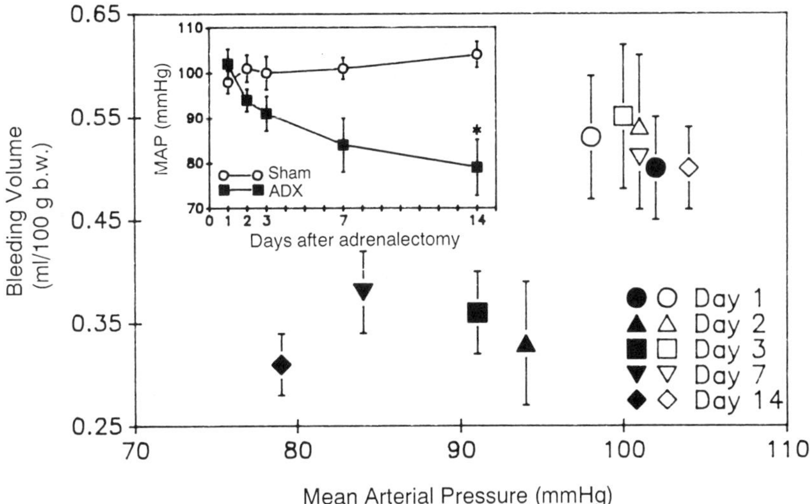


FIGURE 11.1. Time course of the effect of adrenalectomy (closed symbols) on blood pressure of urethane-anesthetized rats as compared to sham-operated controls (open symbols) (*inset*) and on bleeding volume required to reduce blood pressure from 60 to 40 mm Hg. Values represent mean ± SEM, n = 5–8,* $p < 0.05$ as compared with sham-operated rats (student's *t* test).

## *The Pituitary–Adrenal Cortex Axis*

HYPOX prevents the cardiovascular effects of naloxone in rats with endotoxic (Davis et al., 1984) and hemorrhagic shock (Holaday et al., 1981). It has been shown that $\beta$-endorphin and ACTH are released concomitantly under a variety of conditions including hemorrhagic shock in dogs (Tuggle and Horton, 1986) and in foot-shocked rats (Rossier et al., 1978). In intact animals, naloxone might antagonize possible shock-exacerbating effects of increased levels of circulating $\beta$-endorphin. The absence of ACTH rather than the absence of $\beta$-endorphin might be related to the lack of an effect of naloxone in HYPOX animals. Plasma levels of corticosterone decrease markedly after HYPOX (Davis et al., 1984) due to the absence of ACTH. Evidence indicates that corticosteroids are necessary for the effect of naloxone. Patton et al. (1983) have demonstrated that in ADX dogs with hemorrhagic shock, intravenous (i.v.) pretreatment with a high dose of hydrocortisone (50 mg) restored the cardiovascular responses to naloxone. In contrast, in intact dogs subjected to hemorrhagic shock, treatment with dexamethasone (7.5 mg/kg) resulted in an attenuation of naloxone's cardiovascular improving effects (Vargish et al., 1982, 1983). However, no dose-response curves were generated with the steroids in these studies. It is possible that in the studies by Vargish et al. (1982, 1983) the steroid doses were too high. This hypothesis is supported by the observation that hydrocortisone alone decreased survival in hemorrhagic dogs (Patton et al., 1983), indicating a potential exacerbating influence of high doses of steroids.

Besides its corticotropic activity, ACTH might exert an antishock effect that is independent from the adrenal cortex. Evidence to support this notion has been reported by Bertolini and collegues (for review see Bertolini et al., 1989). They showed that the i.v. administration of pharmacological doses of ACTH caused a dose-dependent reversal of the hypotension in rats (Bertolini et al., 1986b) and humans (Bertolini et al., 1987) with hemorrhagic shock. This effect of ACTH could be inhibited by peripheral $\alpha$-adrenoceptor blockade and by reserpine (Guarini et al., 1988a) but not by ADX (Bertolini et al., 1986a). Moreover, fragments of ACTH that are devoid of corticotropic activity can increase blood pressure in hemorrhagic rats (Bertolini et al., 1986c). Thus, the cardiovascular improving response to ACTH is not related to its hormonal effects on the adrenal cortex but is dependent on an intact sympathetic nervous system. It has been suggested that ACTH mobilizes blood from peripheral reserve organs such as the liver (Guarini et al., 1988b) and the spleen (Guarini et al., 1987).

In a recent series of experiments we investigated the importance of corticosterone for the effects of naloxone on the bleeding volumes required to reduce blood pressure in anesthetized ADX rats. Replacement treatment with a 100% corticosterone pellet (100 mg, s.c.), but not with a 12.5% corticosterone pellet (12.5 mg corticosterone and 87.5 mg cholesterol, s.c.), resulted in an increase in the required bleeding volume in naloxone-treated ADX rats as compared to control ADX animals implanted with a 100% cholesterol pellet (Fig. 11.2). Plasma levels of corticosterone are 1 to 3 $\mu$g/ml and approximately 25 $\mu$g/ml in rats with a 12.5% and a 100% corticosterone pellet, respectively (Dallman et al., 1987; Meyer et al., 1979). These values correspond to the circulating levels of corticosterone under resting conditions and after stress, respectively. Apparently, the effect of naloxone on bleeding volumes is present only when the plasma levels of corticosterone are increased.

Two distinct types of rat brain corticosteroid receptors have been identified, the mineralocorticoid (MR or Type 1) and the glucocorticoid (GR or Type 2) receptor (Reul and De Kloet, 1985). It has been shown that in ADX rats low plasma corticosterone levels result in substantial occupation of brain MR whereas GR become occupied only at higher plasma corticosterone concentrations. Therefore, our results with the 100% corticosterone pellet are indicative of an involvement of GR rather than MR in the effect of naloxone on bleeding volumes. This notion is reinforced by the fact that central administration of a specific GR antagonist, RU 38486 (Gagne et al., 1985), resulted in an inhibition of the increased bleeding volume seen in naloxone-treated ADX rats with a 100% corticosterone pellet (Eijgelshoven et al., unpublished data). A high concentration of GR is present in the NTS (Reul and De Kloet, 1986), suggesting that these sites might be

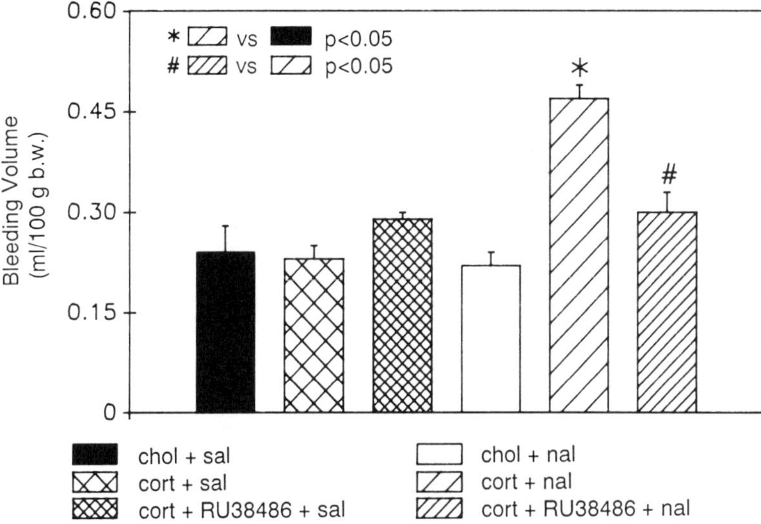



FIGURE 11.2. Effect of corticosterone replacement on the effect of naloxone on the bleeding volume required to reduce blood pressure from 60 to 40 mm Hg in urethane-anesthetized adrenalectomized rats. Adrenalectomy and implantation of pellets was performed 2 days before the bleeding experiments. Values are mean ± SEM, n = 5–7,* $p < 0.05$ as compared with controls with a cholesterol pellet.

involved in cardiovascular regulation. Glucocorticoids have been found to stimulate opioid peptide synthesis (Iglesias and Verbeeck, unpublished observation). However, whether enhanced opioid peptide synthesis is the underlying mechanism for the possible interaction between naloxone and corticosterone is not known at present. Endogenous opioid peptides and glucocorticosteroids might be involved in the control of autonomic nervous activity at the level of the NTS.

## The Sympatho–adrenal Medulla Axis

The bleeding volumes required to reduce blood pressure in naloxone-treated ADX animals with a 100% corticosterone pellet did not reach the volumes measured in SHAM animals injected with the opiate antagonists (Eijgelshoven et al., unpublished data). This finding suggests that other factors besides adrenal steroids are involved in the effects of naloxone; one of these might be the catecholamines of the adrenal medulla. A substantial release of the pressor catecholamines occurs during shock. A 50-fold increase in circulating adrenaline and a 10-fold increase in plasma noradrenaline have been reported in endotoxemic rats (Holaday et al., 1988). In most studies, naloxone does not further augment the release of the catecholamines (Feuerstein et al., 1981; Holaday et al., 1988). However, adrenal demedullation (Holaday et al., 1983) and adrenoceptor antagonists can block the effect of naloxone (Amir, 1984a; Schadt and York, 1982), indicating the importance of the catecholamines. Since naloxone apparently does not influence the release of the pressor substances from the medulla, it was postulated that the opiate antagonist might potentiate the pressor effect of adrenaline and noradrenaline. In rats subjected to endotoxic shock, but not in control animals, naloxone elevated the magnitude and duration of the pressor response to adrenaline by 40% (Holaday et al., 1988). Thus, the increased levels of circulating opioid peptides, as observed during shock, may reduce the efficacy of the also released catecholamines to counteract the shock-related hypotension. The molecular mechanism of this interaction is unknown.

## Comparison of Shock Hypotension with $\alpha$-Methyldopa–Induced and Clonidine-Induced Hypotension

It is interesting to note that several similarities exist between the hemorrhagic hypotension and the fall in blood pressure induced by the centrally acting antihypertensive drugs $\alpha$-methyldopa and clonidine. These compounds lower blood pressure via stimulation of central $\alpha_2$-adrenoceptors, which leads to a decrease of sympathetic nerve activity and/or an increase in parasympathetic tone (for review see Henning, 1984; Kobinger, 1978). Intracisternal pretreatment of rats with naloxone results in inhibition of $\alpha$-methyldopa–induced (Van Giersbergen and De Jong, 1988) and clonidine-induced (Van Giersbergen et al., 1989c) hypotension, indicating an involvement of endogenous opioid peptides in the hypotensive mechanism of action of these antihypertensive drugs (for review and additional references see Kunos et al., Chapter 10 in this volume). The hypotensive response to clonidine is sensitized by hypophysectomy (Conway et al., 1984) and by adrenalectomy (Zandberg and De Jong, 1977). In adrenalectomized rats, naloxone has no effect on the fall in blood pressure induced by clonidine (Dixon and Chandra, 1985). Furthermore, using the same antisera as in the stepwise hemorrhagic hypotension paradigm, we generated experimental evidence that $\beta$-endorphin and dynorphin A(1–13) play a role in the mechanism of action of $\alpha$-methyldopa (Van Giersbergen et al., 1989d) and clonidine (Van Giersbergen et al., 1989c). [Met$^5$]enkephalin appears not to be important and, in contrast to the hypotension induced by stepwise bleeding, $\alpha$-endorphin and $\gamma$-endorphin also have no influence (Van Giersbergen et al., 1989,cd). Finally, the NTS is a possible site of interaction between the endogenous opioids and $\alpha$-methyldopa (Petty and De Jong, 1984; Van Giersbergen et al., 1989b) and clonidine (Mosqueda-Garcia et al., 1986). Thus, endogenous opioid peptides appear to play a role in hypotensive influences of different origins. In conclusion, during a challenge of cardiovascular homeostasis by either blood loss or the administration of centrally acting antihypertensive agents, endogenous opioid peptide systems may become activated exerting a predominantly hypotensive influence. It is apparent that intact pituitary–adrenal medulla and cortex axes are a prerequisite to observe an effect of naloxone on both forms of hypotension. $\beta$-endorphin and dynorphin A(1–13) probably are the most prominent members of the opioid peptide families involved in cardiovascular regulation during a decrease in blood pressure. Although the precise mechanism leading to hypotension is not known, evidence in the literature points toward a possible involvement of these peptides in the control of autonomic nervous activity.

## Summary and Concluding Remarks

There is considerable evidence indicating an involvement of endogenous opioid peptides in the pathophysiology of shock. These peptides may activate opiate receptors in the central nervous system and in the periphery during shock, thereby exacerbating the effects of shock. The exact location of these receptors is still a matter of discussion. In the brain, areas in the medulla oblongata such as the NTS and the rostral ventrolateral medulla are suggested as possible sites. At these sites, stimulation of opiate receptors may result in a decrease in sympathetic and/or an increase in parasympathetic nerve activity. In the periphery, the involved opiate receptors may be located on the heart and on the blood vessels where the opioid peptides may depress heart action and decrease the pressor effects of circulating catecholamines, respectively. Using specific opioid peptide antisera, we demonstrated in a rat model of hemorrhagic shock that dynorphin A(1–13) and $\beta$-endorphin and $\alpha$-endorphin, or closely related peptides, presumably are the endogenous ligands for the brain opiate receptors. Circulating enkephalins or $\beta$-endorphin, released from the adrenal medulla and pituitary, respectively, may stimulate peripheral opiate receptors. Furthermore, in our laboratory we have obtained evidence suggesting an interaction between brain opioid systems and the brain glucocorticoid receptors (GR). Since the NTS contains high numbers of both opiate and GR, this nucleus might be a possible site of interaction. The glucocorticoids and the opioid peptides might interact in an antagonistic fashion in the control of sympathetic and parasympathetic tone. However, these possibilities need to be explored in future work.

The promising results with naloxone in animal models of shock have led to a substantial number of clinical investigations. In the clinic, however, controversial results with the opiate antagonists were obtained (for review see Holaday et al., 1988). Further clinical studies are clearly necessary to evaluate a potential therapeutic value of naloxone in the treatment of shock.

# References


Amir S (1984a): Beneficial effects of i.c.v. naloxone in anaphylactic shock is mediated through peripheral beta-adrenoceptive mechanisms. *Brain Res* 290:191–194.

Amir S (1984b): Naloxone improves, and morphine exacerbates, experimental shock induced by release of histamine by compound 48/80. *Brain Res* 297:187–190.

Amir S, Van Ree JM (1985): Beneficial effect of γ-endorphin-type peptides in anaphylactic shock. *Brain Res* 329:329–333.

Atweh SF, Kuhar MJ (1977): Autoradiographic localization of opiate receptors in rat brain. I. Spinal cord and lower medulla. *Brain Res* 124:53–67.

Bertolini A, Ferrari W, Guarini S (1989): The adrenocorticotropic hormone (ACTH)-induced reversal of hemorrhagic shock. *Resuscitation* 18:253–267.

Bertolini A, Guarini S, Ferrari W (1986a): Adrenal-independent, anti-shock effect of ACTH-(1–24) in rats. *Eur J Pharmacol* 122:387–388.

Bertolini A, Guarini S, Ferrari W, Rompianesi E (1986b): Adrenocorticotropin reversal of experimental hemorrhagic shock is antagonized by morphine. *Life Sci* 39:1271–1280.

Bertolini A, Guarini S, Rompianese E, Ferrari W (1986c): Alpha-MSH and other ACTH fragments improve cardiovascular function and survival in experimental hemorrhagic shock. *Eur J Pharmacol* 130:19–26.

Bertolini A, Guarini S, Ferrari W, Noera G, Massini C, Di Tizio S (1987): ACTH-(1–24) restores blood pressure in acute hypovolaemia and haemorrhagic shock in humans. *Eur J Clin Pharmacol* 32:537–538.

Brakkee JH, Wiegant VM, Gispen WH (1979): A simple technique for rapid implantation of a permanent cannula into the rat brain ventricular system. *Lab Animal Sci* 29:78–81.

Conway EL, Brown MJ, Dollery CT (1984): No evidence for involvement of endogenous opioid peptides in effects of clonidine on blood pressure, heart rate and plasma norepinephrine in anesthetized rats. *J Pharmacol Exp Ther* 229:803–808.

Curtis MT, Lefer AM (1980): Protective actions of naloxone in hemorrhagic shock. *Am J Physiol* 250:H416–H421.

Dallman MF, Akana SF, Cascio CS, Darlington DN, Jacobson L, Levin N (1987): Regulation of ACTH secretion: Variation on a theme of B. *Rec Prog Horm Res* 43:113–173.

Daly T, Beamer KC, Vargish T, Wilson A (1987): Correlation of plasma beta-endorphin levels with mean arterial pressure and cardiac output in hypovolemic shock. *Crit Care Med* 15:723–725.

Davis SD, McDonald WJ, Kendall JW, Potter DM (1984): Endotoxin shock: Prevented by naloxone in intact but not hypophysectomized rats. *Proc Soc Exp Biol Med* 175:380–385.

De Jong W, Petty MA, Sitsen JMA (1982): Endorphins and central cardiovascular regulation. *Br J Pharmacol* 37:333P.

Dixon WR, Chandra A (1985): Effect of naloxone, WIN 44,441-3 and corticosterone on blood pressure responses to clonidine in conscious, unrestrained, intact and adrenalectomized rats. *Fed Proc* 44:2859–2860.

Evans AGJ, Nasmyth PA, Stewart HC (1952): The fall of blood pressure caused by intravenous morphine in the rat and cat. *Br J Pharmacol* 7:542–552.

Faden AI, Holaday JW (1979): Opiate antagonists: A role in treatment of hypovolemic shock. *Science* 205:317–318.

Feldberg W, Paton WDM (1951): Release of histamine from skin and muscle in the cat by opium alkaloids and other histamine liberators. *J Physiol* 114:490–500.

Feuerstein G, Chiueh CC, Kopin IJ (1981): Effect of naloxone on the cardiovascular and sympathetic response to hypovolemic hypotension in the rat. *Eur J Pharmacol* 75:65–69.

Feuerstein G, Powell E, Faden AI (1985): Central effects of $\mu$, $\delta$, and $\kappa$ receptor agonists in hemorrhagic shock. *Peptides* 6:11–13.

Gagne D, Pons M, Philibert D (1985): RU 38486: A potent antiglucocorticoid in vitro and in vivo. *J Steroid Biochem* 23:247–251.

Gaumann DM, Yaksh TL, Dousa MK, Tyce GM, Lucas DL, Hench VS (1987): Effects of hemorrhage and naloxone on adrenal release of methionine-enkephalin and catecholamines in halothane anesthetized dogs. *J Auton Nerv Syst* 21:29–41.

Goldstein A, Tachibana S, Lowney LJ, Hunkapillar M, Hood L (1979): Dynorphin (1–13), an extraordinary potent opioid peptide. *Proc Natl Acad Sci USA* 76:6666–6670.

Guarini S, Ferrari W, Mottillo G, Bertolini A (1987): Anti-shock effect of ACTH: Haematological changes and influence of splenectomy. *Arch Int Pharmacodyn Ther* 289:311–318.

Guarini S, Ferrari W, Bertolini A (1988a): Involvement of the sympathetic nervous system in the cardiovascular effects of ACTH-(1–24) during hemorrhagic shock in rats. *Naunyn-Schmiedeberg's Arch Pharmacol* 337:556–560.

Guarini S, Ferrari W, Bertolini A (1988b): Anti-shock effect of ACTH-(1–24): Influence of subtotal hepatectomy. *Pharmacol Res Commun* 20:395–403.

Guillemin R, Vargo TM, Rossier J, Mininck S, Ling N, Rivier C. (1977). Beta-endorphin and adrenal corticotropin are secreted concomitantly by the pituitary gland. *Science* 197:1367–1369.

Hamilton AJ, Carr DB, LaRovere JM, Black PM (1986): Endotoxic shock elicits greater endorphin secretion than hemorrhage. *Circ Shock* 19:47–54.

Hassen AH, Feuerstein G, Faden AI (1982): Cardiovascular responses to opioid agonists injected into the nucleus of tractus solitarius of anesthetized cats. *Life Sci.* 31:2193–2196.

Henning M (1984). $\alpha$-Methyldopa and related compounds. In: *Handbook of Hypertension, vol. 3, Pharmacology of Antihypertensive Drugs*, Van Zwieten PA, ed. Amsterdam: Elsevier Scientific Publishers.

Hinds CJ, Evans SF, Varley JG, Tomlin S, Rees LH (1985): Neuroendocrine and cardiovascular changes in septic shock and after cardiac surgery: Effect of high-dose corticosteroid therapy. *Circ Shock* 15:61–72.

Holaday JW (1983): Cardiovascular effects of endogenous opiate systems. *Annu Rev Pharmacol Toxicol* 23:541–594.

Holaday JW, D'Amato RJ, Ruvio BA, Feuerstein G, Faden AI (1983): Adrenalectomy blocks pressor responses to naloxone in endotoxic shock: Evidence for sympathomedullary involvement. *Circ Shock* 11:201–210.

Holaday JW, Faden AI (1978): Naloxone reversal of endotoxin hypotension suggests role of endorphins in shock. *Nature* 275:450–451.

Holaday JW, Faden AI (1980): Naloxone acts at central opiate receptors to reverse

150    P.L.M. Van Giersbergen et al.

hypotension, hypothermia and hypoventilation in spinal shock. *Brain Res* 189:295–299.

Holaday JW, O'Hara M, Faden AI (1981): Hypophysectomy alters cardiorespiratory variables: Central effects of pituitary endorphins in shock. *Am J Physiol* 241:H479–H485.

Holaday JW, Malcolm DS, Long JB (1988): Endogenous opioids in the pathophysiology of shock: Sites of action, autonomic failure, and receptor interactions. In: *Opioid Peptides and Blood Pressure Control*, Stumpe KO, Kraft K, Faden AI eds. Heidelberg-Berlin: Springer-Verlag.

Höllt V (1986): Opioid peptide processing and receptor selectivity. *Annu Rev Pharmacol Toxicol* 26:59–77.

Hughes J, Smith TW, Kosterlitz HW, Fothergill LA, Morgan BA, Morris HR (1975). Identification of two related peptapeptides from the brain with potent opiate agonist activity. *Nature* 258:577–580.

Inoue M, Kimura T, Matsui K, et al. (1987): Responses of vasopressin and enkephalins to hemorrhage in adrenalectomized dogs. *Am J Physiol* 253:R467–R474.

Janssen HF (1983): Studies on a central site of action of naloxone in endotoxin shock. *Adv Shock Res* 10:73–81.

Kobinger W (1978): Central $\alpha$-adrenergic systems as targets for hypotensive drugs. *Rev. Physiol. Biochem Pharmacol* 82:39–100.

Lechner RB, Gurll NJ, Reynolds DG (1985): Intracoronary naloxone in hemorrhagic shock: Dose-dependent stereospecific effects. *Am J Physiol* 249:H272–H277.

Lemaire I, Tseng R, Lemaire S (1978): Systemic administration of $\beta$-endorphin: Potent hypotensive effect involving a serotonergic pathway. *Proc Natl Acad Sci USA* 75:6240–6242.

Li CH, Chung D (1976): Isolation and structure of an untriakontapeptide with opiate activity from camel pituitary glands. *Proc Natl Acad Sci USA* 73:1145–1148.

Meyer JS, Micco FJ, Stephenson B, Krey LC, McEwen BS (1979): Subcutaneous implantation method for chronic glucocorticoid replacement therapy. *Physiol Behav* 22:867–870.

Morilak DA, Drolet G, Chalmers J (1990): Cardiovascular effects of opioid antagonist naloxone in rostral ventrolateral medulla of rabbits. *Am J Physiol* 258:R325–R331.

Mosqueda-Garcia R, Eskay R, Zamir N, Palkovits M, Kunos G (1986): Opioid-mediated cardiovascular effects of clonidine in spontaneously hypertensive rats: Elimination by neonatal treatment with monosodium glutamate. *Endocrinology* 118:1814–1822.

O'Benar JD, Hannon JP, Peterson JL, Bossone CA (1987): Beta-endorphin, ACTH, and cortisol response to hemorrhage in conscious pigs. *Am J Physiol* 252:R953–R958.

Olson GA, Olson RD, Kastin AJ (1987): Endogenous opiates: 1986. *Peptides* 8:1135–1164.

Patton ML, Gurll NJ, Reynolds DG, Vargish T (1983): Adrenalectomy abolishes and cortisol restores naloxone's beneficial effects on cardiovascular function and survival in canine hemorrhagic shock. *Circ Shock* 10:317–327.

Pert CB, Snyder SH (1973): Opiate receptor: Demonstration in nervous tissue. *Science* 179:1011–1014.

Petty MA, De Jong W (1982): Cardiovascular effects of $\beta$-endorphin after microinjection into the nucleus tractus solitarii of the anesthetized rat. *Eur J Pharmacol* 81:449–457.

Petty MA, De Jong W (1984): Endorphins and the hypotensive response to stimulation of alpha-receptors in the brainstem by alpha-methylnoradrenaline. *Neuropharmacology* 23:643–648.

Petty MA, De Jong W, De Wied D (1983): The blood pressure changes resulting from the microinjection of fragments of the beta-endorphin molecule into the nucleus tractus solitarii (NTS). *Life Sci* 33 (suppl 1):735–737.

Reul JMHM, De Kloet ER (1985): Two receptor systems for corticosterone in rat brain: Microdistribution and differential occupation. *Endocrinology* 117:2505–2511.

Reul JMHM, De Kloet ER (1986): Anatomical resolution of two types of corticosterone receptor sites in rat brain with in vitro autoradiography and computerized image analysis. *J Steroid Biochem* 24:269–272.

Rios L, Jacob J (1981): Comparisons des effects du chlorhydrate et de l'iodomethylate de naloxone sur le choc endotoxinique chez le rat anesthesie. *Arch Inst Pasteur Tunis* 58:313–327.

Rossier J, French ED, Rivier C, Ling N, Guillemin R, Bloom FE (1978): Footshock induced stress increases beta endorphin levels in blood but not brain. *Nature* 270:618–620.

Sandor P, De Jong W, Wiegant VM, De Wied D (1987): Central opioid mechanisms and cardiovascular control in hemorrhagic hypotension. *Am J Physiol* 253:H507–H511.

Schadt JC, York DH (1982): Involvement of both adrenergic and cholinergic receptors in the cardiovascular effects of naloxone during hemorrhagic hypotension in the conscious rabbit. *J Auton Nerv Syst* 6:237–251.

Schmidt WK, Tam SW, Schotzberger GS, Smith DH, Clark R, Vernier VG (1985): Nalbuphine. *Drug Alcohol Depend* 14:339–362.

Simon EJ, Hiller JM, Edelman I (1973): Stereospecific binding of the potent narcotic analgesic [3]H-etorphine to rat brain homogenate. *Proc Natl Acad Sci USA* 70:1947–1949.

Smith R, Owens PC, Lovelock M, Chan E-C, Falconer J (1986): Acute hemorrhagic stress in conscious sheep elevates immunoreactive $\beta$-endorphin in plasma but not in cerebrospinal fluid. *Endocrinology* 118:2572–2576.

Terenius L (1973): Stereospecific interaction between narcotic analgesics and a synaptic plasma membrane fraction of rat cerebral cortex. *Acta Pharmacol Toxicol* 32:317–320.

Tuggle DW, Horton JW (1986): Beta-endorphin in canine hemorrhagic shock. *Surg Gynecol Obstet* 163:137–144.

Van Giersbergen PLM, Cox-van Put J, De Jong W (1989a): Central and peripheral opiate receptors appear to be activated during controlled haemorrhagic hypotension. *J Hypertens* 7(suppl 6):S26–S27.

Van Giersbergen PLM, De Jong W (1988): Antagonism by naltrexone of the hypotension and bradycardia induced by $\alpha$-methyldopa in conscious normotensive rats. *J Pharmacol Exp Ther* 244:341–347.

Van Giersbergen PLM, Roording P, De Lang H, De Jong W (1989b): Participation of opiate receptors located in the nucleus tractus solitarii in the hypotension induced by $\alpha$-methyldopa. *Brain Res* 498:154–158.

Van Giersbergen PLM, Tierney SAV, Wiegant VM, De Jong W (1989c): Possible involvement of brain opioid peptides in clonidine-induced hypotension in spontaneously hypertensive rats. *Hypertension* 13:83–90.

Van Giersbergen PLM, Wiegant VM, De Jong W (1989d): Possible involvement of beta endorphin(1–31) and dynorphin(1–13) in the central hypotensive mechanism of action of alpha methyldopa. *Neuroendocrinology* 49:71–79.

Vargish T, Beamer K (1985): Hemodynamic effects of naloxone in early canine hypovolemic shock. *Circ Shock* 17:45–57.

Vargish T, Gurll NJ, Reynolds DG, Lutz SA, Ganes EM (1983): Hemodynamic changes following corticosteroid and naloxone infusion in dogs subjected to hypovolemic shock without resuscitation. *Life Sci* 33:489–493.

Vargish T, Reynolds DG, Gurll NJ, Ganes EM, Lutz SA (1982): The interaction of corticosteroids and naloxone in canine hemorrhagic shock. *J Surg Res* 32:289–295.

Zandberg P, De Jong W (1977): Hypotensive action of clonidine after adrenalectomy in the rat. *J Pharm Pharmacol* 29:697–698.

# 12
# Neuropeptides in Central Baroreceptor Reflex Pathways

MIKLÓS PALKOVITS

The baroreceptor pathways are made up of two regulatory circuits: a short-loop reflex arc and a long-loop pathway (Fig. 12.1).

The short-loop baroreceptor reflex arc consists of three neurons: 1) Primary baroreceptor afferents (#1 on Fig. 12.1) from peripheral baroreceptors are conveyed by the carotid sinus nerve (glossopharyngeal nerve) and the aortic depressor nerve (vagal nerve). Neuronal perikarya are located in the petrosal and nodose ganglia. From the ganglia, fibers enter the medulla oblongata and terminate in the nucleus of the solitary tract (NTS), which serves as a primary baroreceptor center. This nucleus is a heterogeneous group of cells that contain 10 subdivisions. Besides baroreception, the NTS serves as a relay center for the regulation of other autonomic functions, such as respiration, taste, and gastric motility. Within the nucleus, afferents from various visceral receptors terminate in specific subnuclei. Baroreceptor afferent fibers make synaptic contacts in cells located mainly in the medial and commissural subnuclei. 2) One group of neurons in the medial and commissural NTS projects to the vagal nuclei (dorsal vagal nucleus and nucleus ambiguus), and few of them, if any, to spinal cord preganglionic neurons in the intermediolateral cell column. These NTS neurons serve as interneurons (#2 on Fig. 12.1) interconnecting the afferent and efferent limbs of the baroreceptor reflex arc. 3) Axons from vagal (parasympathetic—#3 on Fig. 12.1) and spinal (sympathetic—#4 on Fig. 12.1) preganglionic neurons run to the periphery and terminate on vegetative ganglionic cells. (The existence of a two-neuron, vagal-vagal reflex arc, i.e., primary vagal afferents terminating directly on vagal efferent neurons in the dorsal vagal nucleus or nucleus ambiguus, has been observed, but this type of short reflex loop is more likely to carry respiratory or gastric than baroreceptor signals.)

The long-loop reflex pathway receives the same peripheral inputs and has the same outputs as the short-loop pathway, but instead of having direct interconnections with interneurons, secondary baroreceptor signals in the long-loop pathway ascend from the NTS to higher modulatory centers, from where they descend to baroreceptor efferents in the medulla or

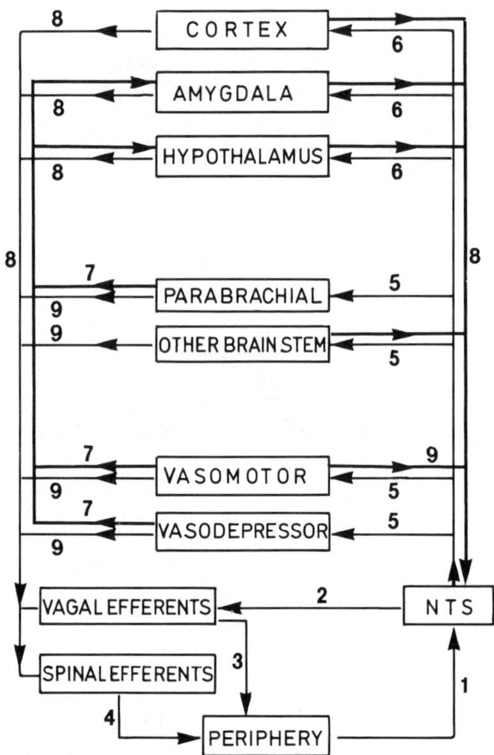



FIGURE 12.1. Short-loop and long- loop baroreceptor reflex pathways: connections among primary (NTS=nucleus of the solitary tract), secondary ($A_1$, $A_5$–$C_1$ catecholaminergic cell groups, also regarded as vasomotor and vasodepressor areas), modulatory (cortex, amygdala, hypothalamus, and pontine-locus coeruleus, parabrachial nuclei) areas and medullary (vagal) as well as spinal cord (intermediolateral cell column) preganglionic efferent neurons. See numbers in text.

the spinal cord (Fig. 12.1). The ascending fibers may terminate on medullary centers (vasomotor and vasodepressor centers in the ventrolateral medulla, which partly correspond to $C_1$–$A_5$ and $A_1$ catecholaminergic cell groups, respectively), in certain pontine-medullary nuclei (raphe nuclei, parabrachial nuclei, locus coeruleus—#5 on Fig. 12.1), and forebrain modulatory centers, such as the hypothalamus, central amygdala, bed nucleus of the stria terminalis (NIST), and the insular and prefrontal cortex (#6 on Fig. 12.1).

Baroreceptor structures receive neuronal inputs not only from the NTS but also from the vasomotor and vasodepressor centers and from the parabrachial nuclei (#7 on Fig. 12.1). The parabrachial nuclei serve as secondary relay centers of autonomic (including baroreceptor) reflex mechanisms.

Long descending axons arise in the cingulate cortex and the central amygdaloid nucleus, and they descend directly or indirectly (relayed by NIST neurons) to the vagal nuclei and the spinal cord. A fairly high number of neurons in the hypothalamic paraventricular, arcuate, and perifornical nuclei project down to the same areas (#8 on Fig. 12.1). Fibers from parabrachial and other ventromedial and ventrolateral medullary neurons also participate in the innervation of preganglionic baroreceptor efferents in the medulla oblongata and the spinal cord (#9 on Fig. 12.1). For references on further neuroanatomical details of baroreceptor reflex pathways see Leslie (1985), Palkovits (1988a, 1989), and Berecek and Hofbauer (1988).

Immunohistochemical evidence indicates that neuropeptides are present as neurotransmitters in each segment of the short-loop and long-loop baroreceptor pathways (see Kalia et al., 1984; Palkovits, 1988b, 1989; Riche et al., 1990 for details or reviews; Sawchenko, 1983; Yamazoe et al., 1984). The presence of the peptide histidine isoleucine amide-27 (PHI-27), which is widely distributed in the central nervous system (Hökfelt et al., 1987), has not yet been explored in the primary baroreceptor centers. In the present study, PHI-27–like neurons and fibers were identified in the NTS by using immunohistochemistry in combination with various types of surgical transections in the lower brain stem.

## Materials and Methods

Adult, male Sprague-Dawley rats (200 ± 10 gm body weight) were maintained under standard laboratory conditions (lights on from 6:00 AM till 6:00 PM, 23 ± 1°C), and were given standard rat chow (pellets) and tap water ad libitum.

## *Experimental Surgery*

Under ether anesthesia, the heads of the animals were fixed in a Kopf stereotaxic device. Four types of surgical interventions with appropriate sham operations (six animals per group) were performed: 1) unilateral, 2mm-wide coronal knife cuts at the diencephalon–mesencephalon border, 2) pontine hemisections with a coronal cut, 8 mm caudal to the bregma. One side of the pons was completely transected; 3) unilateral coronal cut 1.5 mm rostral to the obex, 1.0 mm wide, and 1 mm deep, which severed the direct rostral connections of the NTS and the dorsal vagal nucleus; and 4) intracranial unilateral vagotomy. After transecting the atlanto-occipital membrane, in a maximal (about 40–45°) nose-down position of the head, a 2-mm long, unilateral sagittal knife cut was performed 1.0 mm lateral to the midline, along the lateral edge of the NTS, starting from 1 mm rostral and ending 1 mm caudal to the obex and penetrating to the ventral surface of the medulla. Animals were decapitated on the 3rd or the 14th post-operative day.

## Immunohistochemistry

Intact, colchicine-treated (100 $\mu$g colchicine in 10-$\mu$l vehicle was injected into the lateral ventricle 2 days prior to perfusion) and operated rats were anesthesized with pentobarbital, and the animals were perfused through the ascending aorta with an ice-cold fixative solution containing 4% para-formaldehyde and 0.2% picric acid in 0.167 M phosphate buffer (pH 7.3). The forebrain containing the hypothalamus, the amygdala, and the bed nucleus of the stria terminalis (NIST), the mesencephalon, the pons, and the medulla were dissected separately and placed in the same solution overnight at 4°C. Forty-$\mu$m thick coronal sections were cut with a vibratome and incubated in a 1:1000 dilution of PHI-27 antibody overnight at 4°C (The antiserum was a gift of M.C. Beinfeld, St. Louis, MO). After the sections were rinsed in phosphate buffer they were incubated in biotinylated antirabbit immunoglobulin G (IgG) (1:400) followed by biotinylated avidin-peroxidase complex (1:200) for 1 hr each at room temperature. The sections were placed on gelatine-coated slides, dried, dehydrated, and mounted with a plastic mounting medium. Preabsorption of the antibody with 10 $\mu$g of PHI-27 eliminated the staining. The specificity and cross-reactivity (secretin 0.6%, glucagon 0.05%, no cross-reactivity with VIP, motilin) of PHI-27 antiserum has been reported by Beinfeld et al. (1984).

## Results

PHI-27–like immunoreactive fibers distributed in the entire rostrocaudal extent of the NTS (Fig. 12.2). The highest density of a PHI-27–like network appeared in the commissural part of the NTS. Several fibers crossed over in the nucleus, just below the area postrema (Fig. 12.2D). Moderate or low densities of PHI-27 fibers were seen in the medial, dorsomedial, intermediate, and lateral subnuclei (Figs. 12.2B,C) whereas only scattered fibers were observed in the rostral NTS (Fig. 12.2A).

In colchicine-treated rats, PHI-27–like cell bodies were immunostained exclusively in the commissural part of the NTS. Five to 15 mediolaterally elongated cell bodies per section were seen (Fig. 12.3).

Transection of the diencephalic–mesencephalic border or intracranial vagotomy failed to alter the density of the PHI-27–like network in the NTS. Fourteen days after the operation immunoreactivity was visibly reduced although not eliminated in rats with pontine or medullary coronal cuts ipsilateral to the transections. Major changes were found in the medial and lateral NTS, but only a minor depletion if any was observed in the commissural NTS.

No alterations in the density of immunoreactive networks were seen in the NTS following any of the transections on the third postoperative day.

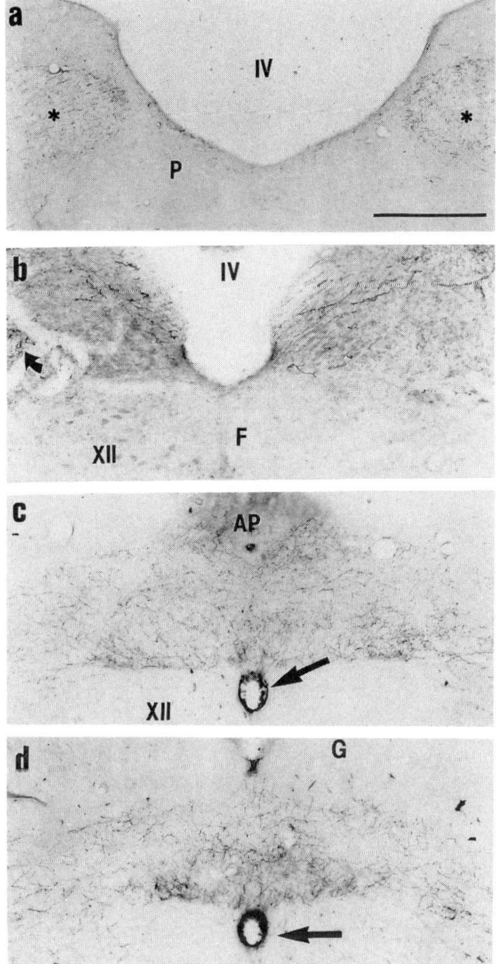



FIGURE 12.2. PHI-27–like immunoreactive nerve fibers in the nucleus of the solitary tract. **A**: rostral NTS (star). **B**: Medial and lateral subdivisions of the NTS, rostral to the obex. **C**: Medial and commissural NTS ventral to the area postrema. **D**: Commissural part of the NTS caudal to the area postrema. Arrows indicate the central canal. AP: area postrema; F: fasciculus longitudinalis medialis; C: gracile nucleus; P: nucleus prepositus hypoglossi; IV fourth ventricle; XII: motor hypoglossal nucleus. Bar scale: 0.4 mm.

However, a retrograde accumulation of PHI-27–like immunoreactivity was seen in certain mesencephalic neurons, ipsilateral to the transection. These were small neurons located on the side of the mesencephalic aqueduct at the level of the colliculus superior. Most of these cells were located in the subependymal layer (Fig. 12.4), with only one to three neurons per section located farther away from the aqueduct but still within the central

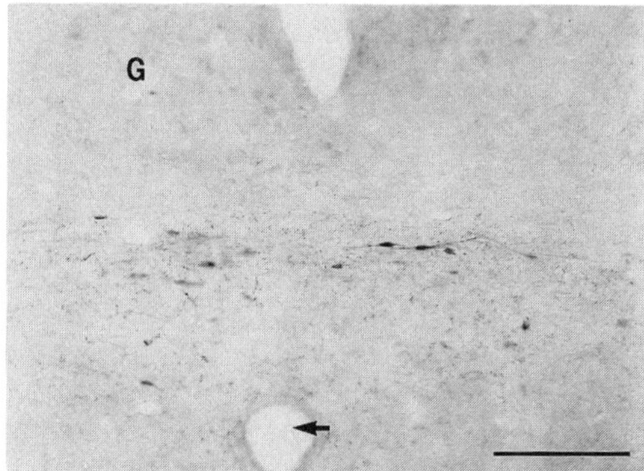


FIGURE 12.3.  PHI-27–like immunoreactive perikarya in the commissural part of the nucleus tractus solitarii. Arrow shows the central canal. G: gracile nucleus. Bar scale: 0.200 $\mu$m.

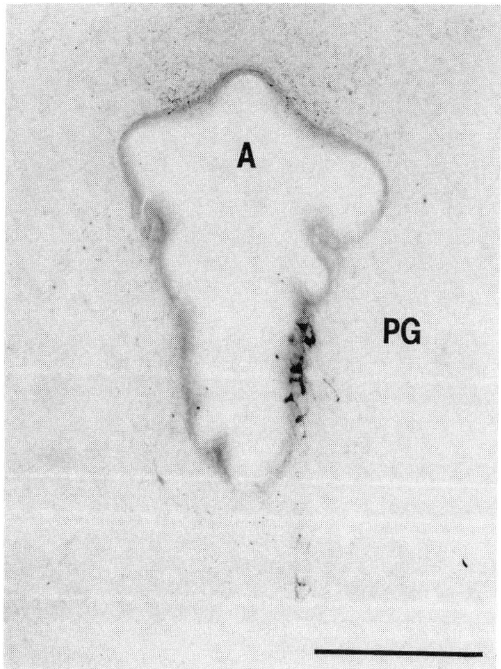


FIGURE 12.4.  Retrograde accumulation of PHI-27–like immunoreactivity in cells located in the mesencephalic central gray matter in rats with medullary hemisection ipsilateral to the knife cut. A: cerebral aqueduct; CG: periaqueductal central gray matter. Coronal section was taken at the level of the superior collicle, 6.3 mm caudal to the bregma. Bar scale: 200 $\mu$m.

gray matter. No retrograde accumulation of PHI-27–like immunoreactivity was seen in hypothalamic, amygdala, or brain stem neurons. Cell bodies containing PHI-27–like material, which were seen in the NTS of colchicine-treated rats, did not appear after any of the surgical transections performed in this study.

# Discussion

Neuropeptides are present in each component of baroreceptor pathways (numbers are shown in Fig. 12.1).

Perikarya of primary baroreceptor neurons (#1) are located in the petrosal and nodose ganglia. Among other neurotransmitters, substance P, cholecystokinin, somatostatin, and calcitonin gene-related peptide (CGRP) are present in the ganglionic perikarya as well as their fibers in the vagal nerve terminating in the NTS (Helke and Hill, 1988). In addition to these, substance P-containing fibers reach the NTS through the trigeminal nerve (South and Ritter, 1986).

More than 20 neuropeptides have been visualized in the NTS (see Palkovits 1988a,b, 1989 for review). Peptidergic neurons give rise to axons to different parts of the baroreceptor reflex arc.

NTS axons to the nucleus ambiguus and the dorsal vagal nucleus (#2) may contain POMC-derived peptides [adrenocorticotropic hormone (ACTH), $\beta$-endorphin, $\alpha$-MSH] (Joseph and Michael, 1988; Palkovits et al., 1987). The somatostatin projection from the NTS to the ambiguus nucleus may subserve the reflex control of esophageal motility (Cunningham and Sawchenko, 1989).

Neurons in the NTS project directly to the ventrolateral medulla (#5). These connections are mainly aminergic and GABAergic, but ACTH-containing projections have also been reported on the basis of immuno-histochemical (Joseph and Michael, 1988) and lesion-combined radio-immunoassay measurements (Palkovits et al., 1987). Recently, an enke-phalin-containing pathway from the NTS to the pressor area of the rostral ventrolateral medulla has been localized in rabbit (Morilak et al., 1989).

Several neuropeptides are present in NTS projections to the parabrachial nuclei (#5). Enkephalin, somatostatin, substance P, cholecystokinin, neurotensin, neuropeptide Y, dynorphin, and bombesin were localized in these axons (Maley and Panneton, 1988; Mantyh and Hunt, 1984; Milner et al., 1984; Riche et al., 1990). They may not all be involved in baroreceptor mechanisms, since the parabrachial nuclei also serve as a secondary respiratory and gustatory center. Among the peptides in NTS-parabrachial connections, neurotensin, neuropeptide Y, and cholecystokinin may be col-ocalized with catecholamines in cells derived from the $A_2$ and $C_2$ catecholaminergic cell groups located in and around the NTS (Hökfelt et al., 1984; Kwai et al., 1988; Sawchenko et al., 1985).

Long ascending fibers from the NTS terminate in the forebrain (#6). The major targets of these axons are the hypothalamic paraventricular and supraoptic nuclei, neurons in the lateral hypothalamus, the bed nucleus of the stria terminalis, and the central amygdaloid nucleus. A number of neuropeptides have recently been localized in all of these projections, like enkephalin, somatostatin, neuropeptide Y, neurotensin, and dynorphin (Riche et al., 1990; Sawchenko et al., 1988, 1990). In addition to these, bombesin-containing and inhibin $\beta$-containing NTS fibers have been observed to terminate in the paraventricular nucleus (Riche et al., 1990; Sawchenko et al., 1990).

Hypothalamic and limbic areas, which receive NTS afferents, project to preganglionic medullary and spinal cord baroreceptor efferents (#8). Descending fibers from the paraventricular nucleus contain oxytocin, vasopressin (Sofroniew and Schrell, 1981), corticotropin-releasing factor (CRF), somatostatin, enkephalin, substance P, and neurotensin (Sawchenko and Swanson, 1982; Strack et al., 1989) and cholecystokinin (Kiss et al., 1984). These fibers terminate in neurons in the dorsal vagal nuclei and in the spinal cord. ACTH/$\beta$-endorphin/$\alpha$MSH axons from neurons in the arcuate nucleus may innervate the intermediolateral cell column in the spinal cord. Substance P-, somatostatin-, neurotensin-, and CRF-containing neurons in the central amygdaloid nucleus as well as in the bed nucleus of the stria terminalis may innervate parabrachial neurons and preganglionic cells in the dorsal vagal nucleus (Gray and Magnuson, 1987; Veening et al., 1984). In addition to forebrain efferents, descending peptidergic fibers to the spinal cord arise from the medulla oblongata (#9). By using tract-tracing techniques in combination with multiple immunostaining, enkephalin- (Sasek and Helke, 1989; Thor and Helke, 1987), substance P-,thyrotropin-releasing hormone (TRH)- (Sasek et al., 1990), and somatostatin-immunoreactive projections (Strack et al., 1989) have been traced from the ventromedial medulla (raphe magnus, raphe pallidus, paragigantocellular reticular nuclei, and parapyramidal area) to the intermediolateral cell column.

Descending fibers to the NTS may also contain PHI-27. Observations in the present study indicate that a portion of PHI-27 fibers and terminals in the NTS may be intrinsic (commissural NTS), whereas another portion may arise from cells located in the periaqueductal gray matter. The existence of descending fibers from such mesencephalic cells to the NTS has been reported by ter Horst et al. (1984) in rat and by Bandler and Törk (1987) in cat based on the use of anterograde and retrograde tract-tracing techniques. In those studies, however, the transmitters contained in these mesencephalic-NTS fibers were not identified. On the other hand, PHI-27 immunoreactivity and VIP immunoreactivity have been detected by Hökfelt et al. (1987) in the periaqueductal gray matter, in almost the same group of cells as those in Fig. 12.4, but the projections of those neurons were not investigated. Retrograde accumulation of PHI-27 in these cells following hemisection indicates that at least a part of these cells project to the NTS.

Additional brain stem efferents that innervate the NTS (#9) include somatostatin-immunoreactive and enkephalin-immunoreactive cells in the ventromedial medulla, mainly in the paragigantocellular nucleus (Millhorn et al., 1987), and TRH-containing neurons in the medullary raphe nuclei (Palkovits et al., 1986), which appear to terminate on NTS neurons.

It was generally believed that vegetative preganglionic cells in the medulla oblongata and the spinal cord were exclusively cholinergic. Recent studies indicate that a certain percentage of preganglionic vagal efferents are noncholinergic. Catecholamines, especially noradrenaline, have been detected in vagal efferent fibers arising in $A_1$ cells in or around the ambiguus nucleus or in $A_2$ cells in or around the dorsal vagal nucleus (Gwyn et al., 1985; Ritchie et al., 1982; Tayo and Williams, 1988). Neuropeptides, like neurotensin (Mezey, Fodor, and Palkovits, unpublished observation) or galanin (Palkovits, Horváth, and Mezey, to be published) may also be present in preganglionic neurons. These neurons may not represent a separate group of cells in the vagal nuclei, but may have the peptides colocalized and coexpressed with catecholamines (Hökfelt et al., 1984; Melander et al., 1986). Neurotensin, which is present in cells of both vagal nuclei (Jennes et al., 1982), accumulates there in preganglionic neurons after intracranial or extacranial vagotomy (Mezey, Fodor, and Palkovits, unpublished observation). Since preganglionic vagal efferent neurons are generally considered to be solely cholinergic in nature, the presence of peptidergic (or aminergic-peptidergic) neurons in the dorsal vagal and ambiguus nuclei is of considerable interest.

It is noteworthy that neurotensin is also present in spinal preganglionic efferent neurons in the intermediolateral cell column (Krukoff et al., 1985), most probably in colocalization with noradrenaline.

Although during the last few years numerous neuropeptides have been localized in baroreceptor pathways in the central nervous system, our neuroanatomical knowledge about the chemical nature of these pathways is far from being complete. Furthermore, it should be considered that neuropeptides represent only one group of neurotransmitters involved in baroreceptor pathways. The functional role of neuropeptides in various portions of the short-loop and long- loop baroreceptor reflex arcs as well as the mechanisms of their action have not yet been clarified.

# References

Bandler R. Tork I (1987): Mibrain periaqueductal grey region in the cat has afferent and efferent connections with solitary tract nuclei. *Neurosci Lett* 74:1–6.
Beinfeld MC, Korchak DM, Roth BI, O'Donohue TL (1984): The distribution and chromatographic characterization of PHI (peptide histidine isoleucine amide)-

27–like peptides in rat and porcine brain. *J Neurosci* 4:2681–2688.

Berecek KH, Hofbauer KG (1988): Neuropeptides as modulators of blood pressure. In : *Progress in Hypertension*, vol. 1, Saito H, Parvez H, Parvez S, Nagatsu T, eds. Utrecht: VSP, pp 231–260.

Cunnignham ET Jr, Sawchenko PE (1989): A circumscribed projection from the nucleus of the solitary tract to the nucleus ambiguus in the rat: Anatomical evidence for somatostatin-28-immunoreactive interneurons subserving reflex control of esophegal motility. *J Neurosci* 9:1668–1682.

Gray TS, Magnuson DJ (1987): Neuropeptide neuronal efferents from the bed nucleus of the stria terminalis and central amygdaloid nucleus to the dorsal vagal complex in the rat. *J Comp Neurol* 262:365–374.

Gwyn DG, Ritchie TC, Coulter JD (1985): The central distribution of vagal catecholaminergic neurons which project into the abdomen in the rat. *Brain Res* 328:139–144.

Helke CJ, Hill KM (1988): Immunohistochemical study of neuropeptides in vagal and glossopharnygeal afferent neurons in the rat. *Neuoscience* 26:539–51.

Hökfelt T, Everitt BJ, Theodorsson-Norheim E, Goldstein M (1984): Occurrence of neurotensin-like immunoreactivity in subpopulations of hypothalamic, mesencephalic and medullary catecholamine neurons. *J Comp Neurol* 222:543–559.

Hökfelt T, Fahrenkrug J, Ju G, et al. (1987): Analysis of peptide histidine-isoleucine/vasoactive intestinal polypeptide-immunoreactive neurons in the central nervous system with special reference to their relation to corticotropin releasing factor- and enkephalin-like immunoreactivities in the paraventricular hypothalamic nucleus. *Neuroscience* 23:827–857.

ter Horst GJ, Luiten PGM, Kuypers F (1984): Descending pathways from hypothalamus to dorsal motor vagus and ambiguus nuclei in the rat. *J Auton Nerv Syst* 11:59–75.

Jennes L, Stumpf WE, Kalivas PW (1982): Neurotensin: Topographical distribution in rat brain by immunohistochemistry. *J Comp Neurol* 210:211–224.

Joseph SA, Michael GJ (1988): Efferent ACTH-IR opiocortin projections from nucleus tractus solitarius: A hypothalamic deafferentation study. *Peptides* 9:193–201.

Kalia M, Fuxe K, Hökfelt T, et al. (1984): Distribution of neuropeptide Y-immunoreactive nerve terminals within the subnuclei of the nucleus of the tractus solitarius of the rat. *J Comp Neurol* 222:409–444.

Kawai Y, Takagi H, Tohyama M (1988): Co-localization of neurotensin- and cholecystokinin-like immunoreactivities in catecholamine neurons in the rat dorsomedial medulla. *Neuroscience* 24:227–236.

Kiss JZ, Williams TH, Palkovits M (1984): Distribution and projections of cholecystokinin-immunoreactive neurons in the hypothalamic paraventricular nucleus of rat. *J Comp Neurol* 227:173–181.

Krukoff TL, Ciriello J, Calaresu FR (1985): Segmental distribution of peptide-like immunoreactivity in cell bodies of the thoracolumbar sympathetic nuclei of the cat. *J Comp Neurol* 240:90–102.

Leslie RA (1985): Neuroactive substances in the dorsal vagal complex of the medulla oblongata: nucleus of the tractus solitarius, area postrema, and dorsal motor nucleus of the vagus. *Neurochem Int* 7:191–212.

Maley BE, Panneton WM (1988): Enkephalin-immunoreactive neurons in the nucleus tractus solitarius project to the parabrachial nucleus of the cat. *Brain Res* 442:340–344.

Mantyh P, Hunt SP (1984): Neuropeptides are present in projection neurons at all levels in visceral and taste pathways from periphery to sensory cortex. *Brain Res* 299:297–311.

Melander T, Hökfelt T, Rökaeus Å, et al. (1986): Coexistence of galanin-like immunoreactivity with catecholamines, 5-hydroxytryptamine, GABA and neuropeptides in the rat CNS. *J Neurosci* 6:3640–3654.

Millhorn DE, Seroogy K, Hökfelt T, et al. (1987): Neurons of the ventral medulla oblongata that contain both somatostatin and enkephalin immunoreactivities project to nucleus tractus solitarii and spinal cord. *Brain Res* 424:99–108.

Milner TA, Joh TH, Miller RJ, Pickel VM (1984): Substance P, neurotensin, enkephalin, and catecholamine-synthesizing enzymes: Light microscopic localizations compared with autoradiographic label in solitary efferents to the rat parabrachial region. *J Comp Neurol* 226:434–447.

Morilak DA, Somogyi P, McIlhinney RAJ, Chalmers J (1989): An enkephalin-containing pathway from nucleus tractus solitarius to the pressor area of the rostral ventrolateral medulla of the rabbit, *Neuroscience* 31:187–194.

Palkovits M (1988a): Neuronal circuits in central baroreceptor mechanism. In: *Progress in Hypertension*, vol 1, H Saito, H Parvez, S Parvez, T Nagatsu, eds. Utrecht: VSP Press, pp 387–409.

Palkovits M (1988b): Neuropeptides in the brain. In: *Frontiers in Neuroendocrinology*, vol 10, Martini L, Ganong WF, eds. New York: Raven Press, pp 1–44.

Palkovits M (1989): Neuropeptides and peptidergic transmission in the nucleus of the solitary tract: Their role in the cardiovascular regulation. In: *Hypertension, Brain Catecholamines and Peptides*. FP Nijkamp, D De Wied, eds. Amsterdam: Elsevier.

Palkovits M. Mezey É, Eskay RL (1987): Pro-opiomelanocortin-derived peptides (ACTH/$\beta$-endorphin/$\alpha$-MSH) in brainstem baroreceptor areas of the rat. *Brain Res* 436:323–338.

Palkovits M, Mezey É, Eskay RL, Brownstein MJ (1986): Innervation of the nucleus of the solitary tract and the dorsal vagal nucleus by thyrotropin-releasing hormone-containing raphe neurons. *Brain Res* 373:246–251.

Riche D, De Pommery J, Menetrey D (1990): Neuropeptides and catecholamines in efferent projections of the nuclei of the solitary tract in the rat. *J Comp Neurol* 293:399–424.

Ritchie TC, Westlund KN, Bowker RM, Coulter JD, Leonard RB (1982): The relationship of the medullary catecholamine containing neurones to the vagal motor nuclei. *Neuroscience* 7:1471–1482.

Sasek CA, Helde CJ (1989): Enkephalin-immunoreactive neuronal projections from the medulla oblongata to the intermediolateral cell column: Relationship to substance P-immunoreactive neurons. *J Comp Neurol* 287:484–494.

Sasek CA, Wessendorf MW, Helke CJ (1990): Evidence for coexistence of thyrotropin releasing hormone, substance P and serotonin in ventral medullary neurons that project to the intermediolateral cell column in the rat. *Neuroscience* 35:105–119.

Sawchenko PE (1983): Central connections of the sensory and motor nuclei of the vagus nerve. *J Auton Nerv Syst* 9:13–26.

Sawchenko PE, Arias c, Bittencourt JC (1990): Inhibin $\beta$, somatostatin, and enkephalin immunoreactivities coexist in caudal medullary neurons that project to the paraventricular nucleus of the hypothalamus. *J Comp Neurol* 291:269–280.

Sawchenko PE, Benoit R, Brown MR (1988): Somatostatin-28-immunoreactive inputs to the paraventricular and supraoptic nuclei: Principal source from nona-minergic neurons in the nucleus of the solitary tract. *J Chem Neuroanat* 1:81–94.

Sawchenko PE, Swanson LW (1982): Immunohistochemical identification of neurons in the paraventricular nucleus of the hypothalamus that project to the medulla or to the spinal cord in the rat. *J Comp Neurol* 205:260–272.

Sawchenko PE, Swanson LW, Grzanna R, Howe PRC, Bloom SR, Polak JM (1985): Co-localization of neuropeptide Y Immunoreactivity in brainstem cate-cholaminergic neurons that project to the paraventricular nucleus of the hypo-thalamus. *J Comp Nuerol* 241:138–153.

Sofroniew MV, Schrell U (1981): Evidence for a direct projection from oxytocin and vasopressin neurons in the hypothalamic paraventricular nucleus to the medulla oblongata: Immunohistochemical visualization of both the horseradish peroxidase transported and the peptide produced by the same neurons. *Neuosci Lett* 22:211–217.

South EH, Ritter RC (1986): Substance P-containing trigeminal sensory neurons project to the nucleus of the solitary tract. *Brain Res* 372:283–289.

Strack AM, Sawyer WB, Platt KB, Loewy AD (1989): CNS cell groups regulating the sympathetic outflow to adrenal gland as revealed by transneuronal cell body labeling with pseudorabies virus. *Brain Res* 491:274–296.

Tayo EK, Williams RG (1988): Catecholaminergic parasympathetic efferents within the dorsal motor nucleus of the vagus in the rat: a quantitative analysis. *Neurosci Lett* 90:1–5.

Thor KB, Helke CJ (1987): Serotonin- and substance P-containing projections to the nucleus tractus solitarii of the rat. *J Comp Neurol* 265:275–293.

Veening JG, Swanson LW, Sawchenko PE (1984): The organization of projections from the central nucleus of the amygdala to brainstem sites involved in central autonomic regulation: a combined retrograde transport-immunohistochemical study. *Brain Res* 303:337–357.

Yamazoe M, Shiosaka S, Shibasaki T, et at. (1984): Distribution of six neuropeptides in the nucleus tractus solitarii of the rat: An immunohistochemical analysis. *Neuroscience* 13:1243–1266.

# 13
# Adenosine in Central Cardiovascular Control

ROGELIO MOSQUEDA-GARCIA, CHING-JIUNN TSENG, CAROL BECK, MICHAEL MCCORMICK, AND DAVID ROBERTSON

The endogenous nucleoside adenosine has been increasingly studied for its potential role as a neuromodulator in a number of autonomic functions, including central cardiovascular regulation. Similar to classical neurotransmitters, adenosine is known to be released by nerve terminals following depolarization (Bender et al., 1981), and more recently the presence of adenosine immunoreactivity within discrete neuronal cell groups of the brain stem and spinal cord has been documented (Braas et al., 1986). After release, adenosine can stimulate specific binding sites that are known to be coupled to adenylate cyclase (Van Calker et al., 1979). A regional distribution of adenosine receptors in the brain has been observed by autoradiographic techniques indicating distribution of adenosine binding sites in relevant autonomic brain nuclei (Goodman and Snyder, 1982).

The presence of both an energy- dependent high affinity uptake system (Bender et al., 1980) (which could provide a mechanism for removal of synaptically released adenosine) and the immunocytochemical localization of adenosine deaminase (Marangos et al., 1982; Nagy et al., 1984) (which is involved in the conversion of adenosine to inosine) have been reported in discrete brain regions. Importantly, the highest density of adenosine uptake sites within the central nervous system (CNS) has been observed in the nucleus of the solitary tract (NTS), which regulates reflex cardiovascular activity (Deckert et al., 1987; Marangos et al., 1982).

Recently, we and others have begun to address the question of the potential role of adenosine in central cardiovascular regulation. The studies support an important role of adenosine in the neural reflex control of the circulation and indicate a novel purinergic regulatory mechanism of neuronal cell activity.

## Central Cardiovascular Actions of Adenosine

Adenosine is a potent vasoactive substance that has been known to be involved in the regulation of cerebral (Rubio et al., 1975), muscle (Bockman et al., 1975), and cardiac blood flow (Berne, 1963). The hypotension present during hypoxic conditions in anesthetized animals is thought to be related to increasing central tissue levels of adenosine (Phillis et al., 1987). Furthermore, adenosine antagonists (such as caffeine or theophylline) prevented or attenuated hypoxia-evoked falls in blood pressure (Simpson et al., 1989). These effects are probably centrally mediated as adenosine antagonists that do not cross the blood-brain barrier do not block the hypotension elicited by hypoxia.

Earlier studies documented that direct administration of adenosine into the brain ventricles produced a marked respiratory depression that was often accompanied by changes in circulatory function (Hedner et al., 1982). Later on, it was shown that injections of adenosine analogs into the cerebral ventricles of rats produced dose-related reductions in blood pressure and heart rate that were antagonized by caffeine (Barraco et al., 1986). Importantly, maximal hypotensive responses to adenosine analogs were obtained in a region of the fourth ventricle proximal to the area postrema (AP) and NTS.

## Cardiovascular Effects of Adenosine in the Brain Stem

Neuronal cell groups in the NTS have afferent and efferent connections with rostral and ventral sites of the medulla oblongata, including the AP and the rostral ventrolateral medulla (RVLM) (Palkovits and Zaborszky 1977). These and other nuclei are of primary importance in the control of autonomic cardiovascular function. Our initial experiments documented the cardiovascular effects of microadministration of adenosine in these critical brain stem sites (Tseng et al., 1988).

Normotensive urethane-anesthetized rats were instrumented for continuous recording of blood pressure (BP), heart rate (HR), and sympathetic renal nerve activity (SNA). The animals were placed in a stereotaxic frame for microinjection of adenosine (0.23–2.3 nmol/60 nl) into the NTS, AP, or RVLM. Microinjection of adenosine into the NTS produced a dose-related decrease in systolic, diastolic BP, HR, and SNA (Fig. 13.1). The hemodynamic changes occurred within 90 sec after injection with maximal decreases in BP, HR, and SNA after the dose of 2.3 nmol of adenosine.

Microinjection of adenosine into the AP had similar cardiovascular effects. A somewhat greater effect in this nucleus, however, was observed with the 2.3-nmol dose in systolic/diastolic BP ($-29/-25 \pm 2/3$ mm Hg), HR ($-50 \pm 8$ bpm), but not in SNA ($-53\%$, Table 13.1). In contrast, similar adenosine doses into the RVLM did not significantly modify cardiovascular activity (not shown).

The specificity of the adenosine response in the NTS and AP was tested with the previous microinjection of the adenosine antagonist 1,3-dipropyl-8-p-sulfophenylxanthine (DPSPX, 0.92 nmol). The injection of DPSPX

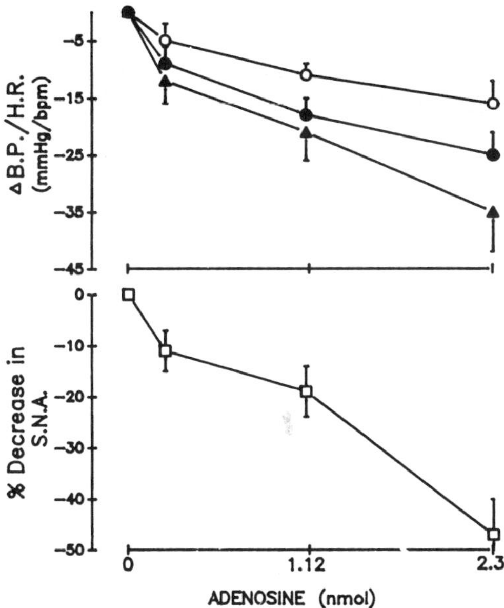

FIGURE 13.1. Cardiovascular effects of increasing doses of adenosine into the NTS. The effects of microinjection of adenosine on systolic BP (open circles), diastolic BP (filled circles), HR (triangles), and sympathetic nerve activity (open squares) were studied in a group of 10 rats.

TABLE 13.1. Effects of the adenosine antagonist DPSPX on the cardiovascular effects of adenosine in the NTS and AP of anesthetized rats.

| | NTS | | AP | |
| | ADO | DPSPX plus ADO | ADO | DPSPX plus ADO |
| --- | --- | --- | --- | --- |
| SBP (mm Hg) | $-25 \pm 4$ | $-3 \pm 2$[a] | $-29 \pm 2$ | $-2 \pm 3$[a] |
| DBP (mm Hg) | $-16 \pm 4$ | $-2 \pm 3$[a] | $-25 \pm 3$ | $-5 \pm 4$[a] |
| HR (bpm) | $-35 \pm 7$ | $-5 \pm 6$[a] | $-50 \pm 8$ | $-6 \pm 3$[a] |
| SNA % | $-47 \pm 7$ | $-8 \pm 4$[a] | $-53 \pm 6$ | $-6 \pm 3$[a] |

Adenosine (2.3 nmol) was injected before and after (15 min) similar administration of DPSPX (0.92 nmol).

n = 10 in the NTS group and 12 in the AP group.

[a] Indicates significant difference ($p < 0.01$) from the corresponding control group.

into the NTS had no effect on basal BP or HR. However, the antagonist abolished the effect of subsequent microinjections of adenosine into the NTS (Table 13.1). The effect of DPSPX on adenosine action lasted for approximately 45 min (Fig. 13.2). Additional specificity of the adenosine response in the NTS was tested with adenosine deaminase. The microinjection of 6 ng of adenosine deaminase (which converts adenosine to inosine,

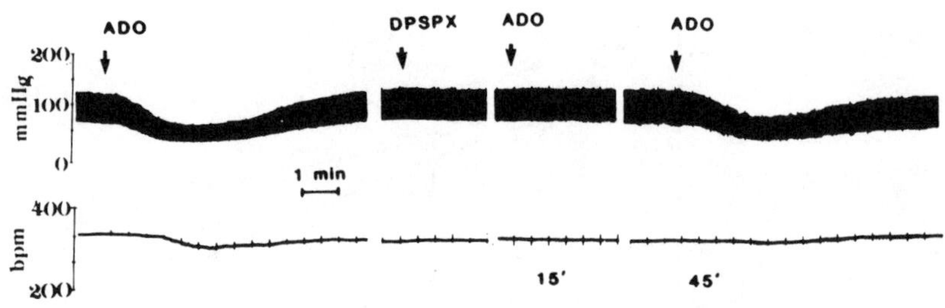


FIGURE 13.2. Actual tracing of the cardiovascular effects of adenosine (ADO, 2.3 nmol) into the area postrema before and after 1-3-dipropyl-8-p-sulfophenyl-xanthine (DPSPX, 0.92 nmol). Upper tracing displays BP recording and HR is shown in the lower one.

an inactive metabolite) prevented the cardiovascular effects of adenosine (Tseng et al., 1988).

Similar cardiovascular effects of adenosine have been reported by Barraco et al (1988), who in addition have documented the regional specificity of the response in the NTS. They have observed that microinjection of adenosine in rostral regions of the NTS were less effective or devoid of cardiovascular responses (Barraco et al., 1987). Moreover, significant cardiovascular effects were not observed after adenosine microinjection in sites lateral or ventrolateral to the caudal NTS (Barraco et al., 1988).

Purinergic cardiovascular effects in the NTS have been further confirmed with the use of adenosine analogs and adenosine 5'-triphosphate (ATP) (Tseng et al., 1988). On an equimolar basis (5'-N-ethylcarboxamido-adenosine NECA) was more potent than PIA [( − )-N$^6$-(R-phenyl-isopropyl)-adenosine], which in turn was more potent than adenosine to produce cardiovascular changes after intra-NTS administration (Table 13.2). Although PIA has relative specificity for $A_1$ and NECA for $A_2$ adenosine receptors, the difference does not allow a definitive characterization of the subtype of adenosine receptor that is involved in the in vivo response. It is interesting to note, however, that microinjection of agents that increase cyclic adenosine monophosphate (cAMP) such as isoproterenol or cAMP itself into the NTS causes a transient decrease in BP and HR (Barraco and Janusz, 1988). Although this would support an $A_2$-mediated response, final characterization of the subtype of adenosine receptor in the NTS awaits the use of more specific agonists or antagonists.

Additional experiments in our laboratory have indicated that ATP and ATP analogs evoked similar potent cardiovascular effects when microinjected into the NTS (Tseng et al., 1988). These effects, however, were probably largely mediated by adenosine receptors rather than by ATP-purinergic receptors ($P_2$) because DPSPX and adenosine deaminase blocked the ATP actions in the NTS.

TABLE 13.2. Cardiovascular effects of NECA and PIA after microinjection into the NTS of anesthetized rats.

|  | NECA | PIA |
|---|---|---|
| SBP (mm Hg) | $-40 \pm 2$ | $-31 \pm 2$ |
| DBP (mm Hg) | $-28 \pm 2$ | $-22 \pm 1$ |
| HR (bpm) | $-45 \pm 2$ | $-38 \pm 1$ |

n = 5; 2.3 nmol of NECA or PIA were microinjected into the NTS as described in the text.

# Intrathecal Effects of Adenosine

Neuronal cell groups located in the spinal cord also participate in cardiovascular function. For instance, the intermediolateral column of the spinal cord receives information from the RVLM and is one of the final relay stations that modulate sympathetic activity (Galosy et al., 1981). The contribution, if any, of purinergic activation on spinal cardiovascular control is largely unknown. In preliminary experiments, we have attempted to characterize the cardiovascular effects of adenosine and one of its analogs after intrathecal (i.t.) administration.

In normotensive Sprague-Dawley rats anesthetized with urethane, an i.t. catheter (PE-10, approximately 36 cm long) was filled with artificial cerebrospinal fluid and inserted into the spinal subarachnoid space. The catheter was positioned so that the inner tip reached the T8–T10 vertebral level. Adenosine (14 $\mu$mol/kg) decreased mean BP by $-17 \pm 3$ mm Hg and HR by $-58 \pm 16$ bpm (n = 4, Fig. 13.3). The hypotensive and bradycardic effects developed gradually with an onset of action between 1 and 2 min after the i.t. injection of adenosine and lasted for approximately 35 min. The adenosine analog, NECA (10 nmol/kg), exhibited more potent cardiovascular effects. Mean BP decreased by $-45 \pm 6$ mm Hg and HR by $-90 \pm 10$ bpm (n = 4, Fig. 3). The cardiovascular effects of i.t. NECA had an onset of action similar to adenosine but lasted for up to 3 hr. Administration of i.t. DPSPX (765 nmol) blocked the cardiovascular responses of similarly microinjected adenosine or NECA, thus indicating a specific adenosine-receptor stimulation.

Regional spinal differences in the response of adenosine may be present since a previous report by Sosnowski et al (1989) did not document significant cardiovascular changes by low doses of NECA at the level of the lumbar spinal cord in conscious animals. Although further characterization is needed (such as ruling out the possibility that the effects of i.t. administered purinergic substances are mediated in part by leaking of the substance to the peripheral circulation), our results suggest that spinal mechanisms of blood pressure control are also susceptible to purinergic modulation.

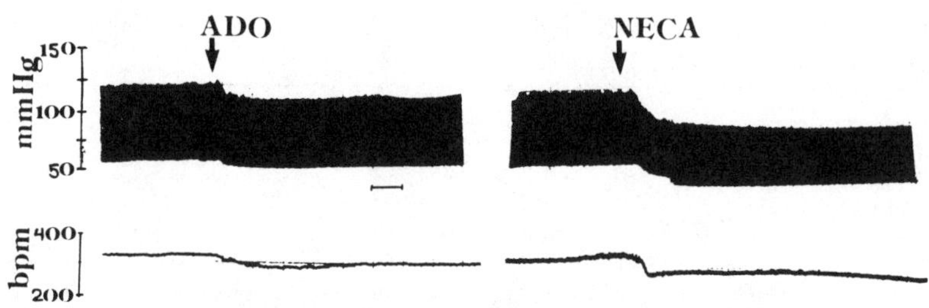


FIGURE 13.3. Cardiovascular effects of adenosine (ADO) or its analog, NECA, after i.t. administration in an anesthetized rat. ADO (14 $\mu$mol/kg) or NECA (10 nmol/kg) were microinjected through an intrathecal line in a total volume of 10 $\mu$l. Horizontal bar represents 2 min.

## Modulatory Effects of Adenosine on Baroreflex Activation

Neuronal cell groups located in the NTS regulate reflex cardiovascular activity (Palkovits, 1977). Afferent fibers that relay baroreceptor information make their first synapse within the NTS from which sympathetic and parasympathetic tone is regulated. The possibility that adenosine is involved in the regulation of baroreflex function was suggested by earlier studies in which infusion of low doses of adenosine evoked a hypotensive effect not followed by a compensatory reflex tachycardia (Von Borstel et al., 1983) and by the potent hypotensive and bradycardic effects of adenosine in the NTS (Tseng et al., 1988). With the use of adenosine antagonists, we have documented the effects of endogenous adenosine in the modulation of the baroreflex in anesthetized and conscious rats (Mosqueda-Garcia et al., 1989a).

Baroreflex activation was evaluated by the bradycardic response to pressor doses of phenylephrine. In urethane-anesthetized rats, administration of saline (60 nl) into the NTS did not modify the reflex bradycardia elicited by phenylephrine and, consequently, the slope of the baroreflex curve ($3.9 \pm 1$ and $4.0 \pm 0.9$ msec/mm Hg for control and saline, respectively, n = 4, Fig. 13.4). In contrast, after microinjection of the adenosine antagonist DPSPX (0.92 nmol), similar increases in BP elicited less bradycardia with a significant inhibition of the baroreflex slope (from $3.5 \pm 0.2$ to $0.8 \pm 0.4$ msec/mm Hg, n = 6, Fig. 13.4). Interestingly, basal BP and HR were not modified by DPSPX.

The effects of intracisternal (i.c.) administration of saline or caffeine on baroreflex sensitivity were studied in another group of anesthetized rats. Baroreflex sensitivity in the control period ($3.9 \pm 1.2$ msec/mm Hg, n = 5, Fig. 13.5) was not different from that in the saline group ($3.6 \pm 0.5$ msec/ mm Hg, n = 4, not shown). Caffeine i.c. did not change basal BP or HR,

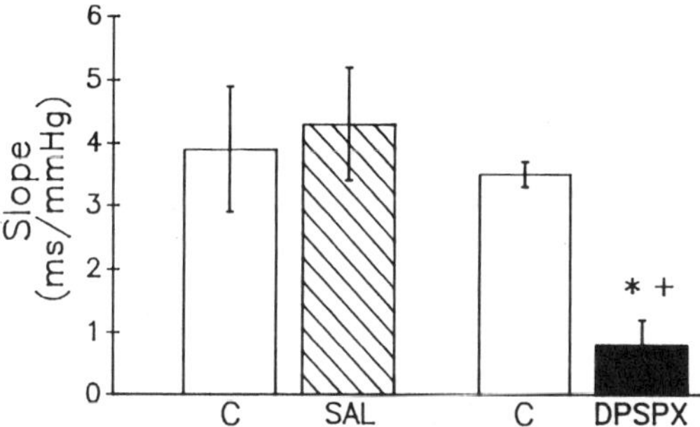

FIGURE 13.4. Effects of DPSPX on baroreflex sensitivity in anesthetized rats. Baroreflex sensitivity was evaluated before (c, open columns) and after 60 nl of intra-NTS saline (sal, hatched bar, n = 4) or 0.92 nmol intra-NTS DPSPX (solid bar, n = 6).

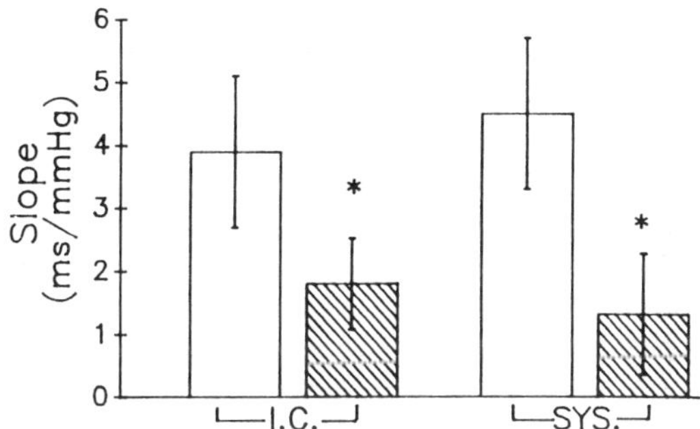

FIGURE 13.5. Effects of caffeine on baroreflex sensitivity in anesthetized rats. Baroreflex response was evaluated before (i.c., open column) and after the intracisternal administration of 6 $\mu$g/10 $\mu$l of caffeine (i.c., hatched bar) in 5 animals or after chronic administration of caffeine (0.1% in drinking water during 7 days; SYS, hatched bar, n = 6) or no treatment (SYS, open bar n = 4), in different groups of animals.

but when baroreflex activation was retested, a significant inhibition was observed (1.5 ± 0.8 msec/mm Hg, Fig. 13.5). In contrast, no significant change was recorded in the saline-treated rats (3.8 ± 0.7 msec/mm Hg).

In a group of rats chronically treated with caffeine (0.1% in drinking water), similar results were obtained. Although basal BP and HR values were not different from the group receiving placebo (control), the slope of the baroreflex curve was significantly less than in the control rats (Fig. 13.5).

Similar effects of ic. caffeine on baroreflex activation were observed in a group of conscious animals. Without caffeine, the pressor effects of phenylephrine were similar to those in anesthetized animals, but the reflex bradycardia was more pronounced and returned more quickly to basal levels. Consequently, the slope of the baroreflex curve was greater in conscious than in anesthetized animals. In contrast to saline, which did not significantly affect the baroreflex slope, the administration of caffeine inhibited the reflex bradycardia and decreased the baroreflex slope (Fig. 13.6). The effects lasted at least 30 min and had fully recovered after a 90-min period.

These results indicate that adenosine antagonists affect baroreflex activation both in couscious and anesthetized rats. The intra-NTS microinjection of DPSPX, a rather selective adenosine antagonist, or the i.c. or systemic administration of caffeine decreased the baroreflex slope, suggesting that endogenous adenosine has a facilitatory role on the baroreflex.

We have recently examined whether the effects of adenosine antagonists observed in animals are also present in humans (Mosqueda-Garcia, et al., 1990). In a group of young normotensive volunteers (21 ± 0.58 yr and caffeine free for 7 days), intraarterial BP and HR were continuously recorded and baroreflex responses were elicited by phenylephrine. Subjects received either 250 mg of caffeine (n = 6) or placebo p.o. (n = 4), and hemodynamic changes including baroreflex responses were obtained at 0, 30, 60, 120, and 180 min after drug administration. At 30 min after caffeine ingestion, BP rose from 127 ± 8/57 ± 4 mm Hg to 136 ± 3/68 ± 5 mm Hg (systolic/diastolic), HR was unchanged, and the baroreflex slope had decreased from 31 ± 7 msec/mm Hg to 11.6 ± 2 msec/mm Hg (Fig. 13.7). Baroreflex sensitivity remained inhibited for the rest of the study period despite BP returning to basal levels. In the placebo subjects. no significant changes were observed in BP, HR, or baroreflex slope. In contrast to the effects of acute caffeine administration in man and the chronic administration in rats,

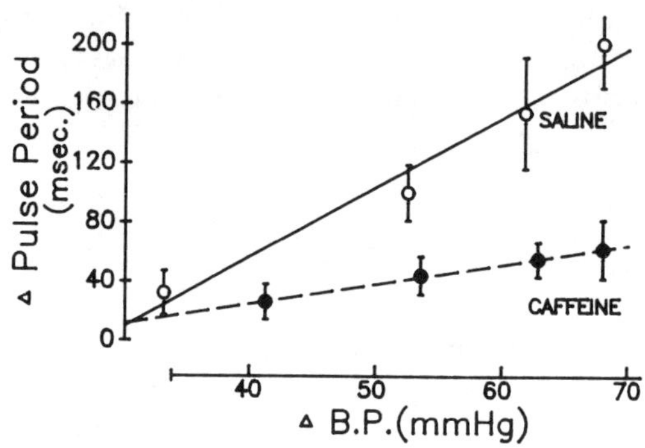


FIGURE 13.6. Inhibition of the baroreflex response to phenylephrine by i.c. administration of caffeine in conscious rats. The animals were pretreated with either saline (i.c., 10 μl, open circles with solid line), or caffeine (6 μg/10 μl, solid circles, dotted line). The lines were derived from linear regression analysis, which yielded slopes of 7.8 ± 2 and 4.3 ± 1.2 msec/mm Hg for saline and caffeine groups, respectively.

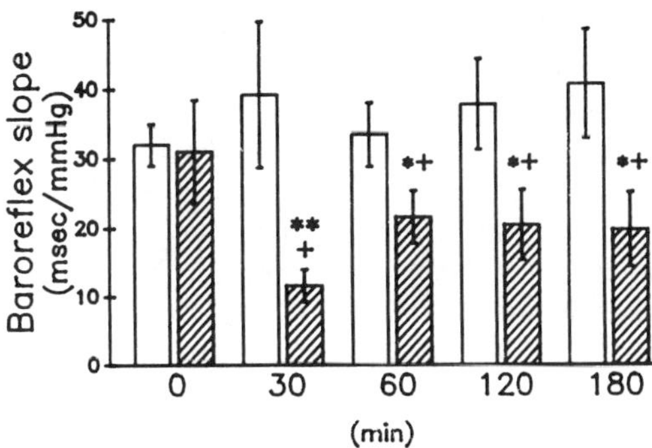



FIGURE 13.7. The effects of acute caffeine administration on baroreflex sensitivity in normotensive volunteers. Baroreflex response was evaluated before (0 min) and after 30, 60, 120, and 180 min of oral acute placebo (open bars, n = 4) or caffeine administration (250 mg, hatched bars, n = 6). Asterisks indicate significant difference from placebo groups (*$p<0.05$, **$p<0.01$) and + significant difference from own control ($p<0.005$).

no significant changes on baroreflex sensitivity were observed after chronic caffeine ingestion in the same group of volunteers. These results confirm that the effects of adenosine antagonists on baroreflex activation (previously observed in animals) are also present in man and suggest that adenosine has an important modulatory role on the reflex control of the circulation. On the other hand the development of tolerance to caffeine in man may explain the absence of effects by chronic caffeine administration on baroreflex function. This implies that the action of caffeine on relvant baroreceptor mechanisms are overcome (with time) by either central or peripheral changes that restore initial hemodynamic conditions. These adaptative mechanisms may be absent or inactive in some species (i.e., rats) in which chronic caffeine administration will maintain significant inhibition of baroreflex sensitivity.

## "Excitatory" Effects of Adenosine in the NTS

Electrophysiological experiments have demonstrated that local application of adenosine has a marked depressant action on the firing of neurons in several brain regions. Spontaneous neuronal cell firing in cerebral cortex, hippocampus, thalamus, cerebellum, and superior colliculus was inhibited by local iontophoretic application of adenosine and related purinergic compounds (Phillis et al., 1974). A receptor-mediated activation was suggested by the specific antagonistic effect of methylxanthines. Similarly, adenosine can depress excitatory synaptic transmission in cortical structures such as the olfactory cortex and the hippocampus (Dunwiddie and Proctor, 1987).

In addition, there have been reports that adenosine can antagonize transmission in inhibitory circuits (possibly GABAergic) (Schubert et al., 1983). Overall, the primary pharmacological influence of purines on the electrical activity of the brain is depressant rather than excitatory.

Adenosine also can depress the release of both excitatory and inhibitory neurotransmitters in the brain. For instance, the release, or in some cases the turnover rate, of different neurotransmitters (including acetylcholine, serotonin, norepinephrine, dopamine, GABA, and glutamate) (Dolphin and Archer, 1983; Fredholm et al., 1987; Phillis and Barraco, 1985) is reduced by adenosine. It remains unclear whether these effects on release are a general feature within the CNS or whether such actions are confined to the systems that have been characterized to date.

We are currently studying whether the cardiovascular effects of adenosine in the NTS may provide the first indication that regional variations in the inhibitory actions of this nucleoside are present in the CNS.

Activation of neuronal cells within the NTS, either by electrical stimulation or by microinjection of excitatory amino acids, results in decreased sympathetic tone, hypotension, and bradycardia (DeJong et al., 1975). On the other hand, inactivation of NTS function by ablation (Doba and Reis, 1973), microinjection of local anesthetics, antagonists of excitatory amino acids (Talman, 1989), or gamma-aminobutyric acid (GABA) agonists results in a sustained increased in BP (Kubo and Kihara, 1988). As mentioned before, within the CNS adenosine has actions opposite to those of excitatory substances, including L-glutamate. Therefore, it is striking that adenosine and L-glutamate have very similar actions in the NTS. First, both substances decrease BP, HR, and SNA when microinjected into the NTS (see Reis et al., 1981; Tseng et al., 1988). Second, both adenosine and L-glutamate antagonists inhibit baroreflex activity in this nucleus Mosqueda-Garcia et al., 1988b, 1989a; Reis et al., 1981). Although it has been proposed that L-glutamate might be the primary neurotransmitter of the first synapse of the baroreflex arc, our previous results indicate a facilitatory role of adenosine in baroreflex regulation. We now have speculated that adenosine and L-glutamate might interact in the reflex control of the circulation.

In preliminary experiments (Mosqueda-Garcia et al., 1988a, 1989b) we explored this hypothesis by testing whether a specific adenosine antagonist is able to inhibit the effects of L-glutamate in the NTS and conversely, if a glutamate antagonist is able to inhibit the effects of intra-NTS adenosine. In urethane anesthetized normotensive rats, we have found that while the intra-NTS administration of the adenosine antagonist DPSPX (0.92 nmol/60 nl) inhibited the cardiovascular effects of intra-NTS adenosine, it had no effect on L-glutamate actions. In contrast, kynurenic acid (KYN), a glutamate antagonist, inhibited in a dose-dependent manner the effects of both adenosine and L-glutamate (Table 13.3). These results suggest that the hemodynamic effects of adenosine may be mediated, at least partially, by an interaction with L-glutamate in the NTS.

TABLE 13.3. Effects of the antagonists DPSPX or kynurenic acid (KYN) on the cardiovascular actions of adenosine (ADO) or L-glutamate (L-Glu) in the NTS of anesthetized rats.

| | Control | | DPSPX | | Control | | KYN | |
| | MBP (mm Hg) | HR (bpm) | MBP (mm Hg) | HR (bpm) | BP (mm Hg) | HR (bpm) | MBP (mm Hg) | HR (bpm) |
|---|---|---|---|---|---|---|---|---|
| L-Glu | −31 ± 5 | −139 ± 11 | −28 ± 6 | −136 ± 14 | −28 ± 3 | −145 ± 19 | −10 ± 3[a] | −23 ± 3[b] |
| ADO | −25 ± 3 | −40 ± 13 | −2 ± 2[a] | −5 ± 8[a] | −24 ± 2 | −30 ± 3 | −7 ± 3[a] | −12 ± 5[a] |

ADO or L-Glu (2.3 nmol) were microinjected into the NTS before and after (10 min) similar microinjection of DPSPX (0.92 nmol) or KYN (33 nmol).
[a,b]Indicate significant difference at 0.5 and 0.1 levels, respectively.
n = 4 in each group.

In further experiments we have considered the following possibilities to explain the above observations:

1. Adenosine produces direct glutamate receptor activation. The possibility that adenosine has a nonspecific interaction with glutamate receptors has not been previously explored. Thus, the observed effects could be explained if adenosine bound to or otherwise interacted with glutamate receptors.
2. Adenosine enhances the release of glutamate. Activation of presumably presynaptic adenosine receptors located in the glutamatergic neuron could increase the release of this excitatory amino acid.
3. Adenosine decreases the release of an inhibitory neurotransmitter. As mentioned before, there is substantial evidence that adenosine inhibits the release of many neurotransmitters. Adenosine effects in the NTS could be explained by the inhibition of the release of an inhibitory substance that in turn inhibits glutamate release.

In preliminary studies (Mosqueda-Garcia et al., 1988b) we observed that in rat brain stem membranes that include the NTS, an analog of adenosine,

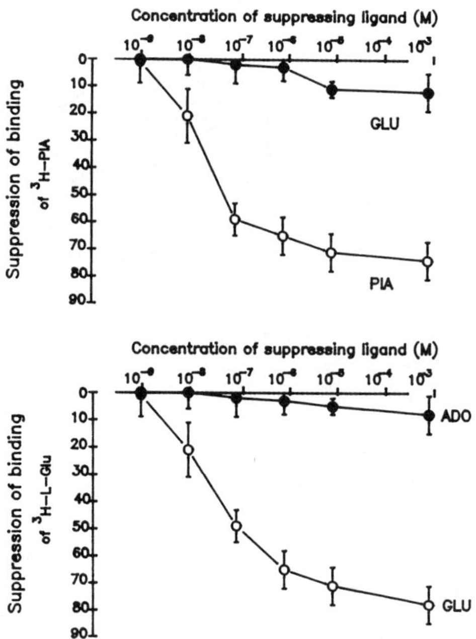


FIGURE 13.8. Interaction of adenosine and glutamate with adenosine and glutamate binding sites in brain stem membranes from normotensive Sprague-Dawley rats. Adenosine receptors were identified by $^3$H-PIA binding. Competition-displacement studies were done incubating the membranes with different concentrations of unlabeled L-glutamate or PIA. Glutamate receptors (*bottom*) were identified by $^3$H-L-glutamic acid, n = 6.

PIA, was not able to displace [3H]-L-glutamic acid. Similarly, "cold gluta-mate" was unable to displace [3H]-PIA from similar experimental prepara-tion (Fig 13.8). These results suggest that the interaction observed between adenosine and glutamate cannot be explained at the level of the receptor.

Alternatively, we have started to study the possibility that adenosine modulates glutamate levels in the NTS. We have used a microdialysis in vivo technique to address this question. Microdialysis is a relatively new bioanalytical method with which it is possible to sample a number of differ-ent extracellular fluid elements, including purines and excitatory amino acids. A microprobe cannula was implanted stereotaxically in the NTS of urethane-anesthetized rabbits. Artificial cerebrospinal fluid (CSF) was per-fused at a rate of 1 $\mu$l/min. After implantation of the probe, a stabilization period of at least 2.5 hr was necessary to obtain stable adenosine and gluta-mate levels. After this period, the NTS was perfused for 60 min with arti-ficial CSF containing no adenosine or an adenosine concentration of $10^{-3}$ M. Samples (60 $\mu$l) were analyzed for their glutamate content using a picotag Waters system for high pressure liquid chromatography (HPLC) analysis of free amino acids.

Using these techniques we have obtained preliminary results indicating that perfusion of adenosine through the dialysis probe increases glutamate levels. A period of 1 to 2 hr was needed to obtain steady levels of glutamate after placement of the microprobe in the NTS. Basal glutamate concentra-tion was 20.44 ± 3.7 $\mu$mol/L, with a relatively wide intersubject variation (range 8.6–28.35 $\mu$mol/L, n = 5). Perfusion of a solution of $10^{-3}$ M adeno-sine through the microdialysis probe increased glutamate levels to 127.4 ± 50 $\mu$mol/L (Fig. 13.9). Although a consistent increase in glutamate levels was observed in each animal with respect to its own basal levels,

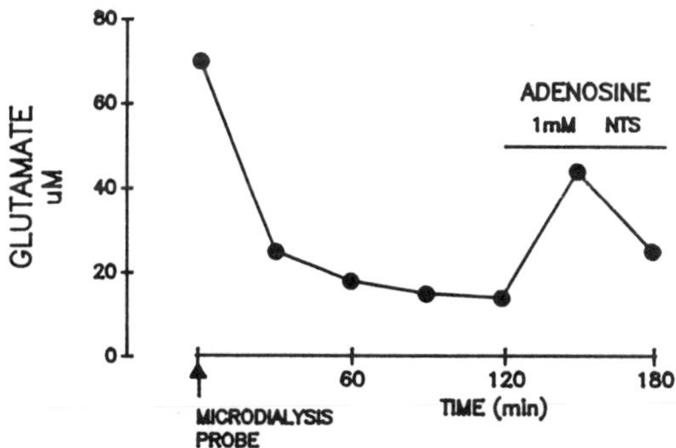


FIGURE 13.9. Effects of adenosine perfusion in the NTS on glutamate levels. A microdialysis probe was implanted into the NTS of an anesthetized rabbit. High levels of glutamate were observed after the microprobe implantation that decline and stabilize between 60 and 120 min. Infusion of $10^{-3}$ M of adenosine through the microprobe evoked an increase in glutamate levels.

considerable variation was observed across the experimental group. In the least responsive animal glutamate increased by 56% whereas in the most responsive the levels increased by 1036%. Overall, these results suggest that adenosine may exert part of its cardiovascular effects by either release of glutamate directly from the NTS or by acting through inhibition of an unidentified inhibitory substance on glutamate release.

## Conclusions

We and others have demonstrated that adenosine affects cardiovascular activity after administration in the brain stem of conscious and anesthetized rats. Potent hypotensive and bradycardic effects and a decrease in SNA have been shown by injection of adenosine into the lateral or fourth ventricle, into the cisterna magna, intrathecally, or directly into the NTS and AP of anesthetized rats.

Adenosine antagonists have proven to be important tools in elucidation of the physiological cardiovascular action of adenosine. The results with caffeine and related methylxanthines have indicated that endogenous adenosine has a facilitatory role on baroreflex activation in both humans and animals.

Finally, the "excitatory" effects of adenosine in the NTS are probably explained by an interaction with L-glutamate. Unlike most sites in the CNS, adenosine in the NTS seems to have a facilitatory role on glutamate release that has not been previously described in the central nervous system. This could explain how purinergic systems in this brain stem nucleus activate, rather than inhibit, cardiovascular neuronal activity.

*Acknowledgments.* This work was supported in part by grants from the National Institutes of Health, HL 34021 and International Life Sciences Institute. Rogelio Mosqueda-Garcia was a Fellow from the American Heart Association, Tennessee Affiliate. David Robertson is a Burroughs Wellcome Scholar in Clinical Pharmacology.

## References

Barraco RA, Janusz CJ (1988): Microinjections of isoproterenol into the nucleus tractus solitarius modulates respiration. *Med Sci Res* 16:977–979.

Barraco RA, Janusz CJ, Polasek PM, Parizon M, Roberts PA (1988): Cardiovascular effects of microinjection of adenosine into the nucleus tractus solitarius. *Brain Res Bull* 20:129–132.

Barraco RA, Phillis JW, Campbell WR, Marcantonio DR, Salah RS (1986): The effects of central injections of adenosine analogs on blood pressure and heart rate in the rat. *Neuropharmacology* 25:675–680.

Barraco RA, Polasek PM, Janusz CJ, Campbell WR, Schoener EP (1987): Parameters affecting microinjections of adenosine and its analogs on blood pressure and heart rate in the rat. *Gen Pharmacol* 18:405–416.

Bender AS, Wu PH, Phillis JW (1980): The characterization of [³H]-adenosine uptake into rat cerebral cortical synaptosomes. *J Neurochem* 35:629–640.

Bender AS, Wu PH, Phillis JW (1981): The rapid uptake and release of [³H]-adenosine uptake into rat cerebral cortical synaptosomes. *J Neurochem* 36:651–660.

Berne RM (1963): Cardiac nucleotides in hypoxia: possible role in regulation of coronary blood flow. *Am J Physiol* 204:317–322.

Bockman EL Berne RM, Rubio R (1975): Release of adenosine and lack of release of ATP from contracting skeletal muscle. *Pflueger's Arch* 355:229–241.

Braas KM, Newby AC, Wilson SV, Snyder SH (1986): Adenosine-containing neurons in the brain localized by immunocytochemistry. *J Neurosci* 6:1952–1961.

Deckert J, Bisserbe JC, Klein E, Marangos PJ (1957): Adenosine uptake sites in brain: Regional distribution of putative subtypes in relationship to adenosine A-1 receptors. *J Neurosci* 8:2338–2347.

DeJong W, Zandberg P, Bohus B (1975): Central inhibitory noradrenergic control. *Prog Brain Res* 42:285–298.

Doba N, Reis DJ (1973): Acute fulminating neurogenic hypertension produced by brainstem lesions in the rat. *Circ Res* 32:584–593.

Dolphin AC, Archer ER (1983): An adenosine agonist inhibits and a cyclic AMP analogue enhances the release of glutamate but not GABA from slices of rat dentate dyrus. *Neurosci Lett* 43:49–54.

Dunwiddie TV, Proctor WR (1987): Mechanisms underlying physiological responses to adenosine in the central nervous system. In: *Topics and Perspectives in Adenosine Research*, Gerlach E, Becker BF, eds. Berlin: Springer-Verlag, pp 499–508.

Fredholm BB, Duner-Engstrom M, Fastbom J, et al. (1987): Interactions between the neuromodulator adenosine and the classic transmitters. In: *Topics and Perspectives in Adenosine Research*, Gerlach E, Becker BF, eds. Berlin: Springer-Verlag, pp 509–520.

Galosy RA, Clarke LK, Vasko MR, Crawford IL (1981): Neurophysiology and neuropharmacology of cardiovascular regulation and stress. *Neurosci Biobehav Rev* 5:137–175.

Goodman RR, Snyder SH (1982): Autoradiographic localization of adenosine receptors in rat brain using [³H]-cyclohexyladenosine. *J Neurosci* 2:1230–1241.

Hedner T, Hedner J, Wessberg P, Jonasson T (1982): Regulation of breathing in the rat: Indications for a role of central adenosine mechanisms. *Neurosci Lett* 33:147–151.

Kubo T, Kihara M (1988): Evidence for γ-aminobutyric acid receptor-mediated modulation of the aortic baroreceptor reflex in the nucleus tractus solitarii of the rat. *Neurosci Lett* 89:156–160.

Marangos PJ, Patel J, Clark-Rosenberg R, Martino AM (1982): [³H]-nitrobenzylthionosine binding as a probe for the study of adenosine uptake sites in the brain. *J Neurochem* 39:184–191.

Mosqueda-Garcia R. Appalsamy M, Robertson D (1989b): Mechanisms of the central cardiovascular effects of adenosine: Interaction with brain L-glutamate. *Neuroscience* 15:1178.

Mosqueda-Garcia R, Tseng CJ, Appalsamy M, Robertson D (1988a): Adenosine and baroreflex control: effects in the nucleus of the solitary tract. *Clin Res* 36:430A.

Mosqueda-Garcia R, Tseng CJ, Appalsamy M, Robertson D (1989a): Modulatory effects of adenosine on baroreflex activation in the brainstem of normotensive rats. *Eur J Pharmacol* 174:119–122.

Mosqueda-Garcia R, Tseng CJ, Biaggioni I, Robertson RM, Robertson D (1990): Effects of caffeine on baroreflex activity in man. *Clin Pharmacol Ther* 48:568–574.

Mosqueda-Garcia R, Tseng CJ, Robertson D (1988b): Modulatory effects of adenosine on baroreflex activation in the nucleus of the solitary tract. *Pharmacologist* 12:198.

Nagy J, Labella LA, Buss M, Daddona PE (1984): Immunohistochemistry of adenosine deaminase: Implications for adenosine neurotransmission. *Science* 224:166–168.

Palkovits M, Zaborszky L (1977): Neuroanatomy of central cardiovascular control. Nucleus tractus solitarii: Afferent and efferent neuronal connections in relation to the baroreceptor reflex arc. *Prog Brain Res* 47:9–34.

Phillis JW, Barraco RA (1985): Adenosine, adenylate cyclase and transmitter release. *Adv Cyclic Nucleotide Protein Phosphorylation Res* 19:243–257.

Phillis JW, Kostopoulou GW, Limacher JJ (1974): Depression of corticospinal cells by various purines and pyrimidimes. *Can J Physiol Pharmacol* 52:1226–1229.

Phillis JW, Walter GA, O'Regan MH, Stair RE (1987): Increases in cerebral cortical perfusate adenosine and inosine concentrations during hypoxia and ischemia. *J Cerebral Blood Flow Metab* 7:679–686.

Reis DJ, Granata AR, Perrone MH, Talman W (1981): Evidence that glutamic acid is the neurotransmitter of baroreceptor afferents terminating in the nucleus tractus solitarius (NTS). *J Auton Nerv Syst* 3:321–334.

Rubio R, Berne RM, Bockman EL, Curnish RR (1975): Relationship between adenosine concentration and oxygen supply in rat brain. *Am J Physiol* 228:1896–1902.

Simpson L, Barraco RA, Phillis JW (1989): A central role for adenosine in the hypotension elicited by hypoxia in anesthetized rats. *Brain Res Bull* 23:37–40.

Sosnowski M, Stevens CW, Yaksh TL (1989): Assessment of the role of $A_1/A_2$ adenosine receptors mediating the purine antinociception, motor, and autonomic function in the rat spinal cord. *J Pharmacol Exp Ther* 250:915–922.

Talman WT (1989): Kynurenic acid microinjected into the nucleus tractus solitarius of rats blocks the arterial baroreflex but not responses to glutamate. *Neurosci Lett* 102:247–252.

Tseng CJ, Biaggioni I, Appalsamy M, Robertson D (1988): Purinergic receptors in the brainstem mediate hypotension and bradycardia. *Hypertension* 11:191–197.

Van Calker P, Muller M, Hamprecht B (1979): Adenosine regulates via two different types of receptors the accumulation of cAMP in cultured brain cells. *J Neurochem* 33:999–1005.

Von Borstel RW, Wurtman RJ, Conlay LA (1983): Chronic caffeine consumption potentiates the hypotensive action of circulating adenosine. *Life Sci* 32:11151–1158.

# Section III
## Control of Sympathetic Tone, Hypertensive Mechanisms

# 14
# Spinal Mechanisms in the Sympathetic Control of Cardiac Function

HREDAY SAPRU

It is well established that sympathetic preganglionic neurons (SPNs) represent the final neuronal pool in the central nervous system (CNS) through which cardiovascular function is regulated. Although SPNs are located primarily in the intermediolateral column (IML) of the thoracolumbar spinal cord, other areas in the spinal cord (central autonomic area and the intercalated nucleus) also have been implicated in this function (Barman, 1984; McCall, 1988). These conclusions are based on electrophysiological (Dembowsky et al., 1985, 1986; Gebber and McCall, 1976) and anatomical (Gilbey et al., 1982; Henry and Calaresu, 1972a) studies. In the electrophysiological studies, SPNs have been identified by antidromic activation following stimulation of corresponding sympathetic nerves. In the anatomical studies, the identification of SPNs was based on retrograde transport of horseradish peroxidase or Fluorogold along the axons in corresponding sympathetic nerves (Strack et al., 1988). In these procedures, it is not possible to identify axons with *specific cardiovascular function* in the sympathetic nerves. Focal electrical stimulation has also been used to identify sympathoexcitatory sites functionally in the spinal cord (Faden and Jacobs, 1980; Henry and Calaresu, 1972b). However, electrical stimulation activates neuronal cell bodies as well as fibers of passage. We have recently used the newly developed L-glutamate microinjection technique to identify neuronal pools regulating cardiac function in the IML (Sundaram et al., 1989b). Glutamate stimulates neuronal cell bodies but not fibers of passage (Fries and Zieglgansberger, 1974). Using this technique it is possible to avoid activation of ascending, descending, and intraspinal fibers of passage that are present in the spinal cord (Barman, 1984; McCall, 1988). We have investigated the effects of various putative transmitters on the cardiac function in this model and have attempted to identify the excitatory transmitter released in the IML in response to the stimulation of the ventrolateral medullary pressor area. This chapter summarizes this information.

## Materials and Methods

### General Procedures

Male Wistar rats (Charles River Farms, MA) weighing 300 to 350 gm were used. Most of the experiments were done in the rats anesthetized with pentobarbital sodium (45–50 mg/kg, i.p.). The trachea was cannulated with a polyethylene tubing (PE-240) and the rats were ventilated artificially using a rodent respirator (Harvard Apparatus, South Natick, MA; model 680). The rats were immobilized with d-tubocurarine (0.2–0.3 mg/kg, i.v.) after the depth of anesthesia was tested. Both femoral arteries were cannulated with a polyethylene tubing (PE-50); one for monitoring pulsatile blood pressure (BP) via a pressure transducer (Statham P23 Db) and the other for withdrawing samples (100 $\mu$l) for measuring blood gases (using IL 1304 blood gas analyzer). The blood gases were maintained at normal levels (PaO$_2$: 88–100 mm Hg, PaCO$_2$: 33–44 mm Hg; pH: 7.30–7.40) by adjusting the tidal volume and respiratory rate on the respirator. The heart rate (HR) was monitored by a tachograph (Grass 7P4) that was triggered by blood pressure waves. One of the femoral veins was cannulated for intravenous (i.v.) administration of various agents. Rectal temperature was monitored by a digital thermometer (Physitemp Instruments, Clifton, NJ; model BAT-8) and maintained at $37 \pm 0.5°C$. The rate of increase in the left ventricular pressure (dP/dt) and contractility index (Lokhandwala et al., 1985) were used as indices of ventricular contractile state. For monitoring maximum ventricular dP/dt, a premeasured catheter (PE 50) was introduced into the right common carotid artery and advanced until it reached the left ventricle. The left ventricular pressure signal was differentiated using a Grass 7P20C differentiator. The isovolumic pressure (IP) in the left ventricle is defined as the pressure at maximum dP/dt minus the left ventricular end-diastolic pressure. The index of contractility was computed as maximum dP/dt/IP. All the tracings were recorded on a polygraph (Grass 7D).

### Identification of the Spinal Autonomic Nuclei

The rat was placed in the prone position and its head fixed in a stereotaxic instrument to which a rat-spinal unit was attached (David Kopf Instruments, model 980). The fifth cervical and eighth thoracic vertebrae and the pelvic bones were fixed rigidly in the spinal unit. Each level of the upper thoracic cord investigated ($T_1$–$T_3$) was identified using $T_2$ vertebra, which has a long spinous process, as a landmark. The dorsal surface of the spinal cord, from $C_7$ to $T_5$ level, was exposed by laminectomy and irrigated by warm (37°C) paraffin oil to prevent it from drying. The coordinates for the midline of the spinal cord were noted. Microinjections of L-glutamate [1.77 nmol in 20 nl of artificial cerebrospinal fluid (CSF) or 0.9% sodium chloride solution, pH 7.4] were used to explore the location of the neurons eliciting positive chronotropic and inotropic effects. Details of this procedure are described elsewhere (Sundaram et al., 1989b,c; Murugaian et al., 1990).

## Microinjection Technique

Single or double barreled glass micropipettes (Frederick Haer & Co, ME) with a tip diameter of approximately 20 to 40 $\mu$m were filled with solutions. The micropipettes were mounted on a micromanipulator and connected via a PE-20 tubing to a 1-$\mu$l microsyringe (Hamilton) mounted on a computerized assembly for microinjections (Buxco Instruments, Sharon, CT, model STC-100). Microinjections (20-nl volume) were delivered in a 5-sec interval. The volume of microinjection, indicated by the displacement of the syringe plunger in the graduated microsyringe, was visually confirmed under an operation microscope. Injections of artificial CSF or the vehicle used for preparing different drugs (see section on "Chemical Agents") into the IML served as controls.

## Histology

After the spinal autonomic nuclei were identified by microinjections of L-glutamate, 20 nl of India ink was microinjected into the site via an adjacent barrel of the micropipette. The spinal cord was frozen *in situ* by a spray of Histo-Freeze (Fisher Scientific Co., Springfield, NJ), removed, and frozen again in liquid nitrogen. Sections were cut (30 $\mu$m) in a cryostat (Hacker Instruments, Caldwel, NJ; Model OTF/AS/MR), mounted, and stained with cresyl violet Histological verification of the site of injection was made using a standard atlas (Paxinos and Watson, 1986).

## Statistical Analyses

Paired *t* test was used when animals served as their own controls and an independent *t* test was used for testing the significance of differences between mean values from different groups of rats. Differences between various means were determined by analysis of variance followed by Duncan's multiple range test. Differences were considered significant at $p < 0.05$. All values were expressed as mean $\pm$ standard error of the mean (SEM).

## Chemical Agents

### Excitatory Amino Acids

L-glutamate monosodium, N-methyl-D-aspartic acid (NMDA), D-2-amino-phosphonoheptanoic acid (D-AP7; specific antagonist of NMDA receptor), quisqualic acid (QA), AMPA (alpha-amino-3-hydroxy-5-methyl-4-isoxazole-propionic acid), kainic acid (KA), glutamic acid diethylester (GDEE), and kynurenic acid were used. GDEE and kynurenic acid are nonselective antagonists for excitatory amino acid receptors. (Collingrdige et al., 1989).

## Cholinergic Agents

Acetylcholine, AFDX-116 (a specific antagonist for $M_2$ muscarinic receptors), carbachol, cis-methyldioxolane (CD; a specific agonist for $M_2$ muscarinic receptors, McN-A343 (a specific agonist for $M_1$ muscarinic receptors), pirenzepine (PZ; a specific antagonist for $M_1$ muscarinic receptors), and scopolamine hydrochloride were used (see Sundaram et al., 1988a,b, 1989a for references).

## Adrenergic Agents

Idazoxan HCl (an alpha-2 adrenergic receptor antagonist), L-norepinephrine bitartrate, and prazosin HCI (an alpha-l adrenergic receptor antagonist) were used.

## Other Agents

Chlorisondamine salicylate (a ganglion blocker), d-tubocurarine chloride (neuromuscular blocker), and dimethyl-phenyl-piperizinium iodide (DMPP; a ganglion stimulant) were used.

## Sources of the Agents Used

The sources of the agents used were as follows: L-glutamate, DMPP, carbachol, acetylcholine; scopolamine, norepinephrine, prazosin and d-tubocurarine chloride (Sigma Chemicals, St. Louis, MO, USA); idazoxan (Reckitt and Colman, Kingston, UK); AFDX-116 and PZ (Boehringer Ingelheim, Ridgefield CT, USA); quisqualic acid, kainic acid, kynurenic acid, and McN-A343 (Research Biochemicals Inc, Natick, MA, USA).

AFDX-116 was dissolved in 0.05N HCI. Ascorbic acid (0.03% solution) was added as an antioxidant in the norepinephrine solutions. Controls for these agents consisted of vehicles containing ascorbic acid. Prazosin was dissolved in dimethylsulfoxide (DMSO) and then diluted in artificial CSF; the percentage of DMSO in the final solution was 1%. Control injections for prazosin consisted of artificial CSF containing 1% of DMSO. All other agents were dissolved in either 0.9% sodium chloride solution or artificial CSF. The pH of all solutions was adjusted to 7.4. The doses of agents microinjected into the IML refer to the salts.

# Results

## *Functional Asymmetry Between the Left and Right Spinal Cord*

On the right side, the microinjections (20 nl) of L-glutamate (1.77 nmol) into the IML at the $T_2$ level elicited an increase in HR that was much greater than that elicited from the left IML. On the left side at the $T_2$ level, microinjections of the same doses of glutamate into the IML evoked an increase in contractility that was much greater than that elicited from the right IML (Sundaram et al., 1989b). No changes in BP were elicited from the IML on either side (Fig. 14.1). The stereotaxic coordinates for the IML on either side were 0.6 to 0.7 lateral to the midline and 0.7 to 0.9 deep from the dorsal surface of the spinal cord. The bar graphs presented in Figure 14.1 are based on the maximum response (i.e., maximum increase in contractility elicited from the left IML and maximum increase in HR elicited from the right IML) derived from eight animals. At the $T_2$ level, the increase in contractility index from the baseline value was $60 \pm 6\%$ when glutamate was microinjected into the left IML. In the right IML at the same level, microinjections of the same dose of glutamate produced only $13.9 \pm 1.2\%$ increase in contractility index. The reverse was true for positive chronotopic effects of glutamate; on the right side at the $T_2$ level, the increase in HR induced by glutamate was $23.2 \pm 1.2\%$ whereas on the left side increase in HR was $8 \pm 0.4\%$. Maximum increase in the contractility was reached within 50 to 80 sec and the effect lasted for 6 to 8 min. The maximum increase in contractility index ($60 \pm 6\%$) was significantly greater ($p<0.05$) than the maximum increase in HR ($23.2 \pm 1.2\%$). Microinjections of L-glutamate into the IML at the $T_1$ and $T_3$ levels produced relatively small responses. For example, microinjections of glutamate into the $T_1$ (n = 7) and $T_3$ (n = 6) levels produced $42 \pm 2\%$ and $45 \pm 1.2\%$ increase in contractility index, respectively. The sites from which maximal responses were elicited were located in the middle of each segment. At $C_8$ and $T_4$ levels no positive inotropic responses could be obtained even when higher doses (4.5 nmol) of glutamate were microinjected. Microinjections of the vehicle (0.9% sodium chloride solution, pH 7.4) did not evoke a response. Control mean arterial pressure (MAP) and heart rate (HR) in these rats were $101 \pm 4.1$ mm Hg and $322 \pm 16$ beats/min (bpm), respectively.

The positive chronotropic effect (elicited predominantly from the right IML; n = 6) and the positive inotropic effect (elicited primarily from the left IML; n = 5) evoked by microinjections of glutamate were mediated via the sympathetic nervous system because pretreatment of the rats by a ganglion blocker (chlorisondamine, 3 mg/kg, i.v.) blocked these effects. The ganglion blockade was confirmed by the lack of response to a ganglion

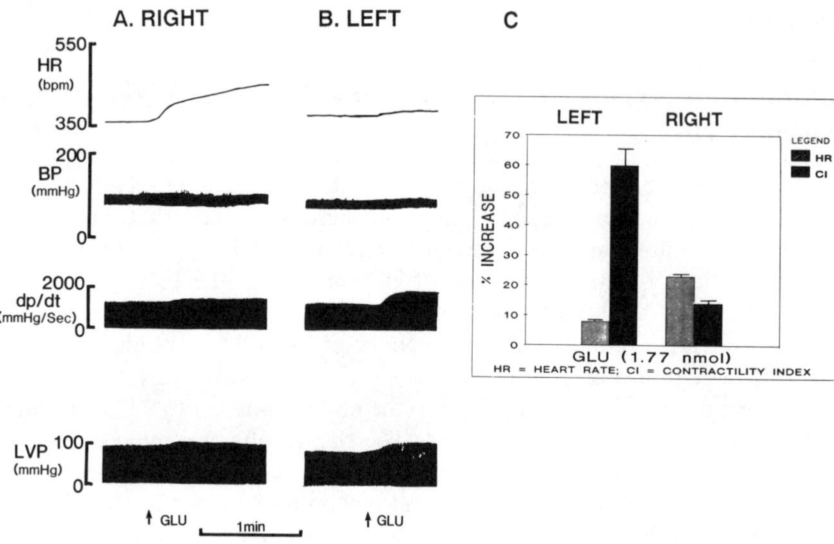



FIGURE 14.1. Asymmetric responses to microinjections of L-glutamate into the right and left IML at the $T_2$ level. In each panel showing polygraph tracings: top trace = heart rate (bpm), second trace = femoral BP (mm Hg), third trace = maximum rate of contraction of the ventricle (dP/dt, mm Hg/sec), and bottom trace = left ventricular pressure (mm Hg). Computation of the contractility index is described in methods. **A**: Microinjection (20 nl) of glutamate (1.77 nmol, arrow) into the right IML produced a predominant increase in HR with a small increase in the left ventricular dP/dt or pressure and no change in BP. **B**: Microinjection (20 nl) of glutamate (1.77 nmol, arrow) into the left IML produced a predominant increase in the left ventricular dP/dt and pressure with a small increase in HR and no change in BP. **C**: Maximum percent increase (compared with the corresponding baseline values) in HR (hatched bars) and contractility index (dark bars) in response to 1.77 nmol of glutamate microinjected into the left and right IML was computed. The contractility index on the left was significantly greater ($p<0.01$) compared to that on the right. The tachycardic effect on the right was significantly greater ($p<0.01$) compared to that on the left. The maximum increase in the contractility index was greater ($p<0.05$) than the maximum increase in HR. (Reproduced with permission from Sundaram et al., 1989b.)

stimulant [dimethyl-phenyl-piperizinium (DMPP) 200 $\mu$g/kg, i.v.]. Chlorisondamine caused a fall in BP that was restored to control levels by i.v. infusions of phenylephrine (10 $\mu$g/min). Intravenous injections of the L-glutamate (0.9–1.77 nmol) did not evoke any response. Bilateral adrenalectomy (n = 5) did not alter the positive chronotropic or inotropic effect induced by microinjections of glutamate on the right or left side, respectively. Spinal transections at $C_2$ (n = 5) or $T_6$ levels (n = 6) did not alter the effects of microinjections of glutamate into the IML. BP was restored to control levels by i.v. infusions of phenylephrine (10 $\mu$g/min) in spinal transected animals.

## *Relative Importance of Different Autonomic Nuclei*

Cytoarchitectonic study of cell groups in the mammalian spinal cord have led to the identification of the following nuclei: nucleus (n.) intermediolateralis thoracolumbalis pars principalis (ILp), the classical lateral horn; n. intermediolateralis thoracolumbalis pars funicularis (ILf), the extension of ILp into the lateral funiculus; n. intercalatus spinalis (IC), the medial extension from the ILp to the central canal zone; and n. intercalatus pars paraependymalis (ICpe), which is generally known as the central autonomic area (CA) (Laskey and Polosa, 1988). The relative contribution of the above-mentioned spinal autonomic nuclei in regulating cardiovascular function was studied by microinjections of L-glutamate (Murugaian et al., 1990). The stereotaxic coordinates for different cell groups in each segment $(T_1-T_4)$ were as follows. The IML (including the ILp and ILf) was located 0.6 to 0.7 mm lateral to the midline and 0.7 to 0.9 mm deep from the dorsal surface of the spinal cord, the IC 0.2 to 0.3 mm lateral to the midline and 1 to 1.1 mm deep, and the CA was at the midline and 1.2 to 1.3 mm deep. The increase in HR and contractility obtained by microinjections of L-glutamate into the right IC and CA at the $T_2$ level was significantly smaller when compared to the responses elicited from the right and left IML in the same segment (Murugaian et al., 1990).

## Putative Transmitters

### *Acetylcholine*

At the $T_2$ level, microinjections of acetylcholine (0.1 nmol) into the right IML produced a marked tachycardic response (Fig. 14.2B). The increase in HR from the base-line was $46 \pm 1.9$, $68 \pm 3.4$ and $29 \pm 1.9$ bpm for 0.01, 0.1, and 1 nmol, respectively (n = 12; Fig. 14.2C). The onset of action was 20 to 30 sec. The duration of action was 4 to 5 min for 0.01 nmol and 6 to 8 min for 0.1 and 1 nmol. Maximum tachycardic response was obtained at the dose of 0.1 nmol. The response at the higher dose of 1 nmol was significantly ($p<0.05$) smaller than that for 0.1 nmol. Although a small increase (5–10 mm Hg) in MAP was observed in a small percentage (5–8%) of animals, in most cases no changes in BP were observed at any of the doses of acetylcholine. Injections of the vehicle (0.9% sodium chloride solution or artificial CSF, pH 7.4) did not evoke a response. Control MAP and HR in these rats were $102 \pm 4$ mm Hg and $338 \pm 32$ bpm, respectively. The specificity of these effects was tested as follows (n = 7). The site eliciting maximum positive chronotropic response ($52 \pm 9$ bpm) was identified by microinjections of glutamate (Fig. 14.2D). Atropine hemisulfate (0.2 nmol) was microinjected at the same site; no significant change in HR was observed (Fig. 14.2E). Fifteen min later, microinjections of acetylcholine (0.1 nmol) at the same site failed to produce the usual increase in HR (Fig.

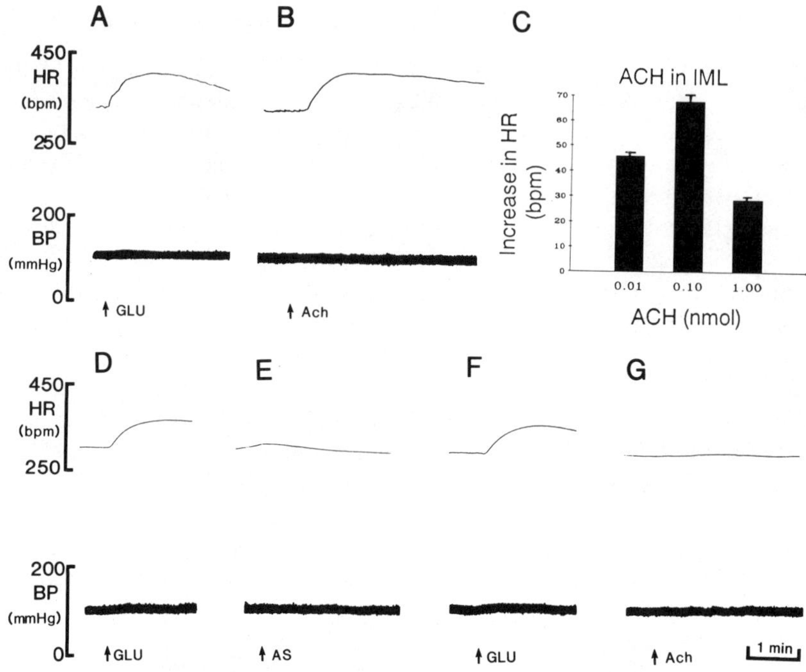



FIGURE 14.2.  Effect of microinjections of acetylcholine into the right IML at the $T_2$ level. In each panel showing polygraph tracings: top trace = heart rate (bpm) and bottom trace = femoral BP (mm Hg). **A**: Microinjection of L-glutamate (1.77 nmol in 20 nl 0.9% sodium chloride solution, pH 7.4) into the right IML produced an increase in HR. Microinjection of 20 nl of 0.9% sodium chloride solution (pH 7.4) produced no response (not shown). **B**: Microinjection of acetylcholine (0.1 nmol) at the same site produced increase in HR. **C**: Tachycardic responses to different doses (0.01–1 nmol) of acetylcholine. **D**: Control tachycardic response to 1.77 nmol of glutamate microinjected into the right IML. **E**: Atropine hemisulfate (0.2 nmol) was microinjected into the same site; no significant change in HR was observed. **F**: Atropine did not alter the effects of glutamate but **G**: it did block the effect of acetylcholinc. (Reproduced with permission from Sundaram et al., 1989c).

14.2G) whereas the positive chronotropic responses to glutamate persisted (Fig. 14.2F). Microinjections of carbachol (a stable analog of acetylcholine; 440 pmol) into the IML elicited responses similar to those of acetylcholine (Sundaram et al., 1989c).

The role of $M_1$ and $M_2$ muscarinic receptors in the IML was investigated by using specific agonists and antagonists for these receptors. Microinjection of cis-methyldioxolane (CD; a specific $M_2$ receptor agonist; 0.8 nmol) into the right IML at the $T_2$ level elicited a dose-dependent (0.2–0.8 nmol; n = 16) tachycardia. Prior microinjections of an $M_2$ receptor antagonist (AFDX-116; 0.8 nmol), but not those of an $M_1$ receptor antagonist (PZ; 2

nmol), prevented the positive chronotropic action of CD. The responses to glutamate, tested 5 min prior to the injection of CD, were not altered by AFDX-116. McN-A343 ($M_1$ agonist) and PZ ($M_1$ antagonist) elicited no response when microinjected into the IML.

## *Norepinephrine*

The effects of microinjections of norepinephrine (NE) into the IML depended on the dose administered. For describing these effects conveniently, the doses of NE were divided into small and large dose ranges. The small dose range consisted of 1, 1.5, and 2 pmol; these doses were contained in 20-nl volumes of 50, 75, and 100 micromolar ($\mu$M) solutions. The large dose range consisted of 0.05, 0.5, 0.8, and 1 nmol; these doses were contained in 20-nl volumes of 2.5, 25, 40, and 50 millimolar (mM) solutions.

Tachycardia induced by small dose range of NE

Relatively small doses of NE ( 1, 1.5, and 2 pmol/20 nl) produced an increase in HR when microinjected into the right IML at the $T_2$ level. Figure 14.3 shows the dose-response relationship for microinjections of NE into the IML at the T2 level. For each dose of NE, n = 5; only one dose was injected in one animal. The maximum increase in HR from the baseline, obtained 4 to 6 min after the microinjection of NE, was $26.7 \pm 1.05$, $36.7 \pm 1.7$, and $23.8 \pm 2.4$ bpm for 1, 1.5, and 2 pmol, respectively. The duration of action was 10 to 15 min for 1 and 2 pmol and 20 to 30 min for 1.5 pmol. Maximum tachycardic response was obtained at the dose of 1.5 pmol. The response to 2 pmol was significantly ($p<0.05$) smaller than that for 1.5 pmol. No changes in BP were observed at any of the doses of NE. Injections of the vehicle (artificial CSF, containing 0.5% ascorbic acid, pH adjusted to 7.4) did not evoke a response. Control MAP and HR in these rats were $96 \pm 8$ mm Hg and $360 \pm 28$ bpm, respectively.

The specificity of the tachycardic effects of NE was tested as follows (n = 10). The site eliciting maximum positive chronotropic response ($54 \pm 8$ bpm) was identified by microinjections of glutamate (1.77 nmol). Prazosin (an alpha-1 adrenergic receptor blocker; 50 pmol) was microinjected at the same site; no change in HR was observed. Five min later, microinjections of NE (1.5 pmol) at the same site failed to produce the increase in HR whereas the positive chronotropic responses to glutamate persisted. In two rats, direct activation of alpha-1 adrenergic receptors by microinjections of phenylephrine (0.1 pmol) elicited tachycardia (35–40 bpm). Microinjections of an alpha-2 adrenergic receptor blocker (idazoxan, 10 pmol) into the IML produced an increase in HR ($43 \pm 3.4$ bpm; n = 5). The onset of the tachycardic effect of idazoxan was 30 to 90 sec and the duration 10 to 15 min. Idazoxan did not block the tachycardic effect

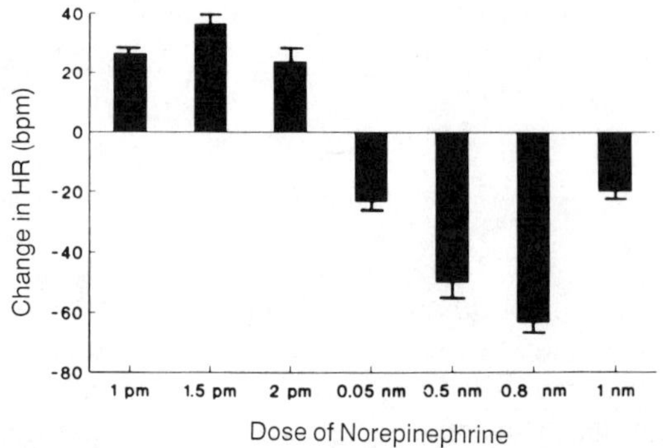


FIGURE 14.3. Dose response of microinjections of norepinephrine into the IML at the $T_2$ level. Norepinephrine was microinjected in different doses in the IML at the $T_2$ level. For each dose n = 5. Only one dose of NE was injected in each animal. Each bar represents mean ± SEM. At lower doses (1, 1.5, and 2 pmol) norepinephrine *increased* HR; maximum increase was observed at 1.5 pmol. These doses represented 20-nl volumes of 50, 75, and 100 $\mu$M solutions of NE. At the higher doses (0.05, 0.5, 0.8, and 1 nmol), a *decrease* in HR was observed. These doses of NE represented 20-nl volumes of 2.5, 25, 40, and 50 mM solutions of NE. Maximum decrease was observed at 0.8 nmol. At 1 nmol, the decrease in HR was less than that induced by 0.8 nmol ($p<0.05$). (Reproduced with permission from Sundaram et al., 1991a).

of NE (1.5 pmol) or L-glutamate (1.77 nmol). These effects of NE were mediated via the sympathetic nervous system because chlorisondamine (3 mg/kg) blocked them.

Bradycardia induced by large dose range of NE

Relatively large doses of NE (0.05, 0.5, 0.8, and 1 nmol/20 nl) produced a dose-dependent decrease in HR when microinjected into the right IML at the T2 level. The decrease in HR from the baseline was 23.3 ± 1.7, 50 ± 2.2, 63.3 ± 1.7, and 20 ± 2.2 bpm for 0.05, 0.5, 0.8, and 1 nmol, respectively. The onset of action was 30 to 90 sec. The duration of action was 20 to 30 min for 0.8 and 1 nmol and 10 to 15 min for 0.05 and 0.5 nmol (Fig. 14.3). Maximum bradycardic response was obtained at the dose of 0.8 nmol; the increase in HR in response to microinjections of L-glutamate (1.77 nmol) was 53 ± 2.5 and 52 ± 3 bpm, before and after the microinjection of NE (0.8 nmol) at the same site. The response to 1 nmole was significantly ($p<0.05$) smaller than that for 0.8 nmol. No changes in BP were observed at any of the doses of NE.

Microinjections of idazoxan (10 pmol) into the IML blocked the bradycardic effect of the subsequent injections of NE (0.8 nmol). Activation of alpha-2 adrenergic receptors by microinjections of clonidine (0.8 nmol) elicited bradycardia (50–60 bpm; n = 2). Microinjections of prazosin (50 pmol) into the IML failed to alter the bradycardic effects of subsequent injections of NE (0.8 nmole).

## Excitatory Amino Acids

### Effect of Quisqualate

Microinjections of quisqualic acid (QA) into the right IML elicited tachycardia. The increase in HR was dose-dependent (doses used were 0.1, 1, 10, and 100 pmol). For each dose of QA, the number of animals was five; only one dose was injected in one animal. The maximum increase in HR from the baseline, obtained 25 to 35 sec after the microinjection of QA, was $28.8 \pm 2.4$, $72.5 \pm 3.2$, $51.2 \pm 1.2$ and $45 \pm 2.9$ bpm for 0.1, 1, 10, and 100 pmol, respectively. The duration of action was 3 to 8 min. Maximum tachycardic response was obtained at the dose of 1 pmol. The response to 10 pmol was significantly ($p<0.05$) smaller than that for 1 pmol. No changes in BP were observed at any of the doses of QA. Microinjections of kynurenate (2 nmol), but not D-AP7 (5 nmol), blocked the actions of QA ($n = 4$). At the dose used, kynurenate (2 nmol) and D-AP7 (5 nmol) did not alter the response to carbachol (0.44 nmol), indicating that they did not exert a local anesthetic-like effect.

### Effect of AMPA

Microinjections of $\alpha$-amino-3-hydroxy-5-methyl-4-isoxazole-propionic acid (AMPA) into the right IML elicited a dose-dependent tachycardia (doses of AMPA used were 0.1, 1, and 10 pmol). Five rats were used for each dose of AMPA and only one dose was injected in one animal. The maximum increase in HR from the baseline, obtained 25 to 35 sec after the microinjection of AMPA, was $46.3 \pm 2.4$, $77.5 \pm 3.2$, and $98.8 \pm 4.3$ bpm for 0.1, 1, and 10 pmol, respectively. The duration of action was 3 to 9 min. No changes in BP were observed at any of the doses of AMPA. Kynurenate (2 nmol) blocked the effects of AMPA whereas D-AP7 (5 nmol) was ineffective.

### Effect of Kainate

Microinjections of kainic acid (KA) into the right IML elicited tachycardia. The maximum increase in HR induced by KA was $31.2 \pm 3.1$, $86.3 \pm 6.3$, and $43.8 \pm 3.8$ bpm for 1, 3, and 10 pmol, respectively. The onset and duration of action were 30 to 40 sec and 3 to 9 min, respectively. Kynurenate (2 nmol) blocked the action of KA whereas D-AP7 (5 nmol) did not alter this response.

### Effect of NMDA

Microinjections of NMDA (100 pmol) into the right IML at the $T_2$ level elicited an increase in HR with no change in BP (Fig. 14.4A). Maximum tachycardic responses were $29 \pm 1.87$, $54 \pm 1.87$, and $78 \pm 1.22$ bpm for 1, 10, and 100 pmol, respectively. The tachycardic effect reached a peak within 40 to 60 sec. The duration of this effect was 4 to 8 min. The effects of NMDA (100 pmol) were tested before (Fig. 14.4C) and after (Fig. 14.4E) microinjections of kynurenate (2 nmol; Fig. 14.4D). Kynurenate blocked the effects of NMDA but not those of carbachol (0.44 nmol; Fig. 14.4F).

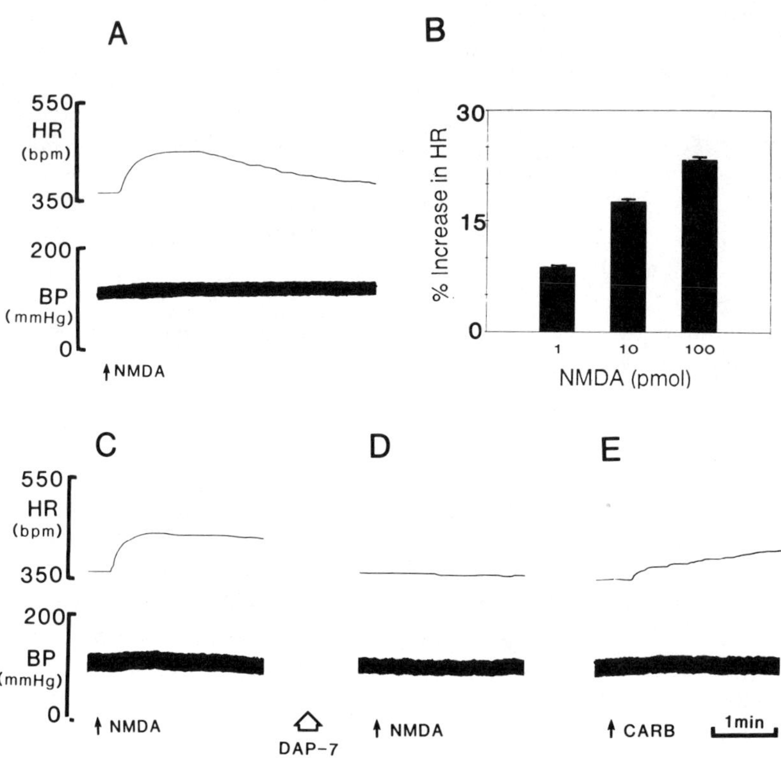


FIGURE 14.4. Effect of microinjections of NMDA (100 pmol in 20 nl of 0.9% sodium chloride solution, pH 7.4) into the right IML at the $T_2$ level. In each panel showing polygraph tracings: top trace = heart rate (bpm) and bottom trace = femoral BP (mm Hg). A: Microinjection of NMDA (arrow) into the right IML produced an increase in HR. Microinjection of 20 nl of 0.9% sodium chloride solution (pH 7.4) produced no response (not shown). B: The tachycardic response was dose (1–100 pmol)-dependent. C: Control tachycardic response to 100 pmol of NMDA microinjected into the right IML. D-AP7 (5 nmol) was microinjected into the same site (large arrow between panels C and D). No response was elicited by D-AP7 (tracings not shown). D: D-AP7 blocked the responses to subsequent microinjections of NMDA (100 pmol). E: D-AP7 did not block the effects of carbachol (0.44 nmol), which was microinjected at the same site within 4 min of the injection of NMDA. (Reproduced with permission from Sundaram et al., 1989b.)

The specificity of the effects of NMDA was further ascertained by testing the tachycardic responses to the microinjections of NMDA (100 pmol) before and after microinjections of D-AP7 (5 nmol) at the same site (n = 7). D-AP7 blocked the action of NMDA (100 pmol) completely but it failed to alter the responses to microinjections of QA (1 pmol), AMPA (10 pmol), or KA (3 pmol); in these experiments the doses of the excitatory amino acids that produced maximum responses were used.

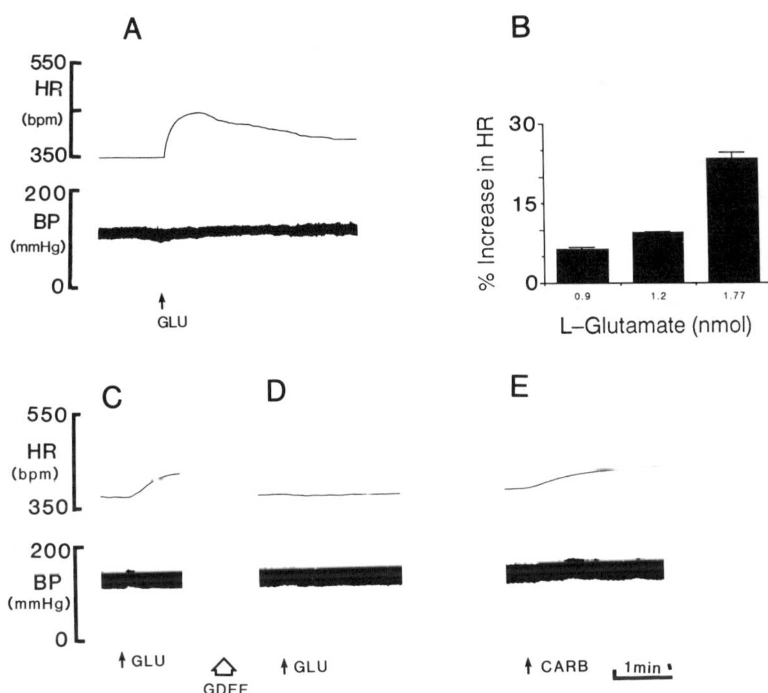


FIGURE 14.5. Effect of microinjections of L-glutamate monosodium (1.77 nmol in 20 nl of 0.9% sodium chloride solution, pH 7.4) into the right IML at the $T_2$ level. In each panel showing polygraph tracings: top trace = heart rate (bpm) and bottom trace = femoral BP (mm Hg). **A:** Microinjection of L-glutamate (arrow) into the right IML produced an increase in HR. Microinjection of 20 nl of 0.9% sodium chloride solution (pH 7.4) produced no response (not shown). **B:** The tachycardic response was dose (0.9–1.77 nmol)-dependent. **C:** Control tachycardic response to 1.77 nmol of glutamate microinjected into the right IML. GDEE (0.08 $\mu$mol) was microinjected into the same site (large arrow between panels C and D). No response was elicited by GDEE (tracings not shown). **D:** GDEE blocked the responses to subsequent microinjections of glutamate (1.77 nmol). **E:** GDEE did not block the effects of carbachol (0.44 nmol), which was microinjected at the same site within 4 min of the injection of glutamate. (Reproduced with permission from Sundaram et al., 1989b.)

Effect of L-Glutamate

Microinjections of L-glutamate (1.77 nmol) into the right IML at $T_2$ level elicited an increase in HR (Fig. 14.5A). Dose-response relationships presented in Fig. 14.5B are based on the maximum tachycardic response elicited from one site in the $T_2$ segment of each rat (n = 8). The increase in HR from the baseline was $19 \pm 1.87$, $27 \pm 1.22$, and $63.12 \pm 4.42$ bpm for 0.9, 1.2, and 1.77 nmol of L-glutamate, respectively. The onset and duration of the tachycardic effect were 40 to 90 sec and 6 to 8 min, respectively.

The specificity of these effects was ascertained by testing the tachycardic responses to the microinjections of glutamate (1.77 nmol) before (Fig. 14.5C) and after (Fig. 14.5D) microinjections of GDEE at the same site (n = 7). In these experiments, GDEE (0.08 $\mu$mol) blocked the action of glutamate completely whereas the responses to microinjections of carbachol (0.44 nmol) at the same site remained unaltered (Fig. 14.5E); the increase in HR induced by carbachol was $56 \pm 3$ bpm before and $53 \pm 3$ bpm after the microinjections of GDEE, respectively. Microinjections of GDEE did not elicit any reponse. Smaller doses of GDEE were ineffective in blocking the responses of glutamate. In another series of experiments (n = 16), kynurenate (2–20 nmol) failed to block the actions of glutamate in the IML.

## *Neurotransmitter Released in the IML at $T_1$–$T_3$ Following the Stimulation of the Ventrolateral Medullary Pressor Area*

The importance of the ventrolateral medullary pressor area (VLPA) in the maintenance of vasomotor tone and reflex regulation of BP has recently been described (Calaresu and Yardley, 1988; Guyenet et al., 1987; Ross et al., 1984; willette et al., 1983). Extracellular recordings *in vivo* and intracellular recordings *in vitro* have shown that the neurons in the VLPA exhibit pacemaker-like activity (Sun et al., 1988a,b) suggesting that the VLPA may be one of the important sources of vasomotor tone. Barman and Gebber (1987) have identified an excitatory input from the lateral tegmental field neurons to the VLPA and have suggested that sympathoexcitatory neurons in the VLPA are driven by this antecedent input. The VLPA includes the $C_1$ adrenergic neurons (Ross et al., 1984). However, the role of $C_1$ neurons in cardiovascular regulation is not yet conclusively established. Anatomic and electrophysiological evidence shows that the neurons (especially $C_1$ neurons) in the VLPA send direct projections to the IML (Ross et al., 1984). Although many neurotransmitters have been implicated in the spinal cord (Laskey and Polosa, 1988; McCall, 1988), conclusive evidence to support the role of any of them in cardiovascular regulation is lacking.

We have recently studied the role of excitatory amino acids as transmitters in the IML at $T_2$ level using microinjection technique. In one group of rats (n = 5), the VLPA was identified by microinjections of L-glutamate using a dorsal approach (Urbanski and Sapru, 1988a,b). Microinjections of glutamate (1.77 nmol) in the left VLPA produced an increase in MAP ($43.75 \pm 4.2$ mmHg) and left ventricular contractility; the contractility index (CI) was increased from the base-line value of $38.3 \pm 1$ to $46.5 \pm 2.76$. In order to avoid the effects of BP changes (induced by chemical stimulation of the VLPA) on CI, the spinal cord was transected at $T_4$; the baseline value for CI ($38.3 \pm 1$; bar 1 in Fig. 14.6A) did change significantly while the MAP decreased to $55 \pm 10$ mmHg. After a stabilization period of 1 hour, the left VLPA was again stimulated by microinjections of glutamate; the increase in the contractility was not significantly ($P > 0.05$) altered; the CI was $47.4 \pm 1.95$ (bar 2 in Fig. 14.6A compared to the value of $46.5 \pm 2.76$ before the spinal transection). The pressor response was significantly ($P < 0.05$) reduced ($7.5 \pm 3.2$ compared to the value of $43.75 \pm 4.2$ mmHg before transection). In the same animals, the IML was bilaterally identified at $T_1$–$T_3$ by injections of L-glutamate (1.77 nmol). Microinjections of 20 nl volumes of 0.9% sodium chloride solution bilaterally into the IML at $T_1$–$T_3$ did not elicit a response. Microinjection of glutamate into the left VLPA 10 min after the microinjections of saline into the IML at $T_1$–$T_3$ increased the CI to $45.5 \pm 2$; this value was not significantly different ($P > 0.05$) from the CI observed before the saline injections into the IML ($47.4 \pm 1.95$) (bar 3 in Fig. 14.6A). Forty-five min later, DAP-7 (5 nmol/20 nl of 0.9% saline) was microinjected into the IML at $T_1$–$T_3$ bilaterally, a significant ($P < 0.05$) reduction in base-line CI (to a value of $30 \pm 1.2$) was observed. Within 5 min, L-glutamate was again microinjected into the left VLPA. No increase in the CI was observed; the CI ($30.25 \pm 1.3$) was not significantly different ($P > 0.05$) from the base-line value of $30 \pm 1.2$ (bar 4 in Fig. 14.6A).

In another group of rats (n = 5), the same procedure was followed except that kynurenate was microinjected into the IML instead of DAP-7. The spinal cord was transected at $T_4$. After a stabilization period of 1 hour, the left VLPA was stimulated by microinjections of glutamate; the CI was significantly ($P < 0.05$) increased ($45.9 \pm 2.5$ compared to the base-line value of $37.5 \pm 1.89$) (first two bars in Fig. 14.6B). In the same animals, the IML was bilaterally identified at $T_1$–$T_3$ by injections of L-glutamate (1.77 nmol). Microinjections of 20 nl volumes of 0.9% sodium chloride solution bilaterally into the IML at $T_1$–$T_3$ did not elicit a response. The CI was increased to $45.2 \pm 2.5$ by the microinjection of glutamate into the left VLPA 10 min after the microinjections of saline into the IML; this value was not significantly ($P > 0.05$) different from that observed before the saline injections in the IML (bar 3 in Fig. 14.6B). Forty-five min later, kynurenate (2 nmol/20 nl of 0.9% saline) was microinjected into the IML at $T_1$–$T_3$ bilaterally; a significant ($P < 0.05$) reduction in CI to a value of $28 \pm 1$ was observed. Within 5 min, L-glutamate was again microinjected

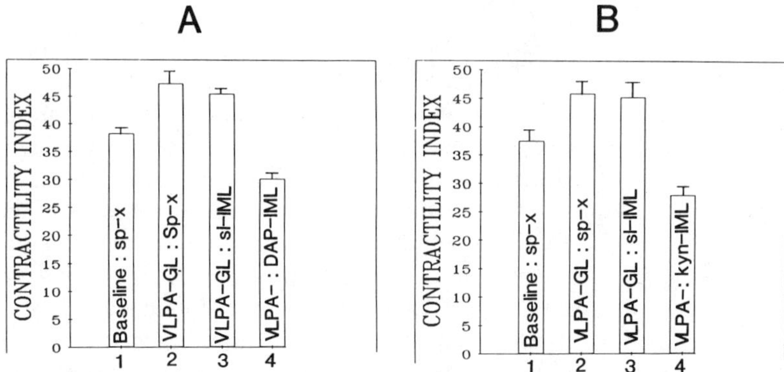



FIGURE 14.6. Changes in contractility index (CI) induced by the stimulation of VLPA. **A**: Bar 1: Base-line CI after spinal transection ($38.3 \pm 1$). Bar 2: Microinjections of L-glutamate (1.77 nmol) into the VLPA significantly ($P < 0.05$) increased the CI to a value of $47.4 \pm 1.95$. Bilateral microinjections of 0.9% sodium chloride solution at $T_1$–$T_3$ did not alter the base-line CI (not shown). Bar 3: stimulation of VLPA by glutamate microinjections increased the CI to a value of $45.5 \pm 2$; this value was not significantly ($P > 0.05$) different from the value in bar 2 ($47.4 \pm 1.95$). Forty-five min later, DAP-7 (5 nmol) was microinjected bilaterally at $T_1$–$T_3$; the base-line CI was decreased to a value of $30 \pm 1.2$ (not shown). Bar 4: Five min later, glutamate was again microinjected into the VLPA; the usual increase in CI was not observed (compare bars 3 and 4). **B**: Bar 1: Base-line CI after spinal transection ($37.5 \pm 1.89$). Bar 2: Microinjections of L-glutamate (1.77 nmol) into the VLPA significantly ($P < 0.05$) increased CI to a value of $45.9 \pm 2.5$. Bilateral microinjections of 0.9% sodium chloride solution at $T_1$–$T_3$ did not alter base-line CI (not shown). Bar 3: stimulation of the VLPA by glutamate microinjections increased the CI to $45.2 \pm 2.5$ which was not significantly ($P > 0.05$) different from the value in bar 2 ($45.9 \pm 2.5$). Forty-five min later, kynurenate (2 nmol) was microinjected bilaterally at $T_1$–$T_3$; the base-line CI was reduced to $28 \pm 1$ (not shown). Bar 4: Five min later, glutamate was again microinjected into the VLPA; the usual increase in CI was not observed (compare bars 3 and 4). Abbreviations: GL = L-glutamate; Sp-x = spinal transection at $T_4$; sl = 0.9% saline; kyn = kynurenate. (Reproduced with permission from Sundaram et al., 1991b).

into the left VLPA; the CI ($28 \pm 1.6$ did not change significantly ($P > 0.05$) from the base-line value of $28 \pm 1$ indicating that kynurenate had blocked the glutamate-induced increase in left ventricular CI (bar 4 in Fig. 14.6B). In separate experiments, microinjections of kynurenate were shown to be devoid of any local anesthetic action because responses to carbachol remained unaltered. Control injections of 20 nl volumes of saline injected in a manner identical to kynurenate microinjections failed to block the responses to glutamate-induced stimulation of the VLPA. Moreover, the responses to the stimulation of the VLPA recovered within 60 min indicating that the IML neurons were intact.

# Discussion

## *Spinal Neuronal Pools Regulating Cardiac function*

In this study, we used the newly developed L-glutamate microinjection technique to identify neuronal pools regulating cardiac function in the IML. Neuronal pools mediating positive chronotropic and inotropic effects were found to be located between $T_1$ to $T_3$ spinal segments. The responses obtained at $T_2$ were greater than those obtained at $T_1$ and $T_3$ levels. Neither the increase in HR nor the increase in contractility could be elicited from segments rostral to $T_1$ or caudal to $T_3$. These results are in agreement with recent anatomic studies in which Fluorogold was injected into the stellate ganglion of the rat and the highest percentage of labeled cells was observed in the IML at the $T_2$ level (Strack et al., 1988). In the rostrocaudal direction, at each of these levels ($T_1$–$T_3$) maximal responses were elicited at the middle of the segment. This is perhaps because SPNs are distributed in clusters in each segment like beads on a string (Laskey and Polosa, 1988). A functional asymmetry was observed in the cardiac responses evoked from the right and left sides of the spinal cord. Microinjections of glutamate into the right side between the $T_1$ and $T_3$ spinal segments produced predominantly tachycardia whereas similar injections into the corresponding sites on the left evoked predominantly an increase in contractility. These observations are in agreement with the reports (Yasunaga and Nosaka, 1979) in which stimulation of the right stellate ganglion of the rat was reported to produce a much greater tachycardic reponse compared to similar stimulation on the left. This asymmetry has been ascribed to the pattern of sympathetic innervation of the heart; the right sympathetic trunk may innervate predominantly the sinoatrial node whereas the left provides innervation to the ventricular muscle (Randall et al., 1963).

Some of the differences between our results and those of others (Faden and Jacobs, 1980; Henry and Calaresu, 1972b) may be because of the electrical stimulation of ascending, descending, or intraspinal pathways. For example, tachycardic responses were elicited from $T_1$ to $L_4$ spinal segments whereas in our studies these responses were restricted to $T_1$ to $T_3$ segments. Inotropic responses have been reported to show right- sided preponderance (Faden and Jacobs, 1980) whereas in our studies increase in cardiac contractility was evoked from the left IML at the $T_1$ to $T_3$ levels. Concomitant pressor responses have been reported by other investigators (Faden and Jacobs, 1980; Henry and Calaresu, 1972b) whereas we observed little or no changes in BP. The lack of BP responses to microinjections of glutamate in our studies may be explained as follows: the vasoconstrictor neurons may be distributed over the entire segment of the IML ($T_1$–$L_4$); activation of only a small percentage of these neurons by microinjections of glutamate into the IML at the $T_1$ to $T_3$ level may be insufficient to elicit a BP response.

Stimulation of the sympathetic preganglionic neurons in the $T_1$ to $T_3$ segments induced positive chronotropic and inotropic effects via the sympathetic nervous system because i.v. injections of chlorisondamine (a ganglion blocker) prevented these responses. Bilateral adrenalectomy did not alter the aforementioned cardiac responses, suggesting that sympathoexcitatory effects were not exerted on this organ even though it receives a minimal (less than 1%) innervation from the above-mentioned sympathetic preganglionic neurons.

Several ascending and descending spinal pathways can influence the function of the sympathetic preganglionic neurons in the IML (Barman, 1984; McCall, 1988). In our study, transections of the spinal cord at levels rostral to $T_1$ and caudal to $T_3$ did not alter the cardiac responses to the microinjections of glutamate excluding the possibility that the aforementioned ascending or descending pathways may have mediated the observed responses. Changes in BP can influence the sympathetic preganglionic neuronal activity via a spinal reflex. Microinjections of glutamate did not induce BP changes. However, BP did fall after spinal transections. In these experiments BP was maintained at control levels by i.v. infusions of phenylephrine.

Sympathetic interneurons have been identified in the vicinity of the IML (Barman, 1984; Gebber and McCall, 1976; McCall, 1988). The possibility that these interneurons were also excited by the microinjections of glutamate and thus contributed to the observed responses cannot be excluded in this study.

It is generally believed that in the thoracolumbar cord different autonomic nuclei [n. intermediolateralis thoracolumbalis pars principalis (ILp), n. intermediolateralis thoracolumbalis pars funicularis (ILf), n. intercalatus spinalis (IC), and the central autonomic area] are involved in regulating sympathoexcitatory functions. The ILf is an extension of ILp into the lateral funiculus (Laskey and Polosa, 1988). Microinjections of even small volumes (10 nl) into the ILp are likely to spread to the ILf. For this reason, responses evoked in this region were described under the general heading "IML." Maximum glutamate-induced responses were elicited from IML; the responses from IC and CA were minimal. These results are generally in agreement with a recent anatomic report (Strack et al., 1988) in which Fluorogold was injected into the inferior cervical (stellate) ganglion.

## Putative Transmitters

### *Acetylcholine*

The presence of muscarinic receptors and neurons that stain for acetylcholine esterase and choline acetyltransferase has been reported in the IML of the rat (see Sundaram et al., 1989c for references). Carbachol (a stable acetylcholine analogue that is not a subtype-selective muscarinic agonist) produced an increase in HR (predominantly on the right side at the $T_2$ level) and contractility (predominantly in the left IML at the $T_2$ level). Since scopolamine blocked these effects, muscarinic receptors must be mediating these responses. Chlorisondamine (a ganglion blocker) prevented the responses of carbachol, indicating that the sympathetic nervous system was involved in these actions. The effect of acetylcholine, the natural transmitter, was similar to that of carbachol except that its action was of shorter duration. At a higher dose (1 nmol/site), the tachycardic responses to acetylcholine were significantly smaller ($p<0.05$) than those observed at a lower dose (0.1 nmol/site). This may be due to the well-known depolarization blockade property of cholinergic agonists.

Although genes encoding four muscarinic acetylcholine receptor subtypes have been isolated (Peralta et al., 1987b), selective agonists and antagonists are available for only two muscarinic receptor subtypes ($M_1$ and $M_2$) (Sundaram et al., 1988a,b, 1989a). Cloning studies have revealed that $M_1$ and $M_2$ receptors represent distinct gene products and have different amino acid sequences (Kubo et al., 1986; Peralta et al., 1987a). At the present time, pirenzepine and McN-A343 are considered the best antagonist and agonist for $M_1$ receptors, respectively. AFDX-116 and CD are the best antagonist and agonist for $M_2$ receptors, respectively (Sundaram et al., 1988a,b, 1989a).

In our study, microinjections of an $M_1$ receptor agonist (McN-A343) failed to evoke a response whereas similar injections of an $M_2$ receptor agonist (CD) evoked cardioacceleratory effects. The specificity of these muscarinic receptor-mediated responses was confirmed by preventing the effects of microinjections of CD into the IML by microinjections of AFDX-116 at the same sites; microinjections of AFDX-116, but not those of PZ, blocked the effects of CD. We have previously reported that microinjections of AFDX-116 (0.8 nmol/site) initially render neurons unresponsive to L-glutamate. However, the responses recover to control levels within 15 to 20 min (Sundaram et al., 1988a,b, 1989a). In this investigation, the muscarinic receptor blocking properties of AFDX-116 were tested only when the responses to glutamate had recovered. At this time, AFDX-116 completely blocked the responses to CD and this effect lasted for 2 hr, suggesting that the muscarinic receptor blocking properties of AFDX-116 outlast its initial depressive effect on neurons. Scopolamine (18 nmol) also produces attenuation of glutamate-induced responses, which lasts for 15 to 20 min. The muscarinic receptor blocking property of scopolamine, as indicated by the lack of responses to carbachol, was tested when the responses to glutamate had recovered.

These results show that muscarinic receptors of $M_2$ subtype are present in the segments of IML that control cardiac function. Activation of muscarinic receptors in the IML at the $T_1$ to $T_3$ level produces increase in the rate and contractility of the heart. Based on the techniques used in our study, it was not possible to ascertain if these receptors are located on the pregang-lionic sympathetic neurons, interneurons, or nerve terminals. Intracellular studies on preganglionic neurons, done in spinal cord slices, show that acetylcholine depolarizes these cells (Laskey and Polosa, 1988). These observations prompt speculations that acetylcholine may be a neurotrans-mitter, subserving sympathoexcitatory function, in as yet unidentified pathways projecting to the IML.

## Norepinephrine

The IML is known to receive a dense noradrenergic innervation from differ-ent supraspinal structures (Coote et al., 1981; Laskey and Polosa, 1988; McCall, 1988). Biochemical and autoradiographic studies have demon-strated the presence of high concentrations of NE (Fleetwood-Walker and Coote, 1981; Zivin et al., 1975) and alpha-2 adrenergic receptors in the IML (Seybold and Elde, 1984), respectively. These reports have prompted suggestions that NE may serve as a neurotransmitter or neuromodulator in the IML (Laskey and Polosa, 1988; McCall, 1988).

In our study (Sundaram et al., 1991), NE in small dose range (1–2 pmol contained in 20-nl volumes of 50–100 $\mu$M solutions) produced an increase in HR. These effects were mediated via alpha-1 adrenergic receptors be-cause prazosin blocked them. At the dose used (50 pmol), prazosin did not exert a nonspecific depression of neurons because the responses to gluta-mate remained unaltered. The tachycardic responses observed in our study can be explained by the electrophysiological changes induced by NE in the SPNs. For example, other investigators have reported depolarization accompanied with repetitive discharge in a population of SPNs when slices of rat spinal cord were superfused *in vitro* with NE solutions (Ma and Dun, 1985; Yoshimura et al., 1987a,b). The highest concentration of the NE solutions (50 $\mu$M) used in the aforementioned *in vitro* studies is within the range of NE concentrations that produced tachycardic responses in our study. Chlorisondamine (a ganglion blocker) prevented the excitatory effects of NE (1.5 pmol), indicating that the sympathetic nervous system was involved in these actions. The existence of a tonic excitatory norad-renergic input to the neurons in the IML is unlikely because microinjec-tions of prazosin alone did not alter HR. Intrathecal injections of NE have also been reported to elicit sympathoexcitatory responses (Shi et al., 1988).

Sympathoexcitatory effects of NE observed in the aforementioned re-ports (Ma and Dun, 1985; Shi et al., 1988; Yoshimura et al., 1987a,b) and this study seem to disagree with microiontophoretic studies in which ap-plication of NE produced inhibition of SPNs (Coote et al., 1981; Guyenet and Cabot, 1981; Guyenet and Stornetta, 1982; Kadzielwala, 1983). This discrepancy may be explained by the concentrations of NE solutions used in different studies. In the present study, 50 to 100 $\mu$M solutions of NE produced tachycardia whereas higher concentrations (2.5–50 mM) produced bradycardia (see next paragraph). It is possible that in the aforementioned microiontophoretic studies high concentrations of NE were ejected; herefore, only inhibitory effects on the neurons were observed. It may be argued that, in the concentration range of 2 mM to 3 M, the amount of drug released by iontophoretic current is essentially independent of solution concentration (Stone, 1985). However, it has been suggested that electrically induced release of ionized substances from micropipettes must involve both iontophoresis and electro-osmosis (Stone, 1985). Because of the latter process, the amount of drug ejected from the micropipette will show clear dependence on concentration of the drug used (Stone, 1985). In addition, ejection by microiontophoresis of an ion that carries a hydration shell will cause movement of drug molecules dissolved in water (Stone, 1985). Keeping these factors in view, it is possible that in the iontophoretic studies mentioned earlier (Coote et al., 1981; Guyenet and Cabot, 1981; Guyenet and Stornetta, 1982; Kadzielwala, 1983), ejection of a high concentration of NE accompanied microiontophoresis.

In the present study (sundaram et al., 1991), larger doses of NE (0.05–1 nmol contained in 20 nl volumes of 2.5–50 mM solutions) produced a decrease in HR when microinjected into the IML. These effects were blocked by idazoxan (alpha-2 adrenergic antagonist) but not prazosin (alpha-1 adrenergic agonist). This observation agrees with the results of direct microiontophoretic application of NE on SPNs (Coote et al. 1981; Guyenet and Cabot, 1981; Guyenet and Stornetta, 1982; Kadzielwala, 1983). Other investigators have shown that superfusion of NE produces inhibition of SPNs, characterized by hyperpolarization and slow inhibitory pustsynaptic potentials (IPSPs), in *in vitro* slices of the spinal cord (Yoshimura and Nishi, 1982; Yoshimura et al., 1987b).

In the doses used, NE, prazosin, or idazoxan did not exert membrane-stabilizing effects since the responses to subsequent microinjections of glutamate remained unaltered.

The slow onset of action of NE (30–90 sec) agrees with the slow time course of NE-induced depolarization or inhibition of SPNs observed in *in vitro* studies (Ma and Dun, 1985; Yoshimura et al., 1986, 1987a,b,c).

In summary, increase as well as decrease in HR can be elicited by microinjections of NE into the IML. The excitatory and inhibitory effects are mediated by alpha-1 and alpha-2 adrenergic receptors, respectively. These observations are in agreement with studies in which NE was administered intrathecally; intrathecal injection of adrenergic receptor agonists elicits inhibitory (Kubo et al., 1987; Sangdee and Franz, 1983; Shi et al., 1988) as well as excitatory (Shi et al., 1988) effects on the sympathetic nervous system. Similar results have been reported in *in vitro* electrophysiological studies on the SPNs (Ma and Dun, 1985; Yoshimura et al., 1986, 1987a,b,c). In these studies, the inhibitory and excitatory effects elicited in response to superfusion of NE solutions have been elicited from the same neurons, suggesting that the alpha-1 and alpha-2 adrenergic receptors may be located on the same neuron (Yoshimura et al., 1987b). Alternatively, alpha-1 and alpha-2 adrenergic receptors may be located on different populations of SPNs or interneurons, which have been identified in the spinal cord. SPNs that control HR seem to be under *tonic inhibitory* influence, which involves alpha-2 adrenergic receptors because idazoxan elicited an increase in HR when microinjected into the IML. Direct activation of alpha-2 adrenergic receptors by microinjections of clonidine elicited bradycardia. Prazosin did not alter HR when injected into the IML, suggesting that alpha-1 adrenergic receptors are not under a tonic control. However, direct activation of alpha-1 adrenergic receptors by microinjection of phenylephrine produced tachycardia. The neuronal pathways that use NE as a transmitter for these functions remain to be identified.

## Excitatory Amino Acids

Several subtypes of excitatory amino acids have been identified. Included in these are NMDA, quisqualate/AMPA, and kainate receptors (Collingridge and Lester, 1989). A specific antagonist (D-AP7) is available only for NMDA receptors. Kynurenate blocks all three amino acid receptors and is therefore a nonselective antagonist. Kynurenate in the dose of 2 to 5 nmol blocked the responses to NMDA (100 pmol), quisqualate (I pmol), AMPA (1 pmol), and kainate (3 pmol). These doses of excitatory amino acids produced maximum increase in HR when injected into the IML. At the doses used, kynurenate did not produce any nonspecific effect because responses to carbachol remained unaltered. Microinjection of kynurenate alone produced a fall in HR or dP/dt, indicating that a tonic excitatory input involving an amino acid may be involved in the IML at the $T_2$ level.

Kynurenate did not block the effects of microinjections of glutamate into the IML. The reason for this action is not clear. It is possible that glutamate may activate interneurons in the IML and release other excitatory transmitters, the actions of which are not susceptible to blockade by kynurenate. GDEE did block the effects of glutamate injections into the IML. At the dose used, GDEE did not block the action of carbachol, thus ruling out the possibility that GDEE might be blocking glutamate-induced release of a muscarinic receptor agonist (e.g., acetylcholine). However, blockade of other excitatory agents such as serotonin by GDEE cannot be ruled out.

## Transmitter Released in the IML Following the Stimulation of the VLPA

Stimulation of VLPA neurons by microinjections of L-glutamate induced an increase in HR and dP/dt. The increase in dP/dt was more consistent and robust compared to the increase in HR. Therefore, alterations in myocardial contractility, instead of HR changes, were investigated in the experiments in which the release of transmitters in the IML following

VLPA stimulation was studied. When the VLPA was stimulated unilaterally (in this case left VLPA), the antagonists for excitatory amino acids were injected bilaterally into the IML at $T_1$–$T_3$ because the VLPA is known to project bilaterally to the IML although with ipsilateral preponderance. Although many substances have been implicated as transmitters in the IML, our studies indicate that an excitatory amino acid, which recognizes NMDA receptors, is released in the IML at $T_1$–$T_3$ level when the neurons in the VLPA are stimulated. This conclusion was based on our observations, in separate experiments, that bilateral microinjections of kynurenate (a non-selective excitatory amino acid receptor antagonist) and DAP-7 (a specific antagonist for NMDA receptors) into the IML at $T_1$–$T_3$ blocked the increase in left ventricular contractility induced by stimulation of the neurons in the left VLPA. Both kynurenate and DAP-7 did not exert any non-specific depression of neurons in the IML because responses to other excitatory agents such as carbachol remained unaltered. DAP-7 (5 nmol) did not alter the responses to KA, QA or AMPA. Blockade of the cardiac responses to the stimulation of the VLPA neurons was not due to the distortion of the neurons in the IML because bilateral injections of 20 nl volumes of 0.9% sodium chloride solution at $T_1$–$T_3$ did not alter these responses. Our results are in general agreement with the reports in which the VLPA was stimulated electrically and kynurenate was administered either intrathecally (Guyenet et al., 1987) or microiontophoretically (Morrison et al., 1989). However, there are some differences between our results and those of other investigators. Since the techniques used in these investigations were different, it is difficult to compare their results with the present studies. For example, Bazil and Gordon (1991) failed to block increase in HR following the chemical stimulation of VLPA when they injected DAP-7 intrathecally; in these experiments, it is possible that DAP-7 did not reach the IML at $T_1$–$T_3$ level in sufficient concentrations. Morrison et al. failed to block the excitation of SPNs in the IML at $T_5$–$T_7$ in response to the electrical stimulation of VLPA when they applied DAP-5 microiontophoretically to SPNs. In this study, it is possible that sufficient concentrations of DAP-5 were not ejected by microiontophoresis to block NMDA receptors.

*Acknowledgments.* This work was supported by the following grants awarded to Dr. H. Sapru: N.I.H. (HL24347) and American Heart Association (NJ). The work presented here was done in collaboration with Drs. K. Sundaram and J. Murugaian.

# References

Barman SM (1984): Spinal cord control of the cardiovascular system. In: *Nervous Control of Cardiovascular Function*, Randall WC ed., New York: Oxford University Press, pp 321–345.

Barman SM, Gebber GL (1987): Lateral tegmental field neurons of cat medulla: a source of basal activity of ventrolateral medullospinal sympathoexcitatory neurons. *J Neurophysiol* 57:1410–1424.

Bazil MK, Gordon FJ (1991): Spinal NMDA receptors mediate pressor responses evoked from the rostral ventrolateral medulla. *Am J Physiol* 260:H267–H275.

Calaresu FR, Yardley CP (1988): Medullary basal sympathetic tone. *Annu Rev Physiol* 50:511–524.

Collingrdige GL, Lester RA (1989): Excitatory amino acid receptors in the vertebrate central nervous system. *Pharmacol Rev* 40:145–210.

Coote JH, Macleod VH, Fleetwood-Walker SM, Gilbey MP (1981): The response of individual sympathetic preganglionic neurons to microelectrophoretically applied endogenous monoamines. *Brain Res* 215:135–145.

Dembowsky K, Czachurski J, Seller H (1985): An intracellular study of the synaptic input to sympathetic preganglionic neurons of the third thoracic segment of the cat. *J Auton Nerv Syst* 13:201–244.

Dembowsky K, Czachurski J, Seller H (1986): Three types of sympathetic preganglionic neurones with different electrophysiological properties are identified by intracellular recordings in the cat. *Pflugers Arch* 406:112–120.

Faden Al, Jacobs TP (1980): Cardiac contractility and the spinal sympathetic neuron. *Neurol Res* 1:227–237.

Fleetwood-Walker SM, Coote JH (1981): Contribution of noradrenaline-, dopamine-, and adrenaline-containing axons to the innervation of different regions of the spinal cord of the cat. *Brain Res* 206:95–106.

Fries W, Zieglgansberger W (1974): A method to discriminate axonal from cell body activity and to analyze "silent" cells. *Exp Brain Res* 21:441–445.

Gebber GL, McCall RB (1976): Identification and discharge patterns of spinal sympathetic interneurons. *Am J Physiol* 231:722–733.

Gilbey MC, Peterson DF, Coote JH (1982): Some characteristics of sympathetic preganglionic neurons in the rat. *Brain Res* 241:43–48.

Guyenet PG, Cabot JB (1981): Inhibition of sympathetic preganglionic neurons by catecholamines and clonidine: Mediation by an alpha-adrenergic receptor. *J Neurosci* 1:908–917.

Guyenet PG, Stornetta RL (1982): Inhibition of sympathetic preganglionic discharges by epinephrine and alpha-methylepinephrine. *Brain Res* 235:271–283.

Guyenet PG, Sun M, Brown DL (1987): Role of GABA and excitatory amino acids in medullary baroreflex pathways. In: *Organization of the Autonomic Nervous System: Central and Peripheral Mechanisms*, Ciriello J, Calaresu FR, Renaud L, Polosa C, eds., New York: Alan R Liss, pp 215–225.

Henry JL, Calaresu FR (1972a): Topography and numerical distribution of neurons of the thoraco-lumbar intermediolateral nucleus in the cat. *J Comp Neurol* 144:205–214.

Henry JL, Calaresu FR (1972b): Distribution of cardioacceleratory sites in intermediolateral nucleus of the cat. *Am J Physiol* 222:700–704.

Kadzielawala K (1983): Inhibition of the activity of sympathetic preganglionic neurones and neurones activated by visceral afferents, by alpha-methyl-noradrenaline and endogenous catecholamines, *Neuropharmacology* 22:3–17.

Kubo T, Fukuda K, Mikami A, et al. (1986): Cloning, sequencing and expression of complementary DNA encoding the muscarinic acetylcholine receptor. *Nature* 323:411–416.

Kubo T, Nagura J, Misu Y (1987): Pharmacological characterization of spinal alpha adrenoreceptor related to blood pressure control in rats. *J Pharmacol Exp Ther*. 240:298–302.

Laskey W, Polosa C ( 1988): Characteristics of the sympathetic preganglionic neuron and its synaptic input. *Prog Neurobiol* 31:47–84.

Lokhandwala MF, Sabouni MH, Jandhyala BS (1985): Cardiovascular actions of an experimental antitumor agent, homoharringtonine, in anesthetized dogs. *Drug Dev Res* 5:157–163.

Ma RC, Dun NJ (1985): Norepinephrine depolarizes lateral horn cells of neonatal rat spinal cord in vitro. *Neurosci Lett* 60:163–168.

McCall RB (1988): Effects of putative neurotransmitters on sympathetic preganglionic neurons. *Annu Rev Physiol* 50:553–564.

Morrison SF, Ernsberger P, Milner TA, Callaway J, Gong A, Reis DJ (1989): A glutamate mechanism in the intermediolateral nucleus mediates sympathoexcitatory responses to stimulation of rostral ventrolateral medulla. In: *Organization of the Autonomic Nervous System: Central and Peripheral Mechanisms*, Ciriello J, Calaresu FR, Renaud L, Polosa C, eds. New York: Alan R Liss, pp 159–169.

Murugaian J, Sundaram K, Krieger AJ, Sapru HN (1990): Relative effects of different spinal autonomic nuclei on cardiac sympathoexcitatory function. *Brain Res Bull* 24:537–542.

Paxinos G, Watson C (1986): *The Rat Brain in Stereotaxic Coordinates*. New York: Academic Press.

Peralta EG, Winslow JW, Peterson GL, et al. (1987a): Primary structure and biochemical properties of an $M_2$ muscarinic receptor. *Science* 236:600–605.

Peralta EG, Ashkenazi A, Winslow JW, Smith DH, Ramachandran J, Capon DJ (1987b): Distinct primary structures, ligand-binding properties and tissue-specific expression of four human muscarinic acetylcholine receptors. *EMBO J* 6.3932–3927.

Randall WC, Priola DV, Ulmer RH (1963): A functional study of distribution of cardiac sympathetic nerves. *Am J Physiol* 205:1227–1231.

Ross CA, Ruggiero DA, Park DH, et al. (1984): Tonic vasomotor control by the rostral ventrolateral medulla: effect of electrical or chemical stimulation of the area containing $C_1$ adrenaline neurons on arterial pressure, heart rate, and plasma catecholamines and vasopressin. *J Neurosci* 4:474–494.

Sangdee C, Franz DN (1983): Evidence for inhibition of sympathetic preganglionic neurons by bulbospinal epinephrine pathways. *Neurosci Lett* 37:167–173.

Seybold VS, Elde RF (1984): Receptor autoradiography in the thoracic spinal cord: correlation of neurotransmitter binding sites with sympathoadrenal neurons. *J Neuosci*. 4:2533–2542.

Shi H, Lewis DI, Coote JH (1988): Effects of activating spinal alpha-adrenoreceptors on sympathetic nerve activity in the rat. *J. Auton Nerv Syst* 23:69–78.

Stone TW (1985): *Microiontophoresis and Pressure Ejection*. New York: John Wiley & Sons, pp 3–64.

Strack AM, Sawyer WB, Marubio LM, Loewy AD (1988): Spinal origin of sympathetic preganglionic neurons in the rat. *Brain Res* 455:187–191.

Sun MK, Hackett JT, Guyenet PG (1988a): Sympathoexcitatory neurons of the rostral ventrolateral medulla exhibit pacemaker properties in the presence of a glutamate-receptor antagonist. *Brain Res* 438:23–40.

Sun MK, Young BS, Hackett JT, Guyenet PG (1988b): Reticulospinal pacemaker neurons of the rat rostral ventrolateral medulla with putative sympathoexcitatory function: An intracellular study in vitro. *Brain Res* 442:229–239.

Sundaram K, Krieger AJ, Sapru HN (1988a): $M_2$ muscarinic receptors mediate pressor responses to cholinergic agonists in the ventrolateral medullary pressor area. *Brain Res* 449:141–149.

Sundaram K, Sapru HN (1988b): Cholinergic nerve terminals in the ventrolateral medullary pressor area: Pharmacological evidence. *J Auton Nerv Syst* 22:221–228.

Sundaram K, Murugaian J, Watson M, Sapru HN (1989a): $M_2$ muscarinic receptor agonists produce hypotension and bradycardia when injected into the nucleus tractus solitarius. *Brain Res* 477:358–362.

Sundaram K, Murugaian J, Sapru HN (1989b): Cardiac responses to microinjections of excitatory amino acids into the intermediolateral cell column of the rat spinal cord. *Brain Res* 482:12–22.

Sundaram K, Murugaian J, Sapru HN (1989c): Microinjections of cholinergic agonists into the intermediolateral cell column of the spinal cord at $T_1$ to $T_3$ increase heart rate and contractility. *Brain Res* 503:22–31.

Sundaram K, Murugaian J, Sapru H (1991a): Microinjections of norepinephrine into the intermediolateral cell column of the spinal cord exert excitatory as well as inhibitory effects on the cardiac function. *Brain Res* 544:227–234.

Sundaram K, Sapru, HN (1991b): NMDA receptors in the intermediolateral column of the spinal cord mediate sympathoexcitatory cardiac responses elicited from the ventrolateral medullary pressor area. *Brain Res* 544:33–41.

Urbanski RW, Sapru HN (1988a): Evidence for a sympathoexcitatory pathway from the nucleus tractus solitarii to the ventrolateral medullary pressor area. *J Auton Nerv Syst* 23:161–174.

Urbanski RW, Sapru HN (1988b): Putative neurotransmitters involved in medullary cardiovascular regulation. *J Auton Nerv Syst* 25:181–193.

Willette RN, Barcas PP, Krieger AJ, Sapru HN (1983): Vasopressor and depressor areas in the rat medulla. *Neuropharmacology* 22:1071–1079.

Yasunaga K, Nosaka S (1979): Cardiac sympathetic nerves in rats: Anatomical and functional features. *Jap J Physiol* 29:691–705.

Yoshimura M, Nishi S (1982): Intracellular recordings from lateral horn cells of the spinal cord *in vitro*. *J Auton Nerv Syst* 6:5–11.

Yoshimura M, Polosa C, Nishi S (1986): Electrophysiological properties of sympathetic preganglionic neurons in the cat spinal cord *in vitro*. *Pflugers Arch Physiol* 406:91–98.

Yoshimura M, Polosa C, Nishi S (1987a): Slow EPSP and depolarizing action of noradrenaline on sympathetic preganglionic neurons. *Brain Res* 414:138–142.

Yoshimura M, Polosa C, Nishi S (1987b): Slow IPSP and the noradrenaline-induced inhibition of the cat sympathetic preganglionic neurons *in vitro*, *Brain Res* 419:383–386.

Yoshimura M, Polosa C, Nishi S (1987c): Noradrenaline induces rhythmic bursting in sympathetic preganglionic neurons. *Brain Res* 420:147–151.

Zivin JA, Reid JL, Saavedra JM, Kopin I. (1975): Quantitative localization of biogenic amines in the spinal cord. *Brain Res* 99:293–301.

# 15
# The Function of Catecholamines in the Control of Sympathetic Preganglionic Neurons

Canio Polosa, Megumu Yoshimura, and Syogoro Nishi

## Fast Transmitters and Modulators

Until recently, chemicals found in axon terminals, released by action potentials, and exerting postsynaptic actions were labeled as transmitters. To transmitters was attributed the role of producing excitation or inhibition by causing short duration depolarization or hyperpolarization of the postsynaptic cell. As the number of putative transmitters has steadily increased and the multiplicity of their actions has become apparent, the concept that transmitters produce only excitation or inhibition has become inadequate. For instance, in the hippocampus at least 20 different putative neurotransmitters have been identified (see review by Nicoll, 1988). Yet few fit the restricted definition of transmitter. Other functional roles for transmitters have begun to be demonstrated. Long-term modulation by transmitters of various potassium or calcium currents has been described. Moreover, some of the transmitters may have a trophic role that may not be revealed by measurement of electrical properties of cells. Thus, whereas some transmitters produce short-lasting ionic currents underlying synaptic excitation or inhibition, other neurotransmitters may exert a tonic control, via multiple mechanisms, of various aspects of cell excitability and function. In the literature, the terms "fast transmitter" and "neuromodulator" are sometimes used to distinguish these two sets of actions. The same chemical may act both as a fast transmitter and as a neuromodulator, for example, acetylcholine acting on nicotinic and muscarinic receptors at autonomic ganglionic synapses.

## Actions of Catecholamines in the Nervous System

Catecholamine-containing axon terminals and catecholamine receptors have been demonstrated in several parts of the central nervous system. As a result of studies of catecholamine actions in different neurons, the generalization can be reached that the actions of catecholamines at synapses are unlike those of classical fast transmitters because they are multiple, long-lasting, and often involve activation of second messenger systems. These actions are, however, quite powerful and therefore changes in the catecholamine level at a synapse may result in marked changes in the output of that synapse. This chapter will survey catecholamine actions on neurons other than the sympathetic preganglionic neuron (SPN). These data will provide a background for the survey of cellular actions of catecholamines on SPNs, studied in vitro, which is the object of this chapter. Although these actions are heterogeneous, an attempt will be made to classify them according to cellular mechanisms. The best described actions of catecholamines on neurons are modulation of potassium and calcium conductance. A single neuron can show many, or even all, of the actions described below.

## Modulation of Potassium Conductances by Catecholamines

Catecholamines hyperpolarize neurons at a variety of sites (e.g., locus coeruleus, Egan et al., 1983; myenteric plexus, Morita and North, 1981; dorsal vagal motor nucleus, Fukuda et al., 1987, substantia gelatinosa, North and Yoshimura, 1984) by an action mediated by an adrenergic alpha-2 receptor. The alpha-2 receptor increases potassium conductance (Williams et al., 1985) and is presumably coupled to the potassium channel through a G protein. The conductance has been characterized in some neurons as an inward rectifying potassium-conductance (Selyanko et al., 1990). This alpha-2–mediated increase in potassium conductance is the basis for the inhibitory action, recorded extracellularly, of catecholamines applied by iontophoresis to various neurons in animals with an intact central nervous system (CNS).

Catecholamines depolarize neurons at a variety of sites (thalamic relay neurons, McCormick and Prince, 1988; dorsal vagal motor nucleus, Fukuda et al., 1987; locus coeruleus, Finlayson and Marshall, 1985; dorsal raphe, Yoshimura et al., 1985; supraoptic nucleus, Randle et al., 1986), by an action mediated by alpha-1 adrenergic receptors. The alpha-1 receptor decreases a resting potassium conductance that has not yet been characterized and may be different in different neurons. This turning off of potassium channels is probably the basis for the increased firing of neurons observed at several sites upon iontophoretic application of catecholamines in earlier studies with extracellular electrodes.

In hippocampal pyramidal neurons catecholamines depress the slow afterhyperpolarization caused by a calcium-activated potassium conductance (Madison and Nicoll, 1986) by an action mediated by beta receptors. This action, which results in a profound change in the properties of repetitive firing of the cells, seems to involve a cyclic adenosine monophosphate (cAMP)-dependent protein kinase.

# Modulation of Calcium Conductance

Catecholamines decrease the calcium current of the spike (cultured dorsal root ganglion cells, Dunlap and Fischbach, 1981; locus coeruleus cells, Williams and North, 1985). This effect seems mediated by an alpha-2 receptor with properties somewhat different from the most common properties of these receptors (Canfield and Dunlap, 1984). The effect seems to involve a G protein and protein kinase. This action is of obvious importance for its secondary effects on calcium-dependent transmitter release at axon terminals and on calcium-dependent potassium conductance.

# Modulation of Transmitter Release by Catecholamines

It is not known yet whether this modulation is through the modulation of conductances already described or through different mechanisms, which may be slow in being identified because of the methodological difficulties in studying axon terminal properties. Data from sympathetic ganglia show that two receptor types are involved, an alpha-2 receptor that depresses release and a beta receptor that enhances release (Brown and Medgett, 1982). The action of the latter receptor seems to involve cAMP.

# Miscellaneous Actions

Beta-receptor–mediated increases in sodium-potassium pump activity (Siggins et al., 1971) and chloride conductance (Segal, 1981) as well as a decrease in a nonspecific cation conductance (Pun et al., 1985) of which the responsible receptor has not yet been characterized are other catecholamine actions that so far have been described in only a few neuron types.

# Catecholamines and SPN

Several lines of evidence suggested, prior to the intracellular work in the slice, that catecholamines may have an important role in the control of SPN function. The intermediolateral (IML) nucleus of the gray matter of the thoracic spinal cord shows intense staining for catecholamines, which disappears below a cord transection (Carlsson et al., 1964). The question of the origin of these catecholamine-containing axon systems is not resolved. Neuron groups in the hypothalamus and brain stem, including the ventrolateral medulla, are the presumed source of this innervation (for review see Coote, 1988; Laskey and Polosa, 1988). Electron microscopic studies have shown that catecholamine-containing axon terminals make synapses with SPNs identified by retrograde horseradish peroxidase (HRP) transport (Chiba and Masuko, 1986; Milner et al., 1988). Binding of adrenergic agonists or antagonists has been demonstrated in the IML, although evidence that the binding is on the SPN is still lacking (Cabot et al., 1984; Dashwood et al., 1985; Seybold and Elde, 1984). In vivo studies with extracellular electrodes have shown that catecholamines applied by iontophoresis produce depressant effects mediated by alpha-2 adrenergic receptors on antidromically identified SPNs (Coote et al., 1981; Guyenet and Cabot, 1981; Kadzielawa, 1983). Studies using various pharmacological agents suggested that catecholamines can also produce excitatory actions on SPNs (Franz et at., 1987; Taylor and Brody, 1976).

## Methods

The results to be reviewed in the next section were obtained in cats anesthetized with alpha-chloralose and Na pentobarbitone (60 and 10 mg/kg i.p., respectively). The piece of spinal cord containing thoracic segments 2 and 3 was excised after laminectomy, desheathed, and cut into 500-$\mu$m

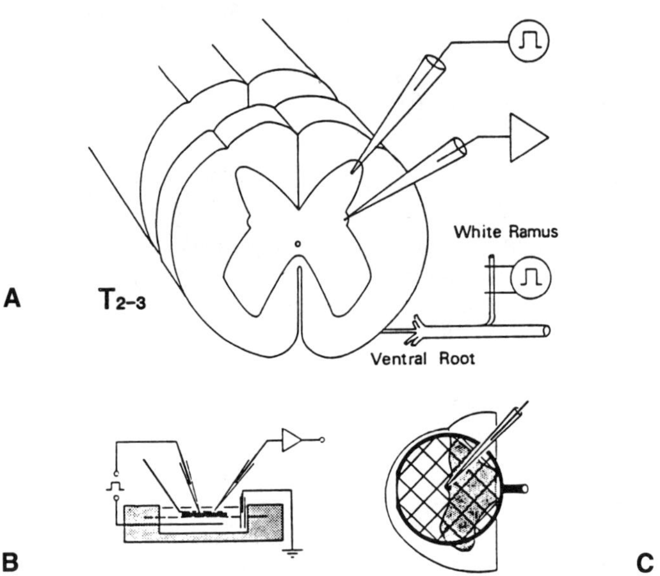


FIGURE 15.1. Details of the slice preparation. **A**: Cross-section of a slice of the T2–T3 segment of the spinal cord, showing position of recording microelectrode in the intermediolateral nucleus. Position of a suction electrode on the segmental white ramus for antidromic identification of SPNs and of a focal stimulation microelectrode for synaptic activation of the SPNs is also shown. **B**: A side view of the perfusion chamber. **C**: View of the perfusion chamber from above.

thick transverse slices. Slices were placed in a recording chamber and superfused with oxygenated Krebs solution at 37°C and pH 7.4. Intracellular recordings were obtained with glass microelectrodes inserted into the IML (Fig. 15.1) (Yoshimura and Nishi, 1982). Recordings were made from SPNs identified antidromically as described earlier (Yoshimura et al., 1986c). Catecholamines and other drugs were added to the superfusing Krebs solution. The catecholamine concentrations used were in the $\mu$M range. In addition to the advantage of permitting stable intracellular recordings for drug studies, the tissue slice has several advantages over the method of in vivo iontophoresis with extracellular microelectrodes. A major advantage is the ability to control drug concentration, thus permitting dose-response curves for agonists and antagonists and allowing a better characterization of the agonist-receptor interaction. Moreover, by using drugs that prevent sodium spikes (tetrodotoxin, TTX) or transmitter release by action potentials (TTX, low calcium), it is possible to distinguish drug actions on the SPN from actions on antecedent neurons. Finally, it is possible with this technique to analyze the mechanism of a drug effect in some detail by exploiting the control of the neuron membrane potential and ionic composition of the medium that is possible in the slice.

# Results

## *Properties of the Neuron*

The SPNs studied had membrane potentials between $-55$ and $-65$ mV at the extracellular potassium concentration of 3.6 mM and input resistance of $65 \pm 5$M$\Omega$. The action potential had a peak amplitude of 70 to 80 mV and showed a characteristic hump on the repolarization phase. The action potential of this neuron results from sodium, calcium, and potassium currents (Yoshimura et al., 1986c). The action potential is followed by a prominent hyperpolarizing afterpotential of long duration and complex configuration. The afterpotential results from a fast and a slow outward potassium current (Yoshimura et al., 1986b) as well as an inward calcium current (Yoshimura et al., 1987e). A transient potassium current (Yoshimura et al., 1987f) may also contribute to spike repolarization and to the afterpotential. Focal electrical stimulation of the slice produces fast and slow excitatory and inhibitory postsynaptic potentials (Nishi et al., 1987; Yoshimura et al., 1986c; Yoshimura et al., 1987b,c).

## *Actions of Catecholamines on Potassium-Currents*

Catecholamines, by an action apparently mediated by an alpha-2 adrenergic receptor (Fig. 15.2A), increase the potassium conductance of the resting SPN membrane (Fig. 15.2C) (Yoshimura et al., 1987c). As a

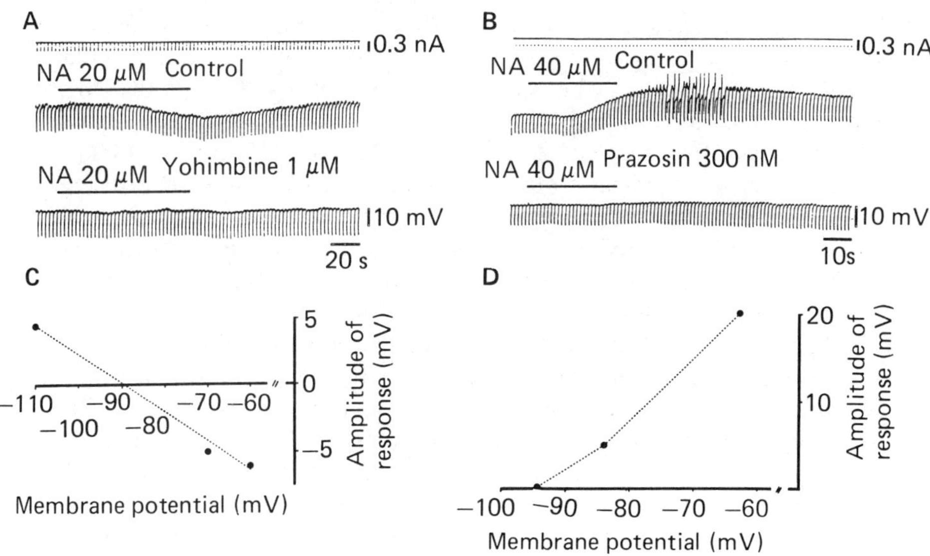



FIGURE 15.2. **A**: The hyperpolarizing action of noradrenaline is yohimbine-sensitive, hence alpha-2–mediated. **B**: The depolarizing action of noradrenaline is prazosinsensitive, hence alpha-1 mediated. **C**. The alpha-2 action of noradrenaline is hyperpolarizing at membrane potential positive to −90 mV, depolarizing at membrane potential negative to −90 mV. **D**. The alpha-1 depolarization action of noradrenaline decreases with membrane hyperpolarization and is nullified at −95 mV. (Reproduced with permission from Ciriello et al., 1987.)

result, the membrane hyperpolarizes (Fig. 15.2A) and the excitability of the neuron is depressed. A secondary mechanism may amplify the inhibitory effect of the alpha-2 receptor. Since the SPN has a transient potassium current that is inactivated at the resting potential (Yoshimura et al., 1987f), even a small hyperpolarization may result in deinactivation of this channel. When an excitatory postsynaptic potential (EPSP) is generated, the transient potassium current can be activated and exert its powerful shunting effect, opposing the depolarizing action of the EPSP. Catecholamines, by an action mediated by an alpha-1 adrenergic receptor, decrease the potassium conductance of the resting SPN membrane (Figs. 15.2B,D) (Yoshimura et al., 1987b). As a result, the membrane depolarizes and, if

FIGURE 15.3. The slow component of the afterhyperpolarization is abolished by the calcium-channel blocker cobalt (**A**, **B**), which abolished the hump, due to the calcium spike, on the repolarization phase of the spike (**D**). The slow component of the afterhyperpolarization is also abolished by superfusion with low calcium (**C**). Intracellular stimulation (2-msec pulses). In **A**, **B**, or **C** the spike is distorted by the pen recorder and the afterpotential is shown at two speeds.

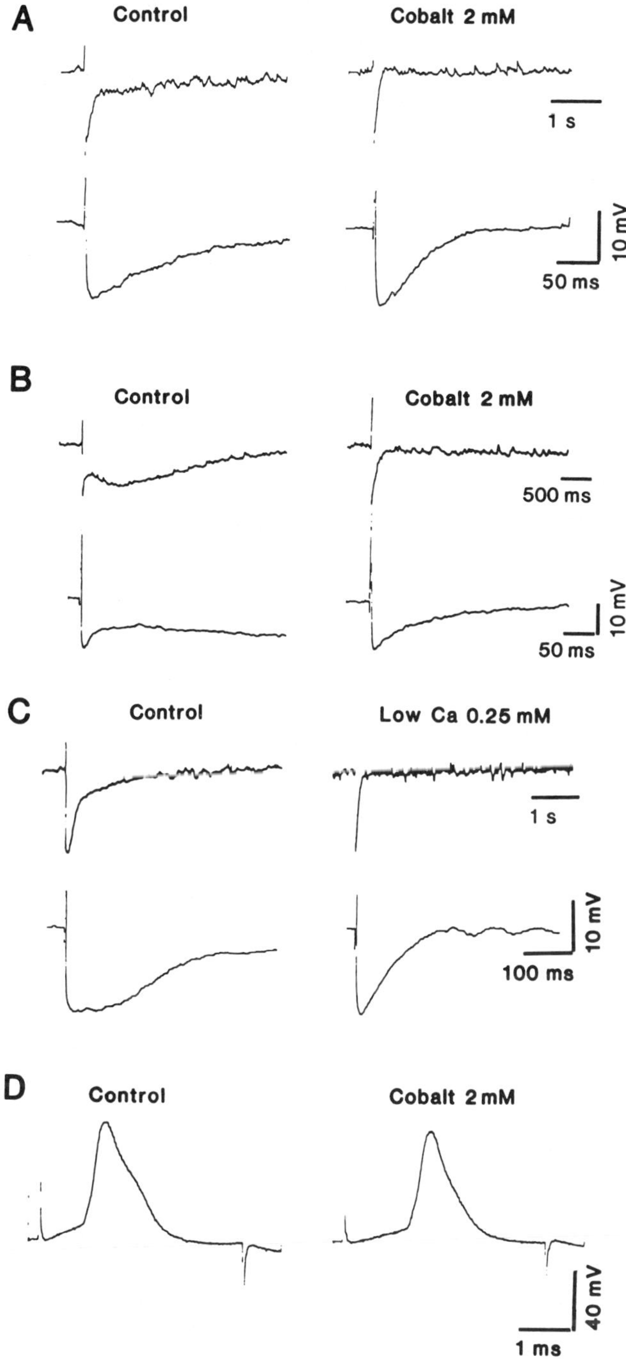
A
Control
Cobalt 2 mM
1 s
10 mV
50 ms
B
Control
Cobalt 2 mM
500 ms
10 mV
50 ms
C
Control
Low Ca 0.25 mM
1 s
10 mV
100 ms
D
Control
Cobalt 2 mM
40 mV
1 ms

threshold is reached, the neuron fires repetitively (Fig. 15.2B). Catecholamines also depress a calcium-activated potassium-conductance. As mentioned above, the SPN spike is followed by an afterhyperpolarization (AHP) (Yoshimura et al., 1986b) which, as in other neurons, has an important role in controlling the frequency of repetitive firing. The AHP has two components, an early component (fast AHP) and a late component (slow AHP). Although both components of the AHP are due to potassium currents, only the slow AHP is due to a calcium-activated potassium conductance. The amplitude and duration of this component are related to magnitude of the calcium component of the spike. Thus, the slow AHP is abolished by superfusion with calcium-free Krebs (Fig. 15.3C) or by the calcium channel blocker cobalt (Fig. 15.3A,B), which abolishes the hump due to the calcium spike on the repolarization phase of the action potential (Fig. 15.3D). The slow AHP is enhanced by the potassium channel blocker TEA, which prolongs the duration of the calcium spike of the SPN (Fig. 15.4). Amplitude and polarity of this component of the AHP depend on the driving force on the potassium ion (Fig. 15.5). We found

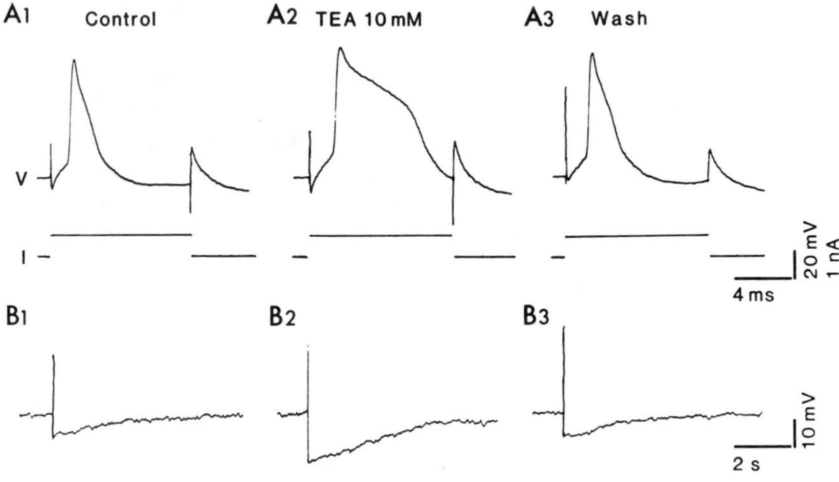


FIGURE 15.4.  Enhancement of the slow component of the afterhyperpolarization by TEA, which broadens the spike by blocking voltage-dependent delayed potassium currents. The broadening is due to prolongation of the calcium spike.

FIGURE 15.5.  Effect of changes in membrane potential (from −65 to −134 mV) on the slow component of the afterhyperpolarization. Spike evoked by a 2-msec intracellular depolarizing current pulse. **A**: Actual records obtained at the indicated values of membrane potential. Spike distorted by pen recorder. **B**: Plot of amplitude of slow afterhyperpolarization shown in **A** (measured 700 msec after the foot of the spike) versus membrane potential. (Reproduced with permission from Yoshimura et al., 1986b.)

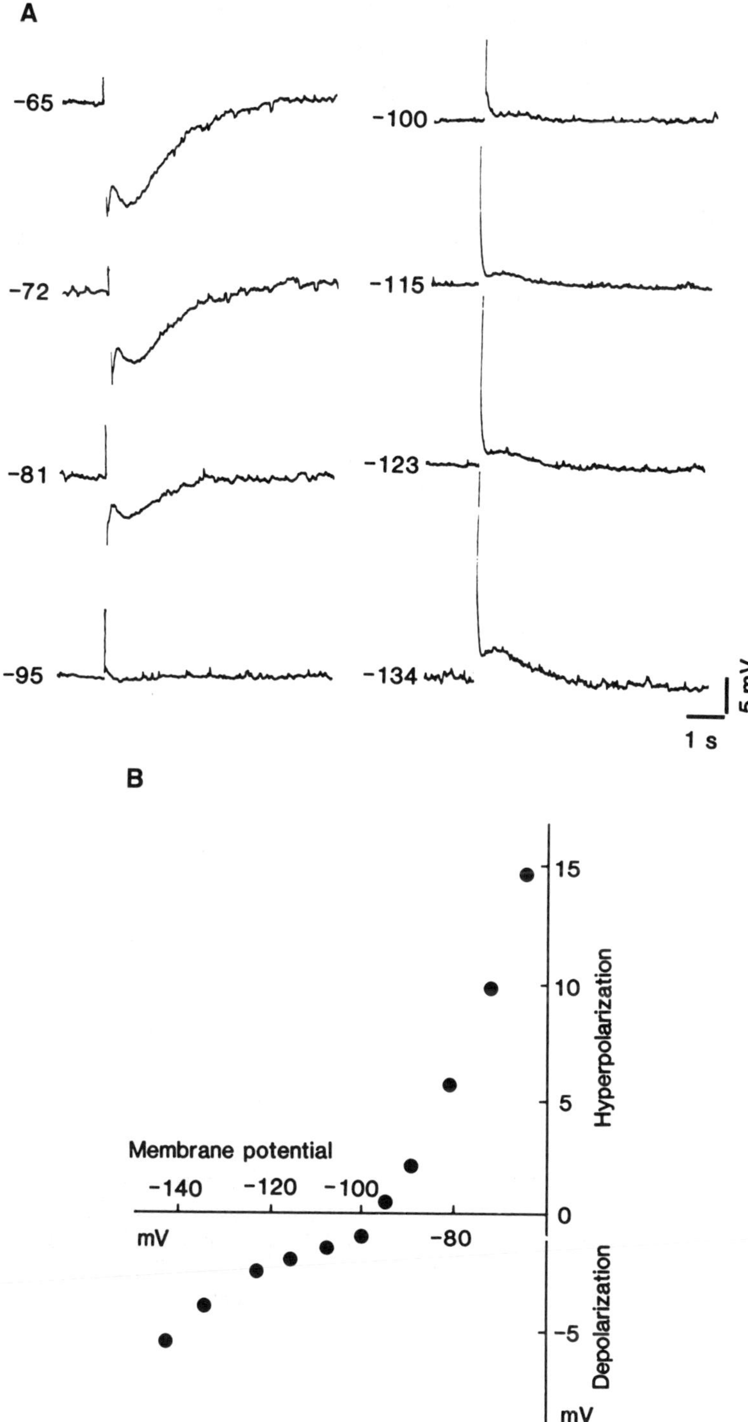


A
-65
-72
-81
-95
-100
-115
-123
-134
5 mV
1 s
B
15
Hyperpolarization
10
5
Membrane potential
-140    -120    -100
mV
-80
0
Depolarization
-5
mV

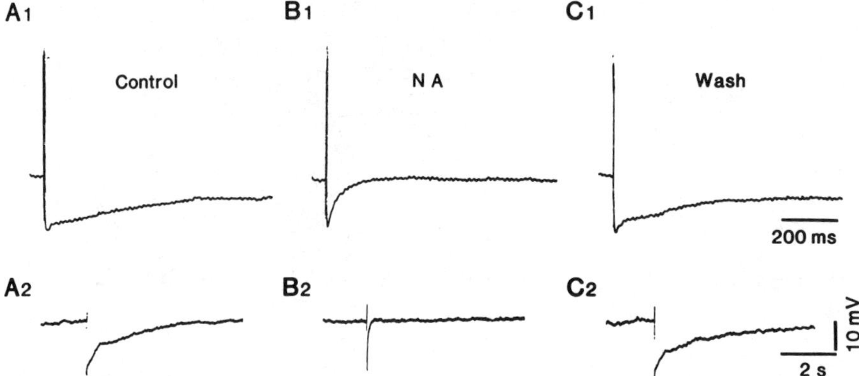



FIGURE 15.6.  Reversible block of the slow component of the afterhyperpolarization by superfusion with noradrenaline [40 $\mu$M (**B**)]. Spike at beginning of sweep evoked by intracellular current injection (2-msec duration) and distorted by pen recorder. (Reproduced with permission from Yoshimura et al., 1986a.)

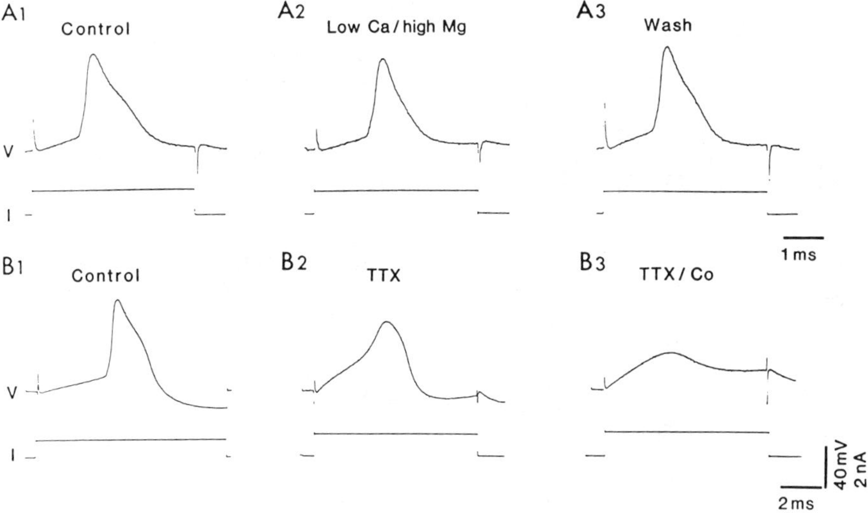



FIGURE 15.7.  Evidence that the SPN spike has a calcium component. Spike evoked by intracellular current injection (2-msec duration). **A** & **B** are recorded in two different SPNs. **A** shows that the shoulder on the repolarizing phase of the spike (A1 and A3) is reversibly lost during superfuson with low calcium (A2). In tetrodotoxin (0.6 $\mu$M, B2) intracellular stimulation evokes a higher threshold, slower rising, spike, which is blocked by cobalt (B3). (Reproduced with permission from Yoshimura et al., 1986c.)

that catecholamines suppress the slow component of the AHP about as effectively as low calcium or cobalt (Fig. 15.6, compare with Fig. 15.3). we have not yet characterized the adrenoreceptor type mediating this effect. As described below, catecholamines depress the calcium component of the SPN spike. We do not know yet whether the depression of the slow AHP by catecholamines can be entirely accounted for by this catecholamine action on the calcium spike or if a depressant action on the potassium conductance of the slow AHP is also involved.

## Actions of Catecholamines on Inward Currents

As mentioned above, the SPN spike has a calcium component that produces a noticeable "hump" on the repolarization phase (Yoshimura et al., 1986a). This hump is eliminated by superfusion with low calcium (Fig. 15.7A) or cobalt. The calcium spike, which has a higher threshold and is slower than the sodium spike, is recorded in isolation during superfusion

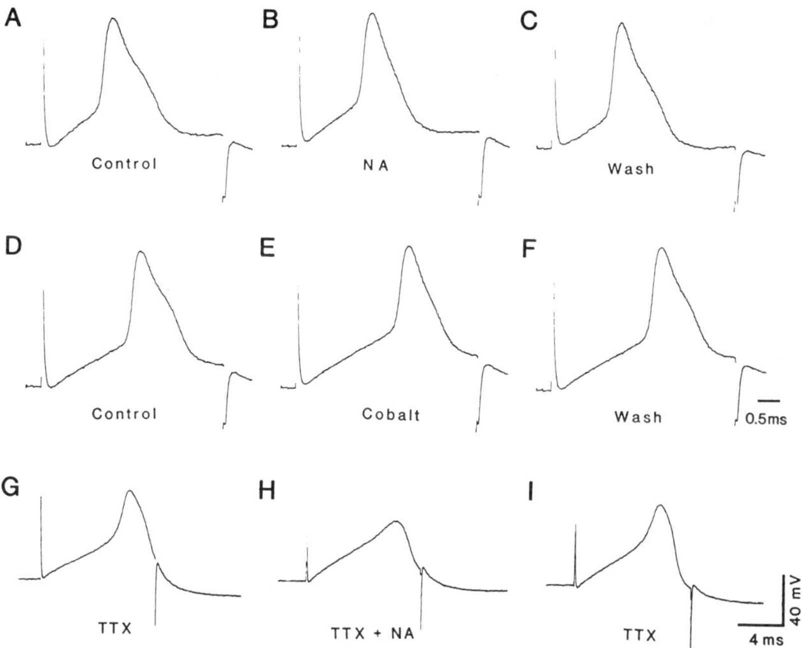


FIGURE 15.8. Spikes evoked by intracellular current injection. Noradrenaline (20 μM, **B**) reversibly eliminates the hump on the repolarization phase of the SPN spike (**A, C**). The effect is similar to that caused, in the same neuron, by cobalt 2 mM (**E**). In another SPN (**G–I**) the calcium spike recorded during superfusion with tetrodotoxin (**G**) is reversibly abolished by addition of noradrenaline (40 μM, **H**). Compare Fig. 15.8H with Fig. 15.7B3. (Reproduced with permission from Yoshimura et al., 1986a.)

with TTX, which blocks the sodium component of the spike (Fig. 15.7B). Noradrenaline has the same effect on the calcium spike as cobalt or low calcium (Yoshimura et al., 1986a). Thus, in normal Krebs, noradrenaline eliminates the hump on the repolarization phase of the spike (Fig. 15.8A–C) as cobalt does (Fig. 15.8D–F). In TTX, noradrenaline eliminates the calcium spike as cobalt does (Fig. 15.8G–I). We have not yet characterized the adrenoceptor (or adrenoceptors) mediating this effect, nor have we established whether the suppression of the calcium spike by noradrenaline is entirely due to a direct action on the calcium channels or is in part secondary to an enhancement of the potassium conductances that repolarize the membrane, which would result in faster repolarization reducing calcium influx because of the voltage dependence of the channels.

Catecholamines cause the appearance in the SPN of a calcium-dependent and voltage-dependent slow sodium current that follows the action potential (Yoshimura et al., 1987a). This postspike inward current depolarizes the membrane, resulting in an afterdepolarization that can produce repetitive (burst) firing. Figure 15.9 shows the development of this afterdepolarization as a function of time after the beginning of perfusion with noradrenaline. This figure shows also the already described depressant effect of noradrenaline on the slow component of the afterhyperpolarization. Figure 15.10 shows that when the noradrenaline afterdepolarization reaches threshold for action potential generation, a burst of action potentials is produced in response to a single short pulse of depolarizing current that, in the absence of noradrenaline, would have produced only a single action potential. The noradrenaline afterdepolarization is markedly

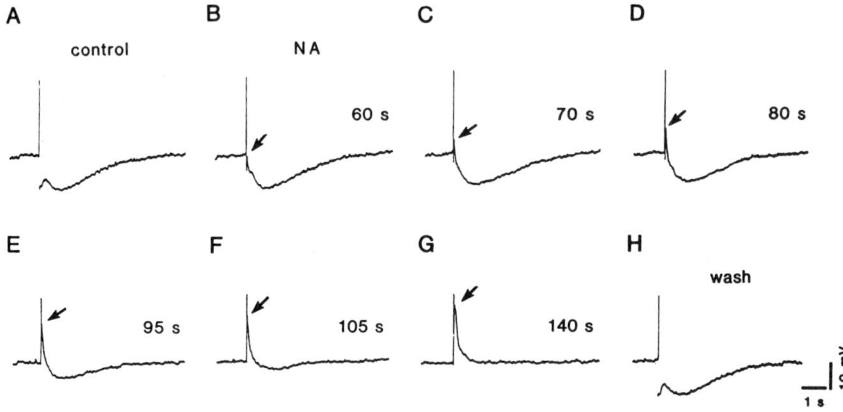



FIGURE 15.9. Modification in the shape of the afterpotential at the indicated times from onset of superfusion with noradrenaline 40 $\mu$M. The arrow points to the afterdepolarization, which reaches maximum amplitude in panel **G**. The spike in each panel is evoked by an intracellular current pulse. Also evident (panels **E–G**) is the depression of the slow component of the afterhyperpolarization. (Reproduced with permission from Yoshimura et al., 1987a.)

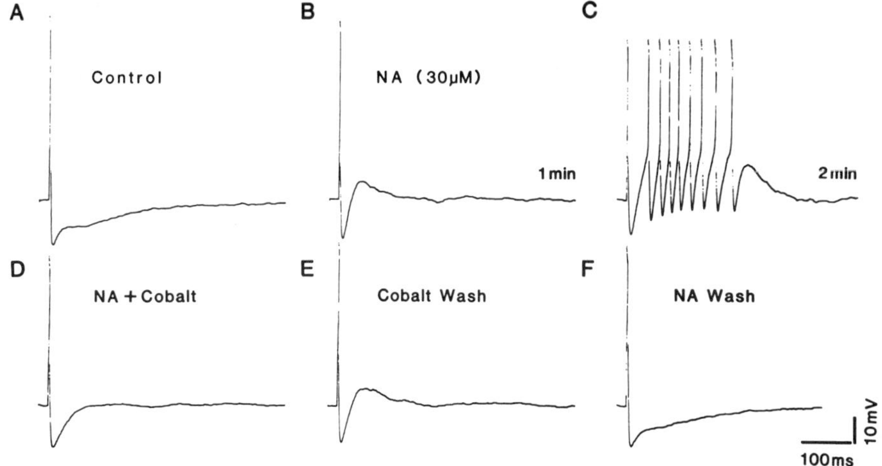

FIGURE 15.10. The depolarizing afterpotential produced by noradrenaline superfusion (30 $\mu$M) causes burst firing of the SPN (**C**). The depolarizing afterpotential is reversibly blocked by cobalt (**D**). The spike at the beginning of each record is evoked by a 2-msec intracellular current pulse. Spikes distorted by pen recorder. (Reproduced with permission from Yoshimura et al., 1986a.)

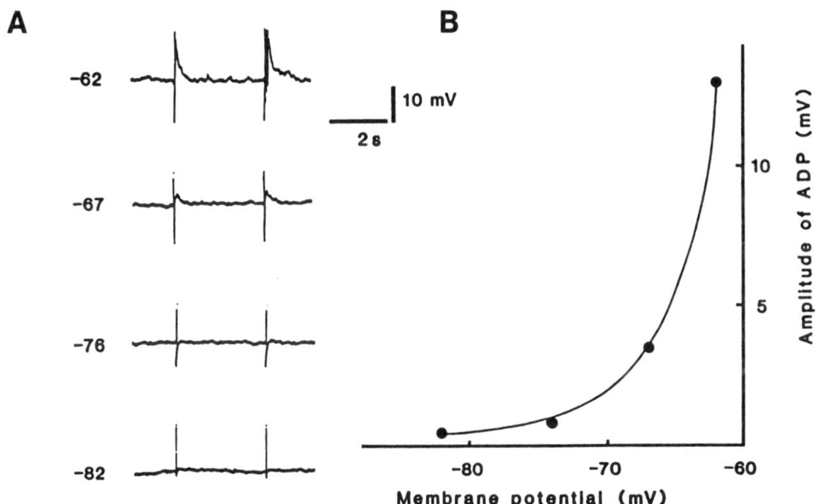

FIGURE 15.11. Voltage dependence of the noradrenaline afterdepolarization. **A:** Records obtained during superfusion with 40 $\mu$M noradrenaline at the indicated membrane potential. Each trace shows two action potentials (evoked by intracellular current pulses and distorted by the pen recorder) and the associated afterpotential. Note that the afterdepolarization decreases in amplitude with membrane hyperpolarization and is abolished at $-76$ mV. The spike undershoot is the fast component of the afterhyperpolarization, which becomes smaller as the membrane potential approaches the potassium equilibrium potential. **B:** Plot of peak amplitude of the noradrenaline afterdepolarization from records in **A** against membrane potential. (Reproduced with permission from Yoshimura et al., 1987a.)

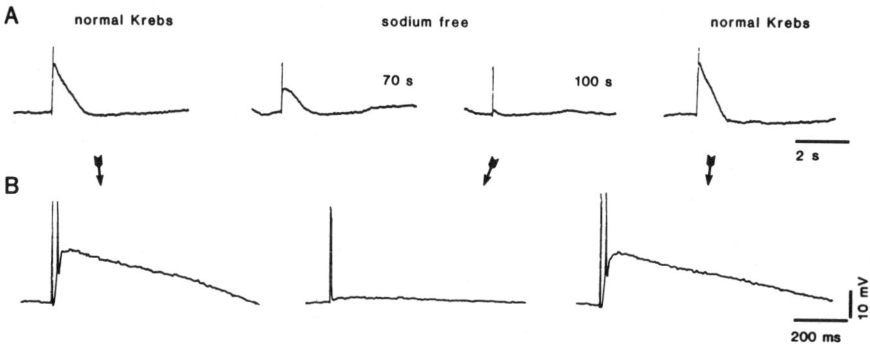

FIGURE 15.12. Sodium dependence of the noradrenaline afterdepolarization. All records obtained during superfusion with 40 $\mu$M noradrenaline. In all records the neuron is made to fire by an intracellular current pulse of 2-msec duration. **A:** Control, sodium-free perfusion, and recovery. **B:** Records with arrow are shown at faster speed. Note disappearance of the noradrenaline afterdepolarization after 100 sec of sodium-free superfusion. (Reproduced with permission from Yoshimura et al., 1987a.)

voltage-dependent (Fig. 15.11). At membrane voltages negative to $-70$ mV, this response becomes very small or disappears. Its size increases with membrane depolarization above this level. The noradrenaline afterdepolarization is calcium-dependent. It is abolished by calcium channel blockers like cobalt (Fig. 15.10D), by superfusion with low calcium Krebs solution, or by intracellular injection of a calcium chelator like EGTA. The noradrenaline afterdepolarization is also sodium-dependent. Superfusion with low sodium Krebs solution abolished this response (Fig. 15.12).

The effects mentioned above, with the exception of the hyperpolarization and depolarization, are seen only when the cell is made to generate action potentials. In addition, catecholamines cause the appearance of a slow, voltage-dependent, inward current, presumably carried by calcium ions. This current is activated in the subthreshold range of membrane potential down to values as low as $-65$ mV. This current produces a spontaneous depolarization of the membrane to threshold (Fig. 15.13). In the absence of spikes (e.g., during superfusion with TTX), presumably in association with a repolarizing current unless the depolarizing current is transient, this current produces a rhythmic spontaneous oscillation of membrane potential (Fig. 15.14). Thus, this is a pacemaker current. This current is abolished in low calcium.

## Evidence of Release of Endogenous Catecholamines

All the above evidence of catecholamine actions on SPNs was obtained under conditions in which exogenous catecholamines were presented to the

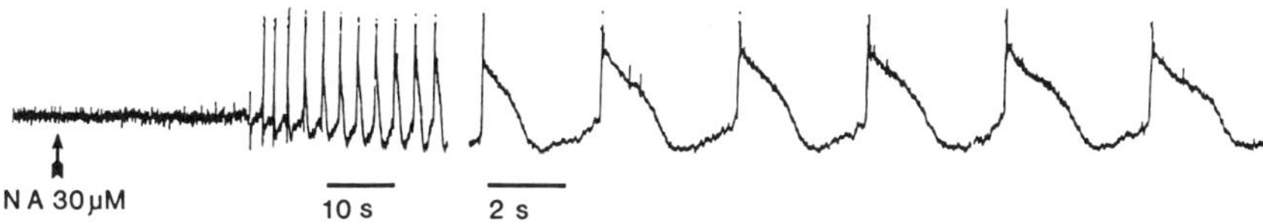


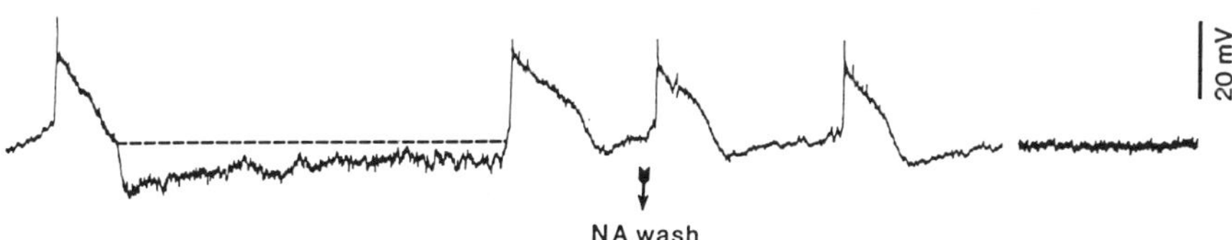


FIGURE 15.13. Pacemaker activity of SPN during superfusion with 30 μM noradrenaline. Thirty sec after the onset of noradrenaline superfusion the neuron starts firing in bursts of two to five spikes in association with the appearance of a large afterdepolarization lasting longer than 1 sec. The bottom record shows that membrane hyperpolarization (by about 10 mV) reversibly stops the bursting. Spikes truncated by pen recorder. (Reproduced with permission from Yoshimura et al., 1987d.)

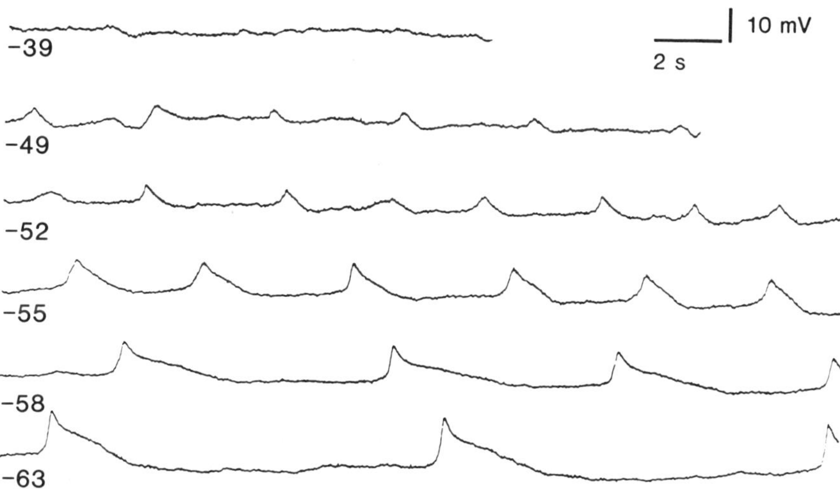


FIGURE 15.14. Superfusion with noradrenaline (40 μM) in the presence of tetrodotoxin (0.6 μM) at the resting membrane potential (−55 mV) resulted in a spontaneous oscillation in membrane potential, presumably responsible for the bursting shown in Fig. 15.13. When the membrane potential was displaced by intracellular current injection, the oscillation decreased in frequency with hyperpolarization and increased with depolarization. The oscillation disappeared when the membrane was depolarized to −39 mV or more positive values and again when the membrane was hyperpolarized to −68 mV or more negative values (not shown). (Reproduced with permission from Yoshimura et al., 1987d.)

preparation. This evidence proves the existence in this neuron of receptors for catecholamines coupled to various membrane conductances. Before assuming that such actions may occur under physiological conditions, two questions must be answered. Is there any evidence that catecholamines are released from axon terminals presynaptic to the SPN? If this question is answered affirmatively, do catecholamines released by the presynaptic axon terminals have access to the receptors activated by the exogenously applied agonists? We have demonstrated that focal stimulation of the slice can evoke slow EPSPs or inhibitory postsynaptic potentials (IPSPs) that are blocked by prazosin and yohimbine, respectively, and are due to ionic mechanisms similar to those underlying the depolarizing and hyperpolarizing action of noradrenaline (Yoshimura et al., 1987b,c). In addition, we have shown that SPN firing produced by a prazosin-sensitive slow EPSP is characterized by spikes that are followed by a triphasic afterpotential, due to a prominent depolarizing component appearing between the early and late component of the AHP (Yoshimura et al., 1987b). These changes in the afterpotential are reminiscent of those observed during superfusion with exogenous noradrenaline.


## Discussion

This survey of catecholamine actions on SPNs shows how many different ionic conductances of the sympathetic preganglionic neuron are controlled by catecholamines. With the exception of the alpha-2 receptor-mediated increase in potassium conductance, which makes the cell less excitable, all other catecholamine actions described so far in this neuron increase the readiness of this neuron to fire. These actions include the alpha-1 receptor-mediated decrease in potassium conductance, the depression of the slow component of the afterhyperpolarization, the afterdepolarization, and the autorhythmicity due to a pacemaker current. On the basis of these actions it appears impossible and inappropriate to classify catecholamines as excitatory or inhibitory transmitters. Clearly, catecholamine actions are more diverse than the effects of glutamate or gamma-aminobutyric acid (GABA). Interestingly, a similar problem of interpretation was faced in early studies of catecholamine actions in the CNS, in the period immediately preceding the adoption of intracellular in vitro analysis, when the methods available were extracellular microelectrode recording and iontophoresis. For example, studies of neurons at various CNS sites innervated by locus coeruleus neurons (the largest noradrenergic cell group in the brain stem) showed that noradrenaline depressed the spontaneous firing of these neurons while enhancing the stimulus-evoked responses of the same neurons. This observation was rationalized with the hypothesis that the specific function of catecholamines at synapses was to increase the signal-to-noise ratio for transmission of information (Woodward et al., 1979). As the concept of neuromodulation became established (for review see Kaczmarek and Levitan, 1987; Nicoll, 1988), it became clear that many neurotransmitters exert a fine control (modulation) of the properties of ionic conductances that control cell excitability, for example, potassium and calcium conductances. Moreover, in a neuron the same conductance may be modified in the same direction by different neurotransmitters (e.g., Selyanko et al., 1990). Thus, catecholamine actions can be explained in terms of the single ion channel behavior. This may be an example of how the chemical composition of the environment of the cell influences cell behavior. Finally, what do catecholamine actions on SPNs have to do with hypertension? The effects of the administration of centrally acting adrenergic agonists in a variety of experimental animal models of hypertension (Chalmers, 1975) as well as the proven efficacy of some of these agonists in the treatment of hypertension in humans (Laverty, 1973) suggest that catecholamines play a critical role in the control of SPN activity and hence of the sympathetic output to the circulation. It therefore seems that an understanding of the mechanisms of catecholamine actions on SPNs is a prerequisite for an understanding of SPN control both in normal conditions and in the hypertensive state.

*Acknowledgment.* This work was supported by the Ministry of Education, Science and Culture of Japan (S.N.) and the Quebec Heart Foundation (C.P.).

# References


Brown DA, Medgett IC (1982): Functional role of presynaptic alpha and beta adrenoceptors in rat isolated superior cervical ganglion. *Br J Pharmacol* 75:18P.

Cabot JB, Edwards E, Bogan N, Schechter N (1984): Alpha-2-adrenergic receptors in avian spinal cord: Increases in apparent density associated with the sympathetic preganglionic cell column. *J Auton Nerv Syst* 11:77–89.

Canfield DR, Dunlap K (1984): Pharmacological characterization of amine receptors on embryonic chick sensory neurons. *Br J Pharmacol* 82:557–563.

Carlsson A, Falck B, Fuxe K, Hillarp NA (1964): Cellular localization of monoamines in the spinal cord. *Acta Physiol Scand* 60:112–119.

Chalmers JP (1975): Brain amines and models of experimental hypertension. *Circ Res* 36:469–480.

Chiba T, Masuko S (1986): Direct synaptic contacts of catecholamine axons on the preganglionic sympathetic neurons in the rat thoracic spinal cord. *Brain Res* 380:405–408.

Coote JH (1988): The organization of cardiovascular neurons in the spinal cord. *Rev Physiol Biochem Pharmacol* 110:147–285.

Coote JH, MacLeod VH, Fleetwood-Walker SM, Gilbey MP (1981): The response of individual sympathetic preganglionic neurons to microiontophoretically applied endogenous amines. *Brain Res* 215:135–145.

Dashwood MR, Gilbey MP, Spyer KM (1985): The localization of adrenoceptors and the opiate receptors in regions of the cat central nervous system involved in cardiovascular control. *Neuroscience* 15:537–551.

Dunlap K, Fischbach GD (1981): Neurotransmitters decrease the calcium conductance activated by depolarization of embryonic sensory neurones. *J Physiol (Lond)* 317:519–535.

Egan TM, Henderson G, North RA, Williams JT (1983): Noradrenaline-mediated synaptic inhibition in rat locus coeruleus neurones. *J Physiol (Lond)* 345:477–488.

Finlayson PG, Marshall KC (1985): Locus coeruleus neurons in culture have a developmentally transient $\alpha_1$-adrenergic response. *Dev Brain Res* 25:292–295.

Franz DN, Steffensen SC, Milner LC, Sangdee C (1987): Neurotransmitter regulation of excitability in sympathetic preganglionic neurons through interactions with adenylate cyclase. In: *Organization of the Autonomic Nervous System: Central and Peripheral Mechanisms*, Ciriello J, Calaresu FR, Renaud LP, Polosa CS, eds. New York: Alan R Liss, pp 121–130.

Fukuda A, Minami T, Nabekura J, Oomura Y (1987): The effects of noradrenaline on neurones in the rat dorsal motor nucleus of the vagus, in vitro. *J Physiol (Lond)* 393:213–231.

Guyenet PG, Cabot JB (1981). Inhibition of sympathetic preganglionic neurons by catecholamines and clonidine: Mediation by an $\alpha$-adrenergic receptor. *J Neurosci* 1:908–917.

Kaczmarek LK, Levitan IB (1987): *Neuromodulation: The Biochemical Control of Neuronal Excitability*. New York: Oxford University Press.

Kadzielawa K (1983): Inhibition of the activity of sympathetic preganglionic neurons and neurons activated by visceral afferents, by alpha-methylnoradrenaline and endogenous catecholamines. *Neuropharmacology* 22:3–17.

Laskey W, Polosa C (1988): Characteristics of the sympathetic preganglionic neuron and its synaptic input. *Prog Neurobiol* 31:47–84.

Laverty R (1973): The mechanisms of action of some hypertensive drugs. *Br Med Bull* 29:152–157.

Madison DV, Nicoll RA (1986): Actions of noradrenaline recorded intracellularly in rat hippocampal CA pyramidal neurones, in vitro. *J Physiol (Lond)* 372:221–244.

McCormick DA, Prince DA (1988): Noradrenergic modulation of firing pattern in guinea pig and cat thalamic neurons in vitro. *J Neurophysiol* 59:978–996.

Milner TA, Morrison SF, Abate C, Reis DJ (1988): Phenylethanolamine N-methyltransferase-containing terminals synapse directly on sympathetic preganglionic neurons in the rat. *Brain Res* 448:205–222.

Morita K, North RA (1981): Clonidine activates membrane potassium conductance in myenteric neurones. *Br J Pharmacol* 74:419–428.

Nicoll RA (1988): The coupling of neurotransmitter receptors to ion channels in the brain. *Science* 241:545–551.

Nishi S, Yoshimura M, Polosa C (1987): Synaptic potentials and putative transmitters actions in sympathetic preganglionic neurons. In: *Organization of the Autonomic Nervous System: Central and Peripheral Mechanisms*, Ciriello J, Calaresu FR, Renaud LP, Polosa C, eds. New York: Alan R Liss, pp 15–26.

North RA, Yoshimura M (1984): The actions of noradrenaline on neurones of the rat substantia gelatinosa in vitro. *J Physiol (Lond)* 349:43–55.

Pun RK, Marshall KC, Hendelman WJ, Guthrie PB, Nelson PG (1985): Noradrenergic responses of spinal neurons in locus coeruleus-spinal cord co-cultures. *J Neurosci* 5:181–191.

Randle JCR, Bourque CW, Renaud LP (1986): Alpha-one adrenergic receptor activation depolarizes rat supraoptic neurosecretory neurons in vitro. *Am J Physiol* 251 (Regulatory Integrative Comp. Physiol. 20): R569–R574.

Segal M (1981): The action of norepinephrine in the rat hippocampus: Intracellular studies in the slice preparation. *Brain Res* 206:107–128.

Selyanko AA, Smith PA, Zidichouski JA (1990): Effects of muscarine and adrenaline on neurones from rana pipiens sympathetic ganglia. *J Physiol (Lond)* 425:471–500.

Seybold VS, Elde RP (1984): Receptor autoradiography in thoracic spinal cord: Correlation of neurotransmitter binding sites with sympathoadrenal neurons. *J Neurosci* 4:2533–2542.

Siggins GR, Hoffer BJ, Oliver AP, Bloom FE (1971): Activation of a central noradrenergic projection to cerebellum. *Nature* 233:481–483.

Taylor DG, Brody MJ (1976): Spinal adrenergic mechanisms regulating sympathetic outflow to blood vessels. *Circ Res* 38 (suppl II):10–20.

Williams JT, Henderson G, North RA (1985): Characterization of alpha two adrenoceptors which increase potassium conductance in rat locus coeruleus neurons. *Neuroscience* 14:95–101.

Williams JT, North RA (1985): Catecholamine inhibition of calcium action potentials in rat locus coeruleus neurons. *Neuroscience* 14:103–109.

Woodward DJ, Moises HC, Waterhouse BD, Hoffer BJ, Freedman R (1979): Modulatory actions of norepinephrine in the central nervous system. *Fed Proc* 38:2109–2116.

Yoshimura M, Higashi H, Nishi S (1985): Noradrenaline mediates slow excitatory synaptic potentials in rat dorsal raphé neurons in vitro. *Neurosci Lett* 61:305–1310.

Yoshimura M, Nishi S (1982): Intracellular recordings from lateral horn cells of the spinal cord in vitro. *J Auton Nerv Syst* 6:5–11.

Yoshimura M, Polosa C, Nishi S (1986a): Noradrenaline modifies sympathetic preganglionic neuron spike and afterpotetial. *Brain Res* 362:370–374.

Yoshimura M, Polosa C, Nishi S (1986b): Afterhyperpolarization mechanisms in cat sympathetic preganglionic neuron in vitro. *J Neurophysiol* 55:1234–1246.

Yoshimura M, Polosa C, Nishi S (1986c): Electrophysiological properties of sympathetic preganglionic neurons in the cat spinal cord in vitro. *Pflügers Arch* 406:91–98.

Yoshimura M, Polosa C, Nishi S (1987a): Noradrealine-induced afterdepolarization in cat sympathetic preganglionic neurons in vitro. *J Neurophysiol* 57:1314–1324.

Yoshimura M, Polosa C, Nishi S (1987b): Slow EPSP and the depolarizing action of noradrenaline on sympathetic preganglionic neurons. *Brain Res* 414:138–142.

Yoshimura M, Polosa C, Nishi S (1987c): Slow IPSP and noradrenaline-induced inhibition of the cat sympathetic preganglionic neuron in vitro. *Brain Res* 419:383–386.

Yoshimura M, Polosa C, Nishi S (1987d): Noradrenaline induces rhythmic bursting in sympathetic preganglionic neurons. *Brain Res* 420:147–151.

Yoshimura M, Polosa C, Nishi S (1987e): After depolarization mechanism in the in vitro, caesium-loaded, sympathetic preganglionic neuron of the cat. *J Neurophysiol* 57:1325–1337.

Yoshimura M, Polosa C, Nishi S (1987f): A transient outward rectification in the cat sympathetic preganglionic neuron. *Pflügers Arch* 408:207–208.

# 16
# Contribution of Forebrain Structures to the Development of Neurogenic Hypertension

JOHN CIRIELLO AND TING-XIN ZHANG

During the last three decades a considerable amount of experimental evidence has been obtained suggesting that an imbalance in the normal operation of the autonomic nervous system contributes to the development or maintenance of high blood pressure (Abboud, 1982; Brody et al., 1980; Ciriello, 1987; Reis, 1981). This suggestion is based primarily on the observation that a rise in sympathetic nerve activity, resulting from increased activity of central or peripheral components of the autonomic nervous system, is normally accompanied by an increase in vascular resistance, cardiac rate and output, renin release, and sodium retention; factors that have been shown to contribute to a chronic elevation in systemic arterial pressure (Abboud. 1982). Increases in sympathetic nervous system activity may result from several factors including decreased activity of inhibitory reflex pathways, increased activity of excitatory reflex pathways, or changes in the excitability of neurons in the central nervous system that are components of sympathoexcitatory or sympathoinhibitory pathways. Recently, it has been shown that the selective removal of the reflex inhibitory influences on central vasomotor neurons from aortic baroreceptor results in a persistent elevation in systemic arterial pressure (Ciriello et al., 1980; Fink et al., 1980, 1981; Ito and Scher, 1978, 1979; Kline et al., 1983; Krieger, 1964; Werber and Fink, 1981). This increased arterial pressure after selective deafferentation of aortic baroreceptors is associated with increased adrenergic activity to several peripheral organs, including the kidney (Fink et al., 1980; Kline et al., 1983; Patel et al., 1981; Werber et al., 1984). The sympathetic drive to the kidney has been shown to alter both renal blood vessels (Werber et al., 1984) and the release of renin (Ciriello et al., 1991; Zhang and Ciriello, 1990).

The observation that aortic baroreceptor deafferentation results in an increased plasma renin activity suggests the possibility that through the renin-angiotensin II system, central sympathoexcitatory pathways involved in the control of arterial pressure are activate and their increased activity contributes to the development of the chronic elevation in arterial pressure. The location and function of structures in the central nervous system responsible for the development and maintenance of the increased arterial pressure in this or other experimental models of hypertension are not well established. Supramedullary structures have been suggested to be necessary for the expression of the neurogenic hypertension following sinoaortic denervation or after lesions of the nucleus of the solitary tract (Doba and Reis, 1973; Mow et al., 1978; Reis and Cuenod, 1964), the primary site of termination of baroreceptor afferent fibers (Ciriello, 1983), as midcollicular decerebration or lesions of the region of the anteroventral third ventricle prevent the development of the hypertension. In addition, sinoaortic denervation has been shown to result in an increase in the metabolic activity in the paraventricular (PVH) and supraoptic nuclei of the hypothalamus (Ciriello et al., 1983). Furthermore, aortic baroreceptor deafferentation has been shown to be associated with increased activity of noradrenergic neurons in the hypothalamus (Patel et al., 1981).

This chapter summarizes data obtained in a series of experiments aimed at identifying the location and function of some forebrain structures involved in the development and maintenance of neurogenic hypertension as a result of the removal of baroreceptor inputs into central nervous system circuits controlling vasomotor tone. All studies reported here were done in conscious rats, and arterial pressure was measured using the indirect tail cuff method (Bunag and Butterfield, 1981).

## Identification of Forebrain Structures Associated with Neurogenic Hypertension

To identify the location of forebrain regions associated with the hypertension after aortic baroreceptor deafferentation, experiments were done using the hexokinase histochemical method (Simon et al., 1989; Turton et al., 1986). After control recordings of arterial pressure were taken the rats were subjected to either bilateral aortic depressor nerve (ADN) or sham denervation. The ADN in the rat has been shown to carry only aortic baroreceptor afferent information (Sapru et al., 1981; Sapru and Krieger, 1977). Three days after transection of the ADN (tADN) arterial pressure was elevated significantly by approximately 21 mm Hg compared with sham denervated animals. Increases in hexokinase activity were observed in the paraventricular nucleus of the hypothalamus, nucleus circularis, supraoptic nucleus, median preoptic nucleus, subfornical organ (SFO), and central nucleus of the amygdala (Fig. 16.1).

The most pronounced changes were observed in both the SFO and PVH. In the SFO the elevated metabolic activity was associated with both neurons and the surrounding neuropil, primarily in the ventral aspect of the structure.

The SFO is thought to be primarily involved in homeostatic mechanisms to maintain body fluid balance (Mangiapane and Simpson, 1980; Man-

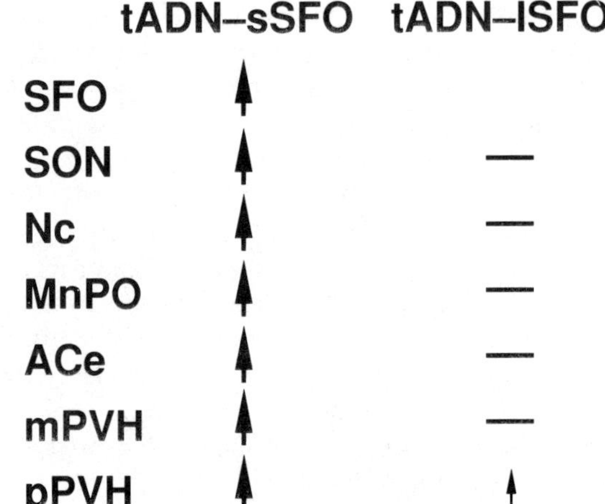


FIGURE 16.1. List of forebrain structures in which changes in the density of hexokinase reaction product were observed after tADN combined with either sham lesion or electrolytic lesion of the SFO. Note that in animals with lesions of the SFO (lSFO) changes in hexokinase activity were reversed to levels not different from control animals except in the parvocellular component of the PVH (pPVH), where it remained elevated compared to control but lower than in tADN-sham SFO (sSFO) animals. ACe: central nucleus of the amygdala; MnPO: median preoptic nucleus; mPVH: posterior magnocellular component of the PVH; Nc: nucleus circularis; SON: supraoptic nucleus.

giapane et al., 1984). In addition, this structure has been shown to be involved in mechanisms controlling arterial pressure in response to circulating levels of angiotensin II (ANG II) (Gutman et al., 1985, 1988; Mangiapane and Simpson, 1980). Injections of ANG II into the SFO and electrical or glutamate stimulation of SFO neurons have been shown to elicit increases in arterial pressure (Gutman et al., 1985; Mangiapane and Simpson, 1980) and the release of vasopressin (Ferguson and Kasting, 1986). As plasma renin activity has been shown to be elevated in rats after tADN (Ciriello et al., 1991; Zhang and Ciriello, 1990), the possibility exists that tADN results in an increased circulating level of ANG II that in turn acts at the SFO to activate a central neuronal circuit involved in the neural and humoral control of arterial pressure. It is interesting to note that the SFO has been shown to project directly to the PVH and several other forebrain structures (Miselis, 1981) shown in this study to have increased metabolic activity after tADN (Turton et al., 1986).

The increased metabolic activity in the PVH was localized to both the neurons and the neuropil surrounding these neurons throughout the dorsal and medial parvocellular and the posterior magnocellular components of the nucleus. The dorsal parvocellular component of the PVH has been shown to contain neurons that project directly to the intermediolateral cell column (Caverson et al., 1984; Swanson and Kuypers, 1980), the site of origin of sympathetic preganglionic axons (Rando et al., 1981). Electrical and chemical stimulation of the PVH has been shown to elicit increases in arterial pressure (Ciriello and Calaresu, 1980; Graham and Nelson, 1983; Porter and Brody, 1986) as a result of increased sympathetic activity and the increased release of vasopressin (Lawrence et al., 1984). Taken together, this evidence suggests that the increased metabolic activity observed in the parvocellular components of the PVH represents the increased activity of terminal axons, some of which likely originate in the SFO, and of paraventriculospinal neurons that contribute to the increase in arterial pressure after tADN. In addition, increase in metabolic activity

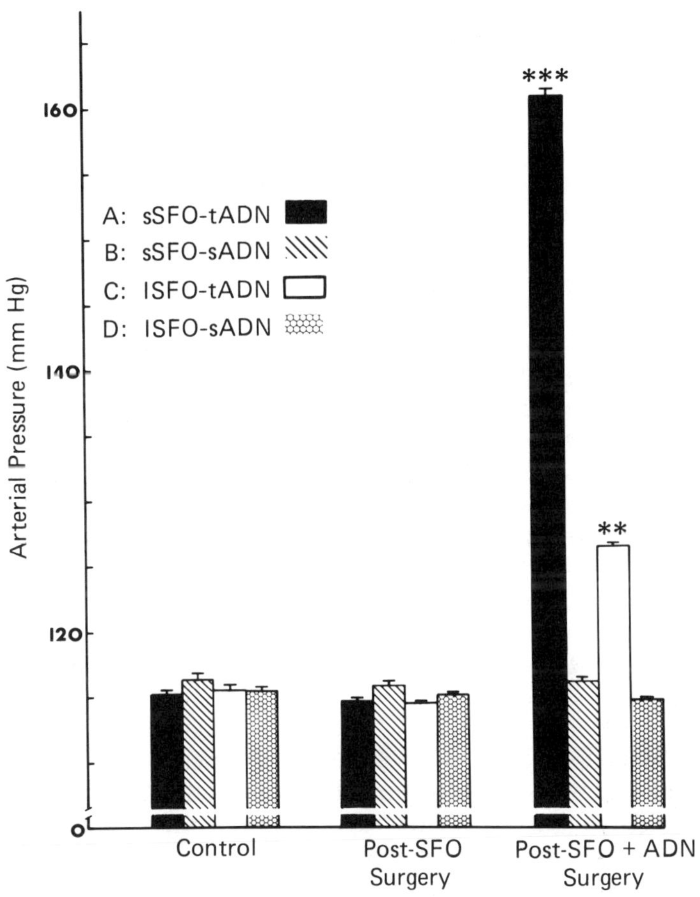


FIGURE 16.2. Histogram showing the effect of SFO lesions on arterial pressure when done before tADN. Note that the arterial pressure in the SFO lesioned (lSFO)-tADN animals does not increase to the same level as that in the sham SFO (sSFO) lesioned tADN animals.

was associated with magnocellular neurons in the posterior PVH. It was apparent that not all magnocellular neurons were activated, indicating a preferential effect on some neurons. This observation is consistent with the demonstration of increased circulating levels of vasopressin after tADN (Bond and Trank, 1970), which may also contribute to the elevated arterial pressure.

## Effect of Lesions of the Subfornical Organ on Neurogenic Hypertension

To investigate the contribution of the SFO to the development and maintenance of the increased arterial pressure resulting after tADN, two series of experiments were done (Caverson et al., 1986; Ciriello et al., 1986). In the first series, after control measurements of arterial pressure were taken, the rats were first subjected to either SFO lesions or sham SFO lesions and second to either bilateral or sham tADN. This was done to determine the contribution of this structure in the development of the hypertension resulting after tADN. Lesions of the SFO did not alter the resting level of arterial pressure. However, the arterial pressure ($161 \pm 2$ mm Hg) in the sham SFO lesioned tADN group was significantly higher than in the other three groups. In addition, arterial pressure in the SFO lesioned tADN rats ($128 \pm 1$ mm Hg) was significantly lower than in sham lesioned tADN rats, but significantly higher compared with SFO lesioned sham tADN ($115 \pm 1$ mm Hg) and sham SFO lesioned sham tADN rats ($117 \pm 1$ mm Hg). These data are summarized in Figure 16.2.

In the second series of experiments to determine the contribution of the SFO to the maintenance of the elevated arterial pressure after tADN, the rats were subjected to either bilateral or sham tADN. These animals were later subjected to either lesions of the SFO or sham lesions of the SFO. As shown in Figure 16.3 arterial pressure was significantly elevated in only the tADN group ($161 \pm 1$ mm Hg). Lesions of the SFO significantly reduced the arterial pressure ($129 \pm 1$ mm Hg) in the tADN animals to a level that remained significantly higher than sham tADN-sham SFO lesioned rats ($118 \pm 1$ mm Hg).

These data indicate that neurons in the SFO play a minor role in maintaining normotensive levels of arterial pressure in the conscious rat. On the other hand, the integrity of these neurons is essential for the development and maintenance of the elevated arterial pressure resulting after tADN. In addition, these data indicate that lesions of the SFO do not completely prevent or reverse the increase in arterial pressure, which suggests that other central or peripheral mechanisms are involved in the hypertensive process.

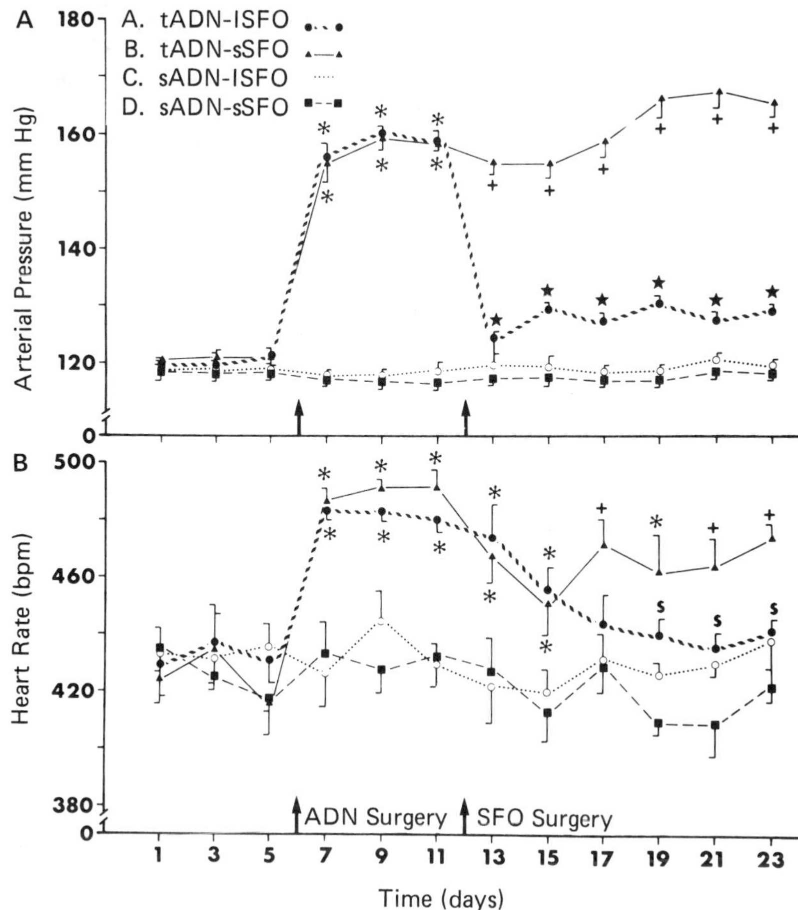


FIGURE 16.3.  **A**: Effect of lesions of the SFO on the arterial pressure and **B**: heart rate after bilateral tADN. Note that lesion of the SFO before tADN prevented the full expression of the hypertension observed in sham SFO lesioned tADN animals. Similarily, lesions of the SFO after tADN reduced the elevated arterial pressure.

# Effect of Subfornical Organ Lesions on Metabolic Activity of Forebrain Structure in Neurogenic Hypertension

To investigate the possibility that other forebrain structures may have contributed to the residual increase in arterial pressure in the tADN animals after lesions of the SFO by maintaining increased metabolic activity, at the completion of the second series of experiments, the brains of the rats were processed for hexokinase histochemistry. In the tADN-sham SFO lesioned rats increased metabolic activity compared to controls was observed in the same six forebrain structures previously described. The density of hexokinase reaction product in these forebrain structures in the normotensive control sham tADN-sham SFO lesioned animals was not altered compared to that in the sham tADN-SFO lesioned animals. On the other hand, lesions of the SFO significantly reduced the metabolic activity in all six structures in the tADN animals to levels not different from those observed in control animals, except for the dorsal parvocellular component of the PVH in which the metabolic activity was significantly reduced compared to tADN-sham SFO lesioned animals but remained significantly elevated compared to the sham tADN-sham SFO lesioned and sham tADN-SFO lesioned animals (Fig. 16.1).

These data, combined with those obtained in the previous study, suggest that parvocellular neurons in the dorsal component of the PVH, which are known to project directly to sympathetic preganglionic neurons in the intermediolateral cell column and to sympathetic premotor neurons in the ventrolateral medulla, likely contribute to the increase in arterial pressure remaining after lesions of the SFO in these neurogenic hypertensive animals.

## Effect of Lesions of the Paraventricular Nucleus of the Hypothalamus on Neurogenic Hypertension

On the basis of the hexokinase histochemical data showing increased metabolic activity in the PVH reported above, three series of experiments were done to investigate the contribution of the PVH in the development and maintenance of the hypertension resulting from tADN (Zhang and Ciriello, 1985a). In the first series, rats were subjected to either bilateral lesions of the PVH or sham PVH lesions and later to either bilateral or sham tADN. Lesions of the PVH did not alter resting level of arterial pressure in the conscious animal. However, arterial pressure in the tADN animals was significantly higher in the sham PVH lesioned rats compared with the PVH lesioned tADN, PVH lesioned sham tADN, and sham PVH lesioned sham tADN animals (Fig. 16.4).

In the second series, the rats were subjected to bilateral or sham tADN and later to bilateral or sham PVH lesions. Arterial pressure was significantly elevated in the tADN group only, compared to the other three groups (Fig. 16.5). Bilateral lesions of the PVH significantly reduced the arterial pressure in the tADN animals compared to tADN-sham PVH lesioned animals, to a level not significantly different from pre-tADN levels, and from sham tADN-PVH lesioned and sham tADN-sham PVH lesioned animals (Fig. 16.5).

Taken together, these data indicate that the elevated arterial pressure

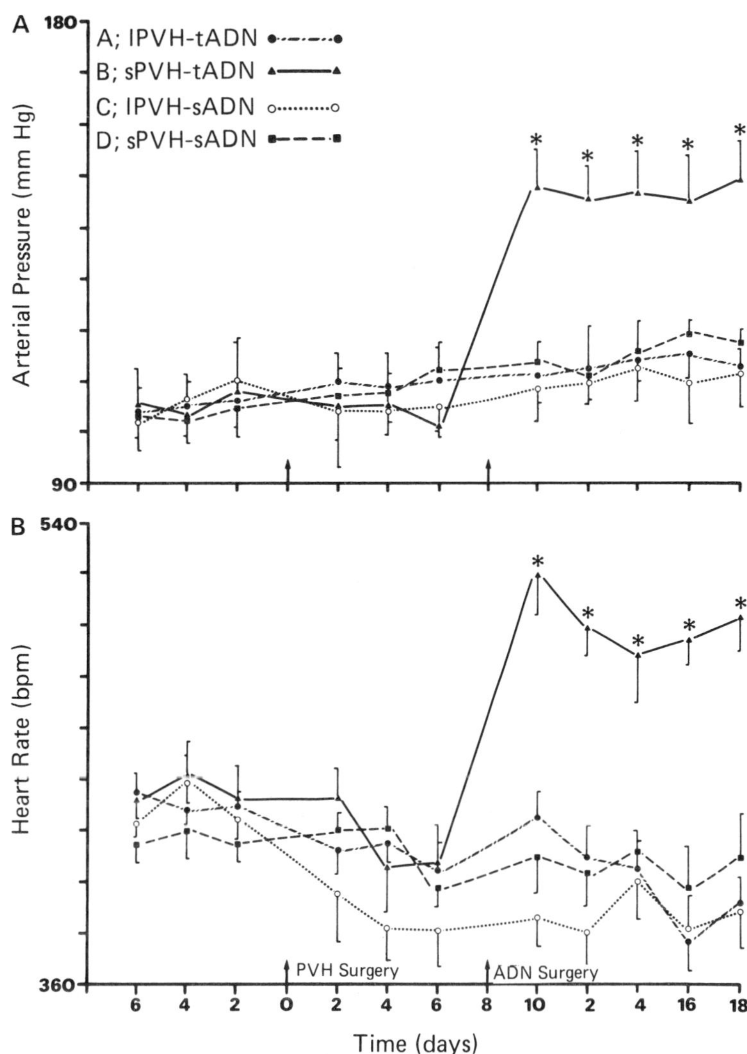


FIGURE 16.4. **A**: Effect of bilateral tADN on the arterial pressure and **B**: heart rate after bilateral PVH lesions. Lesions or sham lesions of the PVH were made on day 0 of the study and tADN or sham tADN was done on day 8. *: Significantly different from experimental groups A, C, and D. Note that the arterial pressure (A) was elevated only in group B when tADN was combined with sham PVH lesions and not in group A that was also subjected to tADN, but further subjected to PVH lesions. (Reproduced with permission from Zhang and Ciriello, 1985a.)

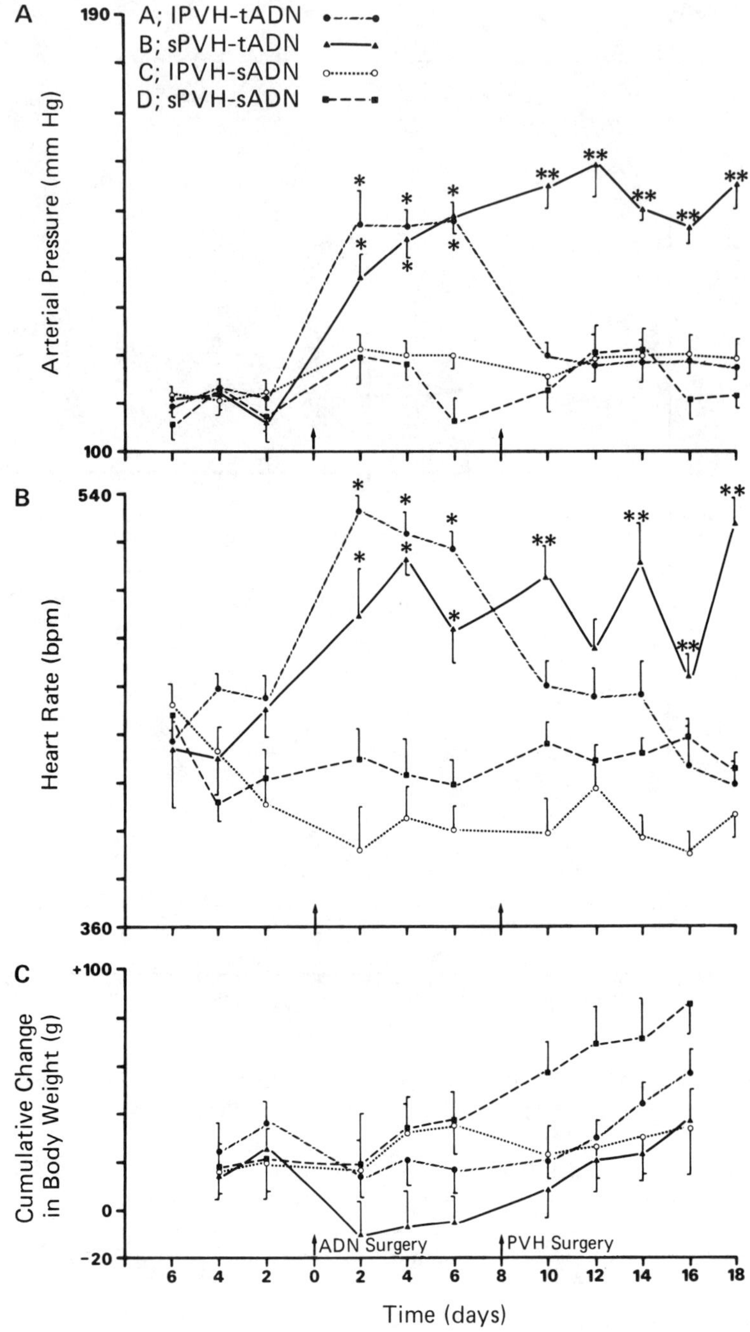

A; IPVH-tADN
B; sPVH-tADN
C; IPVH-sADN
D; sPVH-sADN
190
A
100
Arterial Pressure (mm Hg)
540
B
360
Heart Rate (bpm)
+100
C
0
-20
Cumulative Change
in Body Weight (g)
ADN Surgery
PVH Surgery
6  4  2  0  2  4  6  8  10  12  14  16  18
Time (days)

resulting after tADN is dependent on the integrity of neurons within the PVH. PVH neurons function in both the development and maintenance of the elevated arterial pressure, although these neurons appear to contribute little to normal resting levels of arterial pressure in the conscious animal. However, it remains to be determined whether magnocellular vasopressin-secreting or parvocellular sympathoexcitatory PVH neurons contribute to the hypertensive process.

In the third series of experiments parvocellular PVH neurons were selectively destroyed using the neurotoxin kainic acid (Zhang and Ciriello, 1985b). Following bilateral tADN in two groups of animals, arterial pressure was significantly elevated compared to sham tADN animals (Fig. 16.6). Bilateral microinjection of kainic acid into the PVH significantly reduced the elevated arterial pressure in tADN animals to a level not significantly different from either sham tADN animals that received PVH injections of kainic acid or from pre-tADN levels. However, as can be seen in Figure 16.6 there appears to be a general trend toward a small increase in arterial pressure several days after kainic acid microinjections into the PVH, although this rise in arterial pressure was not significant. As magnocellular neurosecretory neurons of the PVH have been shown to be resistant to the neurotoxic effects of kainic acid, these data indicate that parvocellular neurons in the PVH are components of sympathoexcitatory pathways and are required for the maintenance of the elevated arterial pressure. In addition, the trend toward an increase in arterial pressure following kainic acid lesions may represent an increase in the secretion of vasopressin into the circulation, which is known to be elevated after tADN (Bond and Trank, 1970).

## Conclusions

The neural and humoral components that are likely involved in the development and maintenance of the hypertension resulting after tADN are schematically summarized in Figure 16.7.

The data suggest that removal of the inhibitory reflex control exerted by

◁├─────────────────────────────────

FIGURE 16.5.  **A**: Effect of bilateral lesions of the PVH on the elevated arterial pressure and **B**: heart rate, and **C**: on the cumulative change in body weight after bilateral tADN. ADN surgery was done on day 0 (arrow) of the study and PVH surgery was done on day 8 (arrow). Control measurements were obtained for the 6 days before ADN surgery. *: Significantly different from experimental groups C and D but not from each other; **: Significantly different from groups A, C, and D. Note the increase in arterial pressure after tADN in groups A and B and the reversal of this change in group A after PVH lesions. (Reproduced with permission from Zhang and Ciriello, 1985a.)

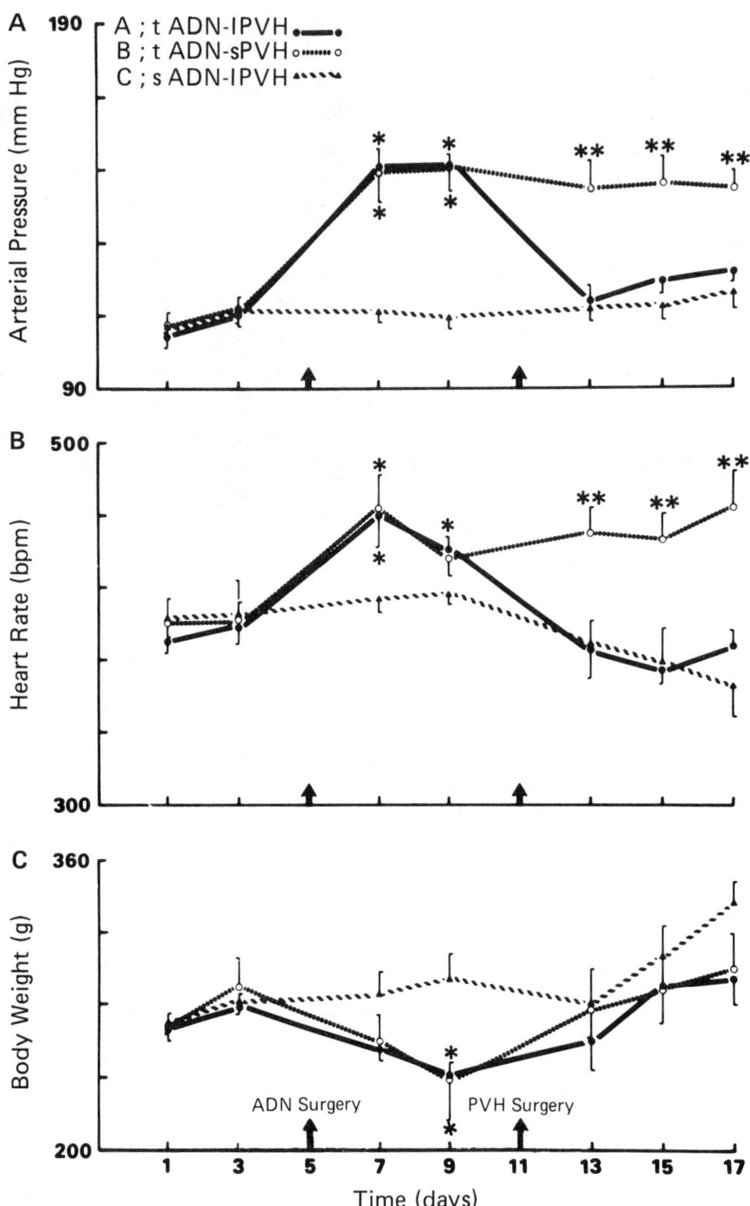



FIGURE 16.6. **A**: Effect of bilateral injections of kainic acid into the PVH on the elevated arterial pressure, **B**: heart rate, and **C**: on the body weight resulting after bilateral tADN. ADN surgery was done on day 5 of the study and PVH injections were made on day II. Control measurements were obtained for the 6 days before ADN surgery. Note the reversal of the increased arterial pressure (A) after injections of kainic acid into the PVH. *: Significantly different from experimental group C but not from each other; ** Significantly different from experimental groups A and C. (Reproduced with permission from Zhang and Cirielo, 1985b.)

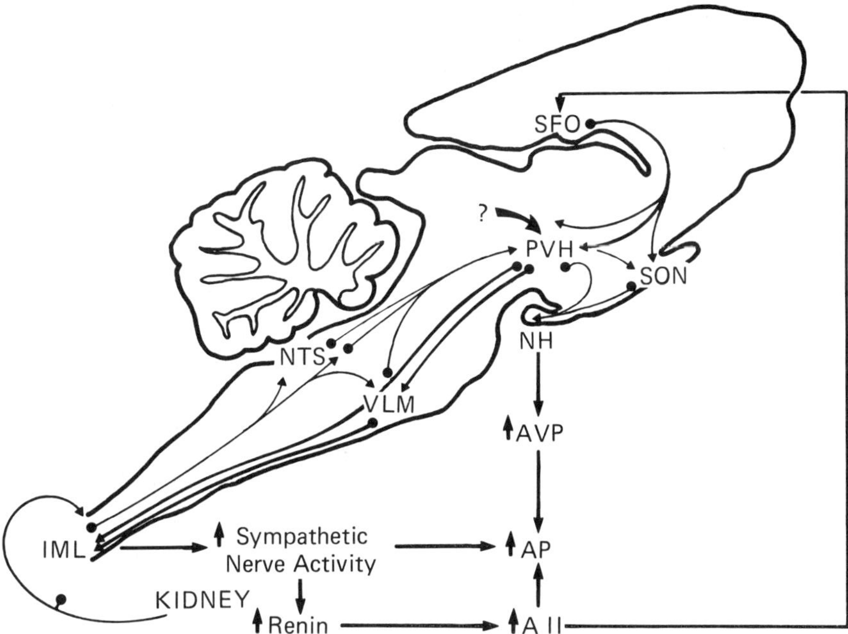


FIGURE 16.7. Schematic representation of the neural and humoral pathways that may be involved in the hypertensive process after tADN. AII: angiotensin II; Ace: central nucleus of the amygdala; AP: arterial pressure; AVP: arginine vasopressin; IML: intermediolateral nuclei; MnPO: median preoptic nucleus; Nc; nucleus circularis; NH: neurohypophysis; NTS: nucleus of the solitary tract; PVH: paraventricular nucleus of the hypothalamus; SFO: subfornical organ; SON: supraoptic nucleus; VLM: ventrolateral medulla.

aortic baroreceptors on magnocellular neurosecretory neurons in the PVH, supraoptic nucleus, and nucleus circularis, and on parvocellular neurons in the PVH and neurons of the central nucleus of the amygdala, results in a chronic elevation in arterial pressure as a result of increased vasopressin release from the neurohypophysis and increased sympathetic activity. The increased sympathetic activity mediated through either direct pathways to sympathetic preganglionic neurons, through a relay in the ventrolateral medulla or through both, would cause peripheral vasoconstriction and the release of renin, which in turn would produce vasoconstriction owing to increased circulating levels of ANG II. Blood-borne ANG II could also further activate sympathoexcitatory pathways and the release of vasopressin by stimulating the SFO, which in turn projects directly to PVH and supraoptic nucleus magnocellular neurons and PVH parvocellular neurons. This positive feedback circuit would continue to maintain the elevated arterial pressure even though carotid and cardiopulmonary baroreceptors reflex mechanisms, which remain in intact in this experimental model of hypertension, would contribute to restoring arterial pressure to normotensive levels. In fact, it has been demonstrated by Doba and Reis (1973) that these remaining inhibitory reflex mechanisms are essential for maintaining some control on this positive feedback circuit, as lesions of the nucleus of the solitary tract, which removes all baroreceptor feedback mechanisms, results in fulminating hypertension.

It is also interesting to note that lesions of the SFO did not completely return to elevated arterial pressure in the tADN animals to normotensive levels, whereas PVH lesions restored the arterial pressure to control levels. This finding suggests that there is at least one other mechanism that provides an excitatory drive to PVH parvocellular neurons and contributes to the hypertensive process. This excitatory input may originate in the kidney because it has been shown recently that activation of renal receptors elicits an increase in arterial pressure (Caverson and Ciriello, 1987; Patel and Knuepfer, 1986) due to the release of vasopressin (Caverson and Ciriello, 1987, 1988; Day and Ciriello, 1985, 1987; Simon and Ciriello, 1989) and activation of PVH sympathoexcitatory neurons (Caverson and Ciriello, 1987, 1988). In addition, similar forebrain structures have been shown to be associated with the hypertension after tADN and involved in the integration of afferent renal nerve inputs and that these sites of interaction may be involved in the maintenance and the reversal of the neurogenic hypertension (Simon et al., 1989).

*Acknowledgment*. This work was supported by the Heart and Stroke Foundation of Ontario. Dr. J. Ciriello is a Career Investigator of the Heart and Stroke Foundation of Ontario.

# References

Abboud FM (1982): The sympathetic system in hypertension. *Hypertension (Dallas)* 4(suppl II):II-208–II-225.

Bond GC, Trank JW (1970): Effect of bilateral aortic nerve section on plasma ADH titer *Physiologist* 13:152 (Abstract).

Brody MJ, Haywood JR, Touw KB (1980): Neural mechanisms in hypertension. *Annu Rev Physiol* 42:441–453.

Bunag RD, Butterfield J (1981): Tail cuff pressure measurement without external preheating in awake rats. *Hypertension (Dallas)* 4:898–903.

Caverson MM, Ciriello J (1987): Effect of stimulation of afferent renal nerves on plasma levels of vasopressin. *Am J Physiol* 252:R801–R807.

Caverson MM, Ciriello J (1988): Contribution of paraventricular nucleus to afferent renal nerve pressor response. *Am J Physiol* 254:R531–R543.

Caverson MM, Ciriello J, Calaresu FR (1984): Paraventricular nucleus of the hypothalamus: an electrophysiological investigation of neurons projecting directly to intermediolateral nucleus in the cat. *Brain Res* 305:380–383.

Caverson MM, Macchi A, Ciriello J (1986): Subfornical organ (SFO) lesions alter the development of hypertension resulting after aortic baroreceptor denervation in the rat. *Proc Fed Am Soc Exp Biol* 45:876 (Abstract).

Ciriello J (1983): Brainstem projections of aortic baroreceptor afferent fibers in the rat. *Neurosci Lett* 36:37–42.

Ciriello J (1987): Forebrain mechanisms in neurogenic hypertension. *Can J Physiol Pharmacol* 65:1580–1583.

Ciriello J, Calaresu F R (1980): Role of paraventricular and supraoptic nuclei in central cardiovascular regulation in the cat. *Am J Physiol* 239:R137–R142.

Ciriello J, Macchi A, Caverson MM (1986): Lesions of the subfornical organ (SFO) attenuate the increase in arterial pressure after aortic baroreceptor denervation. *Proc Fed Am Soc Exp Biol* 45:876 (Abstract).

Ciriello J, Palmer EMJ, Calaresu FR (1980): Arterial pressure and heart rate in the rat after section of the aortic depressor or the carotid sinus nerves. *Proc Can Fed Biol Soc* 23:103 (Abstract).

Ciriello J, Rohlicek CV, Polosa C (1983): Aortic baroreceptor reflex pathway: A functional mapping using [$^3$H] 2-deoxyglucose autoradiography in the rat. *Auton Nerv Syst* 8:111–128.

Ciriello J, Simon JK, Mercer PF (1991): Effect of renal denervation on plasma renin activity after aortic baroreceptor deafferentation. *Can J Physiol Pharmacol* (in press).

Day TA, Ciriello J (1985): Afferent renal nerve stimulation excites supraoptic vasopressin neurons. *Am J Physiol* 249:R368–R371.

Day TA, Ciriello J (1987): Effects of renal receptor activation on neurosecretory vasopressin cells. *Am J Physiol* 253:R234–R241.

Doba N, Reis DJ (1973): Acute fulminating neurogenic hypertension produced by brainstem lesions in the rat. *Circ Res* 32:584–593.

Ferguson AV, Kasting NW (1986): Electrical stimulation in subfornical organ increases plasma vasopressin concentration in the conscious rat. *Am J Physiol* 251:R425–R428.

Fink GD, Bryan WJ, Mann M, Osbom J, Weiber A (1981): Continuous blood pressure measurement in rats with aortic baroreceptor deafferentation. *Am J Physiol* 241:H268–H272.

Fink GD, Kennedy F, Bryan WJ, Werber A (1980): Pathogenesis of hypertension in rats with chronic aortic baroreceptor deafferentation. *Hypertension (Dallas)* 2:319–325.

Graham CA, Nelson DO (1983): Effects of stimulation of paraventricular nucleus on arterial pressure. *Proc Fed Am Soc Exp Biol* 42:584 (Abstract).

Gutman MB, Ciriello J, Mogenson GJ (1985): Effect of paraventricular nucleus lesions on cardiovascular responses elicited by stimulation of the subfornical organ in the rat. *Can J Physiol Pharmacol* 63:816–824.

Gutman MB, Ciriello J, Mogenson GJ (1988): Effect of plasma angiotensin II and hypernatremia on subfornical organ neurons. *Am J Physiol* 254:R746–R754.

Ito CS, Scher AM (1978): Regulation of arterial blood pressure by aortic baroreceptors in the unanesthetized dog. *Circ Res* 42:230–236.

Ito CS, Scher AM (1979): Hypertension following denervation of aortic baroreceptor in unanesthetized dogs. *Circ Res* 45:26–34.

Kline RL, Patel KP, Ciriello J, Mercer PF (1983): Effect of renal denervation on arterial pressure in rats with aortic nerve transection. *Hypertension (Dallas)* 5:468–475.

Krieger EM (1964): Neurogenic hypertension in the rat. *Circ Res* 15:511–521.

Lawrence D, Ciriello J, Pittman QJ, Lederis K (1984): The effect of the vasopressin antagonist d(CH₂)5 d Tyre-VAVP on the cardiovascular responses to stimulation of the paraventricular nucleus. *Proc West Pharmacol Soc* 27:15–17.

Mangiapane ML, Simpson JB (1980): Subfornical organ: forebrain site of pressor and dipsogenic action of angiotensin II. *Am J Physiol* 239:R382–R389.

Mangiapane ML, Thrasher TN, Keil LC, Simpson JB, Ganong WF (1984): Role of the subfornical organ in vasopressin release. *Brain Res Bull* 13:43–47.

Miselis RR (1981): The efferent projections of the subfornical organ of the rat: A circumventricular organ within a neural network subserving water balance. *Brain Res* 230:1–23.

Mow MT, Haywood JR, Johnson AK, Brody MJ (1978): The role of the antero-ventral third ventricle (AV3V) in development of neurogenic hypertension. *Soc Neurosci Abstr* 4:23.

Patel KP, Ciriello J, Kline RL (1981): Noradrenergic mechanisms in brain and peripheral organs after aortic nerve transection. *Am J Physiol* 240:H481–H486.

Patel KP, Knuepfer MM (1986): Effect of afferent renal nerve stimulation on blood pressure, heart rate and noradrenergic activity in conscious rats. *J Auton Nerv Syst* 17:121–130.

Porter JP, Brody MJ (1986): A comparison of the hemodynamic effects produced by electrical stimulation of subnuclei of the paraventricular nucleus. *Brain Res* 375:20–29.

Rando TA, Bowers CW, Zigmond RE (1981): Localization of neurons in the rat spinal cord which project to the superior cervical ganglion. *J Comp Neurol* 196:73–83.

Reis DJ (1981): The brain and arterial hypertension: Evidence for a neural-imbalance hypothesis. In *Disturbances in Neurogenic Control of Circulation*. Abboud FM, Fozzard HA, Gilmore JP, Reis RJ, Bethesda: Am. Physiol. Soc., pp 87–104.

Reis DJ, Cuenod M (1964): Tonic influence of rostral brain structures on pressure regulating mechanisms in cat. *Science* 145:64–65.

Sapru HN, Gonzalez E, Krieger AJ (1981): Aortic nerve stimulation in the rat: Cardiovascular and respiratory responses. *Brain Res Bull* 6:393–398.

Sapru HN, Krieger AJ (1977): Carotid and aortic chemoreceptor functions in the rat. *J Appl Physiol* 42:344–348.

Simon, JK, Ciriello J (1989): Contribution of afferent renal nerves to the metabolic activity of central structures involved in the control of the circulation. *Can J Physiol Pharmacol* 67:1130–1139.

Simon JK, Zhang TX, Ciriello J (1989): Renal denervation alters forebrain hexaki-nase activity in neurogenic hypertensive rats. *Am J Physiol* 256:R930–R938.

Swanson LW, Kuypers HGJM (1980): The paraventricular nucleus of the hypotha-lamus: cytoarchitectonic subdivisions and organization of projections to the pituitary, dorsal vagal complex and spinal cord as demonstrated by retrograde fluorescent double labelling methods. *J Comp Neurol* 194:555–570.

Turton WE, Ciriello J, Calaresu FR (1986): Changes in forebrain hexokinase activ-ity after aortic baroreceptor denervation. *Am J Physiol* 251:R274–R281.

Werber AH, Bryan WJ, Fink GD (1984): Hemodynamic and neural mechanisms of acute neurogenic hypertension in the rat. *Am J Physiol* 247:H991–H998.

Werber AH, Fink GD (1981): Cardiovascular and body fluid changes after aortic baroreceptor deafferentation.

Zhang TX, Ciriello J (1985a): Effect of paraventricular nucleus lesions on arterial pressure and heart rate after aortic baroreceptor denervation in the rat. *Brain Res* 341:101–109.

Zhang TX, Ciriello J (1985b): Kainic acid lesions of paraventricular nucleus neurons reverse the elevated arterial pressure after aortic baroreceptor denervation in the rat. *Brain Res* 358:334–338.

Zhang TX, Ciriello J (1990): Effect of paraventricular nucleus of the hypothalamus on plasma renin activity in neurogenic hypertension. *Soc Neurosci Abstr* 16:638.

# 17
# Mechanisms of Differential Cardiovascular Responsiveness to 2-Deoxyglucose–Induced Central Glycopenia in Conscious Spontaneously Hypertensive and Wistar Kyoto Rats

OLEG S. MEDVEDEV, ALEXANDER I. KUZMIN, VLADIMIR N. SELIVANOV, MICHAEL B. BOGDANOV, OLGA A. TJURMINA, ARARAT D. GJULUMJAN, AND AZIZUL M. HOQUE

It is well established that a variety of emotional stresses provoke release of catecholamines from the sympathoadrenal medullary system (Cannon, 1929; Kvetnansky et al., 1979), but the relationship between stress, adrenal catecholamines, and high blood pressure remains controversial.

According to the "adrenaline hypothesis" of hypertension (Majewski and Rand, 1986; Majewski et al., 1982), repeated exposures to stressful stimuli increase the release of epinephrine from the adrenal glands, which can then activate presynaptic beta$_2$-adrenoceptors and, consequently, facilitate the release of norepinephrine from the sympathetic terminals (Adler-Graschinsky and Langer, 1975).

Evidence supporting this hypothesis has been presented along two lines. First, chronic epinephrine treatment led to an accumulation of epinephrine in peripheral tissues and to development of hypertension in rats (Johnson et al., 1983; Majewski et al., 1981a,b; Schwartz and Eikenburg, 1986). Second, it was shown that epinephrine can activate prejunctional beta–adrenoceptors on sympathetic terminals to enhance norepinephrine release either directly (Stjärne and Brundin, 1975) or after its uptake into sympathetic nerve transmitter stores and its release as a co-transmitter (Majewski et al., 1981c). However, a critical issue that has not been explored is whether experimental hypertension develops as a consequence of increased endogenous epinephrine secretion.

A number of substances like insulin (Holzbauer and Vogt, 1954), 2-deoxy-D-glucose (2-DG) (Hokfeld and Bydgeman, 1961), or fusaric acid (Racz et al., 1985) cause pronounced increases in the concentration of epinephrine in peripheral blood. To test the adrenaline hypothesis of hypertension, we studied the effects of the administration of 2-DG in normotensive Wistar Kyoto (WKY) rats and spontaneously hypertensive rats (SHR).

2-DG induces central nervous system (CNS) glucoprivation because of the competitive inhibition of glucose transport and phosphohexoisomerase activity (Brown, 1962; McDougal et al., 1990). This activates hypothalamic-glucosensitive centers (Smithe et al., 1984) which, in turn, stimulate the sympathetic discharge to the adrenal gland (Katafuchi et al., 1985; Medvedev et al., 1988a, Niijima, 1975). Stimulation of the adrenal medulla leads to increased epinephrine secretion (Hokfeld and Bydgeman, 1961). Thus, 2-DG causes increased epinephrine secretion via efferent nervous pathways, which is similar to the increased epinephrine secretion triggered by stress stimuli. It has also been shown that repeated administration of 2-DG leads to an increase in arterial blood pressure (Medvedev et al., 1989). Mechanisms of 2-DG–induced hypertension, therefore, seem to be different from the mechanisms proposed by the authors of the adrenaline hypothesis of hypertension (Majewski and Rand, 1986).

The aims of our study were to clarify in more detail the endocrine and hemodynamic mechanisms of 2-DG action in awake normotensive animals, to investigate 2-DG–induced responses in SHR and in normotensive WKY rats.

## 2-DG–Induced Changes in Plasma Catecholamine Concentrations

Intravenous (i.v.) administration 2-DG (500 mg/kg) to awake WKY rats resulted in a significant increase in plasma epinephrine and norepinephrine concentrations determined by high performance liquid chromatography (HPLC) with electrochemical detection (Medvedev et al., 1988b; 1989). Within 15 and 40 min of 2-DG injection epinephrine and norepinephrine concentrations were increased 15-fold and 1.7-fold, respectively. Similar changes have been observed by others in rats (Amann and Lembeck, 1986; Okajima et al., 1984; Sun et al., 1979) and in humans (Thompson et al., 1981). On average, plasma epinephrine concentration increased by 2.2 to 2.5 ng/ml in our experiments as a response to 2-DG administration (Medvedev et al., 1989). The same increase in plasma epinephrine levels was observed in rats during the i.v. infusion of epinephrine at the rate of 400 ng/kg/min (Zabludowski et al., 1984). The intensity of adrenal gland stimulation by 500 mg/kg 2-DG is rather strong, since 3 hours after its administration the epinephrine content in the gland is decreased by 64% (Amann and Lembeck, 1986).

A common conclusion of all the papers cited above is the ability of 2-DG to stimulate the release of epinephrine from the adrenal medulla. The mechanism of interrelationship between the high plasma levels of epinephrine and norepinephrine remains unclear. According to the authors of the adrenaline hypothesis of hypertension, epinephrine released from the adrenal medulla acts as an appropriate stimulus for prejunctional beta-adrenoceptors to enhance nerve stimulation-induced release of norepinephrine (Majewski and Rand, 1986). However, it has not been demonstrated convincingly that physiological levels of epinephrine will modulate norepinephrine release either in intact animals or in humans. Physiological concentrations of circulating epinephrine did not facilitate nerve stimulation-evoked overflow of norepinephrine in canine bloodperfused muscle (Kahan et al., 1987). Alternative explanations of the 2-DG–evoked increase in norepinephrine plasma concentration might be that 1) the higher level of norepinephrine is a consequence of increased secretion of this catecholamine by the adrenal medulla, 2) it is a result of an increased firing of sympathetic neurons, or 3) it is the result of altered clearance of norepinephrine from plasma. In the following studies we attempted to differentiate between these three possible mechanisms.

Norepinephrine plasma kinetics were measured in awake rabbits according to the method described by Esler et al. (1988). We found that despite of the small decrease in plasma clearance of norepinephrine (from $76.9 \pm 4.1$ to $66.3 \pm 2.7$ ml/kg/min), the increase in norepinephrine concentration depended mainly on the increase of its release from $20.5 \pm 2.5$ to $38.6 \pm 6.2$ ng kg/min during 2-DG–induced central glucopenia (Medvedev et al., 1990).

Plasma dihydroxyphenylglycol (DHPG), the deaminated metabolite of norepinephrine, can provide information about sympathetic nervous activity, as an alternative to estimates based on plasma norepinephrine kinetics. Since DHPG is produced within noradrenergic neurons, its plasma concentrations relative to those of norepinephrine provide information about neuronal reuptake of norepinephrine, the principal means of terminating the actions of the neurotransmitter at the nerve terminal (Eisenhofer et al., 1988). Plasma concentrations of DHPG increased significantly ($p<0.01$) from $815 \pm 110$ to $1560 \pm 280$ pg/ml during 2-DG–induced glucopenia in awake rabbits (Medvedev et al., 1990). In response to 2-DG, the plasma DHPG response was $201 \pm 25\%$ of the noradrenaline response, significantly more than during nitroprusside-induced hypotension, where the plasma DHPG response was only $79 \pm 15\%$ of the noradrenaline response. The results of the experiments on awake rabbits established that 2-DG–induced changes in norepinephrine release to plasma were predominantly of sympathetic neuronal origin rather than from the adrenal medulla.


## 2-DG–Induced Changes in Systemic and Regional Hemodynamics

2-DG administration (500 mg/kg, i.v.) resulted in a significant decrease in blood pressure in WKY rats by $4.5 \pm 1.3$ mm Hg. Heart rate decreased by $101 \pm 10$ beats/min. Cardiac output was increased by 20%, as determined by an ultrasound Doppler device (the probe was implanted on the ascending aorta) (Medvedev et al., 1989). In a separate group of seven rats, the

TABLE 17.1. 2-DG–induced (500 mg/kg) changes in the regional hemodynamic in the conscious WKY rats (n = 10).

| Organs | 2-DG–induced % change in blood flow | | |
| --- | --- | --- | --- |
| | Baseline blood flow (ml/min/gm) | After 15 min | After 40 min |
| Skin | $0.24 \pm 0.03$ | $-13.2 \pm 9.3$ | $-21.3 \pm 6.2$ |
| Muscles | $0.23 \pm 0.05$ | $-35 + 10.5$[a] | $-38.8 \pm 14.5$[a] |
| Brain | $1.98 \pm 0.18$ | $105.3 \pm 16.2$[b] | $-11.8 \pm 8.3$ |
| Intestine | $3.04 \pm 0.30$ | $72.3 \pm 17.8$[a] | $84.8 \pm 18.6$[a] |
| Spleen | $2.34 \pm 0.37$ | $30.8 \pm 23.3$ | $150.5 \pm 43.5$[a] |
| Heart | $7.94 \pm 1.04$ | $53.9 \pm 12.1$[a] | $92.5 \pm 21.8$[a] |
| Kidney | $6.74 \pm 0.62$ | $6.0 \pm 7.5$ | $23.9 \pm 13.8$ |
| Adrenal glands | $4.70 \pm 0.42$ | $114.6 \pm 20.5$[b] | $131.0 \pm 18.6$[b] |

[a] $p < 0.05$.
[b] $p < 0.01$ when compared with the resting values.

2-DG–mediated decrease in heart rate was blocked completely by atropine sulphate (1 mg/kg i.v.), suggesting that increased vagal activity was the main cause of the bradycardia.

2-DG–induced changes in regional hemodynamics were measured in awake WKY rats with the microsphere technique as described previously (Medvedev and Hoque, 1986). It was shown that after 15 min of 2-DG administration, blood flow was increased in the brain, heart, adrenal gland, stomach, intestine, liver, and spleen whereas blood flow decreased in muscle, skin, diaphragm muscle and testis (Table 17.1).

To our knowledge, this is the first study in which 2-DG–induced changes in cardiac output and regional hemodynamics have been demonstrated in the conscious rat. High levels of plasma epinephrine may be reponsible for the elevation of cardiac output since epinephrine increases cardiac contractility and venous return. The hemodynamic response to 2-DG–induced metabolic stress closely resembles the response to natural stressful stimuli. The 2-DG–induced increase in cardiac output is similar to the increase in cardiac output caused by restraint stress (Medvedev et al., 1986) or transfer of a rat from its home cage to a new one (Iriuchijima and Teranishi, 1982). High plasma epinephrine concentrations can also cause dilatation of brain blood vessels and an increase in brain blood flow (Iadecola et al., 1986).

## 2-DG–Induced Changes in the Activity of Sympathomedullary System in SHR and WKY Rats

2-DG was administered intravenously (500 mg/kg) into conscious unrestrained male SHR and WKY rats. One and a half milliliters of blood was withdrawn through an arterial catheter; this volume was replaced by an equal amount of blood from a conscious donor rat of the same strain. Details of the HPLC determination of catecholamines were described previously (Medvedev et al., 1989).

2-DG–induced changes in plasma catecholamines are presented in Figure 17.1. Baseline values for norepinephrine were 381 ± 66 and 481 ± 121 pg/ml in WKY and SHR rats, respectively. Resting concentrations of epinephrine were 281 ± 80 and 512 ± 122 pg/ml, respectively. As shown in Figure 17.1, at 15 and 45 min after 2-DG injection, the percent changes in SHR plasma norepinephrine and epinephrine levels were half the percent changes in WKY rats. The higher resting levels of plasma epinephrine in SHR compared with WKY rats, as determined in our study , are in good agreement with the results of Sato et al. (1986), who demonstrated increased basal firing rates in single fibers of efferent adrenal nerves and increased secretion rates of catecholamines from the adrenal gland in SHR rats.

Sympathetic responses to 2-DG administration were analyzed in SHR and WKY rats by recording renal sympathetic nerve activity. Rats were initially anesthetized with methohexital sodium (Brietal, Lilly) 75 mg/kg body weight intraperitoneally. The right jugular vein was cannulated. Arterial blood pressure was measured by means of a Statham 23 DC pressure transducer, connected to a PE-50 catheter in the right femoral artery or in the tail artery. Heart rate was measured from the pulse pressure by means of a rate meter.

Sympathetic nerve activity was recorded from the renal nerve (renSNA) with a thin stainless steel electrode. When an optimal recording was achieved, the nerve and the electrode were isolated with silicone rubber (SilGel 604, Wacker), as described by Ricksten and Thoren (1980). The electrode wires and the arterial and venous catheters were tunneled under the skin and exteriorized on the back of the neck. The renSNA was amplified (Grass P 511) and displayed on an oscilloscope. The signal was also

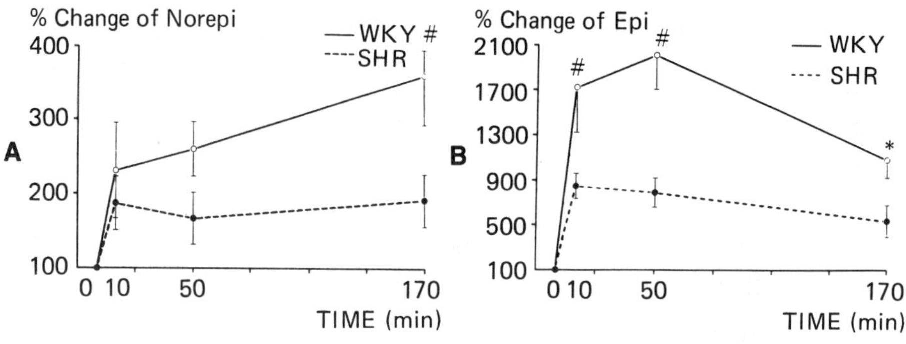


FIGURE 17.1. Percent changes of **A**: norepinephrine and **B**: epinephrine concentrations in blood during i.v. administration of 2-DG (500 mg/kg) in SHR and WKY rats.

TABLE 17.2. Sympathetic renal nerve activity responses to 2-DG administration into the awake SHR and WKY rats.

| | WKY rats (n = 6) | SHR rats (n = 8) |
|---|---|---|
| Baseline | 100 | 100 |
| *After 125 mg/kg i.v. 2-DG administration* | | |
| 5 min | $-9.2 \pm 3.5$ | $+4.4 \pm 8.9$ |
| 15 min | $-2.5 \pm 3.1$ | $+4.3 \pm 8.2$ |
| *After additional 375 mg/kg i.v. 2-DG administration* | | |
| 5 min | $-2.5 \pm 3.1$ | $+29.9 \pm 6.7$[b][d] |
| 15 min | $+20.8 \pm 8.6$[a] | $+33.3 \pm 13.8$[a] |

Values are means $\pm$ SEM
[a] $p < 0.05$.
[b] $p < 0.01$, when compared with respective baseline values.
[c] $p < 0.05$.
[d] $p < 0.01$, when compared with respective WKY group values.

rectified and the average rectified signal was recorded on a Grass polygraph (model 7) together with the mean arterial pressure and heart rate. The post mortem signal was recorded 45 to 60 min after death in all animals as a measure of the noise level, which was then subtracted from the mean rectified signal recorded in the living animal.

2-DG–induced changes in renSNA are presented in Table 17.2. Renal nerve activity had a tendency to decrease in WKY rats after injection of the first dose of 2-DG (125 mg/kg). Five min after injection of a dose of 375 mg/kg to provide a cumulative dose of 2-DG of 500 mg/kg, renSNA was significantly higher in SHR than in WKY rats.

## 2-DG–Induced Hemodynamic Changes in SHR and WKY Rats

2-DG administration ($125 + 375$ mg/kg, i.v.) led to a more prominent blood pressure increase in conscious SHR than in WKY rats. The results of the experiments are given in Table 17.3.

2-DG–evoked pressor response in normotensive WKY rats mainly depends on the increase in cardiac output (Medvedev et al., 1989). One of the factors influencing cardiac output is the venous tone. An increase in venous tone alone can increase venous return and thereby increase cardiac output (Greenway, 1982). Because little is known about the effect of 2-DG on total body venous tone in conscious animals, we performed a series of experiments in SHR and WKY rats in an attempt to answer this question.

One method available to assess total body venous tone is the determination of mean circulatory filling pressure (MCFP) (Guyton et al., 1973).

TABLE 17.3. Blood pressure responses to 2-DG administration into awake SHR and WKY rats.

| | Mean arterial pressure (mm Hg) | |
| | SHR (n = 14) | WKY (n = 6) |
| --- | --- | --- |
| Baseline | 144.4 ± 2.45 | 115.0 ± 1.8 |
| *Changes after 125 mg/kg i.v. 2-DG administration* | | |
| 5 min | −2.6 ± 1.73 | −0.3 ± 1.5 |
| 15 min | −1.8 ± 2.65 | +0.6 ± 1.6 |
| *After additional 375 mg/kg i.v. 2-DG administration* | | |
| 5 min | +9.1 ± 2.76[a] | +4.2 ± 1.8 |
| 15 min | +20.2 ± 4.72[a] | +2.0 ± 1.3[b] |

Values are means ± SEM.
[a]$p < 0.01$, when compared with baseline values.
[b]$p < 0.05$, when compared with the response in SHR group.

MCFP is a function of blood volume, unstressed vascular volume, and venous and arterial compliances. However, venous compliance is many times greater than arterial compliance (Guyton et al., 1973), and therefore has a correspondingly greater influence on MCFP. Thus, at a given blood volume, MCFP should reflect mostly venous rather than arterial tone.

MCFP was determined in conscious SHR and WKY rats according to Yamamoto et al., (1980). Briefly, the circulation is stopped for 5 to 6 sec of the inflation of a balloon-tipped catheter introduced into the right atrium through the external jugular vein. By injecting 0.3 ml of saline into the balloon all blood flow through the right atrium could be stopped, thereby completely arresting the circulation. Arterial blood pressure and central venous pressure were measured during the experiment.

Baseline values of the MCFP in SHR and WKY rats were 9.29 ± 0.20 and 7.43 ± 0.24 mm HG, respectively. Similar MCFP values were found in SHR (9.5 ± 0.3 mm Hg) by Trippodo et al. (1981).

Administration of 500 mg/kg of 2-DG did not change MCFP in SHR, but significantly increased MCFP in the WKY rats (Fig. 17.2). However, as control MCFD values showed a time-dependent decline in SHR, values obtained in 2 DG treated SHR were significantly higher than control values at the later time points (60–120 min) (Fig. 17.2).

The 2-DG–evoked increase in MCFP in WKY rats correlates well with the increase in cardiac output observed in the same animals. The absence of 2-DG–induced changes in MCFP in SHR argues against a possible increase in cardiac output in these animals. As the pressor response to 2-DG was greater in SHR than in WKY rats, we assume that in SHR the pressor response is mainly caused by the increase in peripheral vascular resistance. The more prominent response of the sympathetic nerve activity to 2-DG in SHR than in WKY rats also supports this possibility.

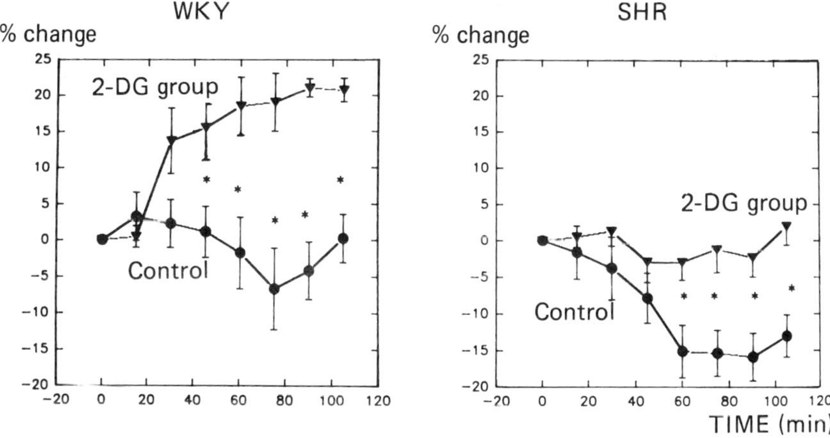


FIGURE 17.2. 2-DG–induced changes in MCFP in awake SHR and WKY rats.

## Conclusions

1. Experimental 2-DG–induced central neuroglycopenia evokes pressor response in SHR but does not alter (or slightly decreases) arterial pressure in WKY rats.

2. The pressor response to 2-DG in SHR is due, primarily, to an increase in sympathetic nerve activity.

## References

Adler-Graschinsky E, Langer S (1975): Possible role of a beta-adrenoceptor in the regulation of noradrenaline release by nerve stimulation through a positive feedback mechanism. *Br J Pharmacol* 53:43–50.

Amann R, Lembeck (1986): Capsaicin sensitive afferent neurons from peripheral glucose receptors mediate the insuline-induced increase in adrenaline secretion. *Naunyn-Schmiedeberg's Arch Pharmacol* 334:71–76.

Brown J (1962): Effects of 2-deoxyglucose on carbohydrate metabolism: Review of the literature and studies in the rat. *Metabolism* 11:1098–1112.

Cannon W (1929): *Bodily Changes in Pain, Hunger, Fear and Rage*. New York: WW Norton.

Eisenhofer G, Goldstein D, Ropchak T, Nguyen H, Keiser H, Kopin I (1988): Source and physiological significance of plasma 3,4-dihydroxyphenylglycol and 3-methoxy-4-hydroxyphenylglycol. *J Auton Nerv Sys* 24:1–14.

Esler M, Jennings G, Korner P, Willet I, Dudley F, Hasking G, Anderson W, Lambert G (1988): Assessment of human sympathetic nervous system activity from measurements of norepinephrine turnover. *Hypertension* 11:3–20.

Greenway C (1982): Mechanism and quantitative assessment of drug effects on cardiac output with a new model of the circulation. *Pharmacol Rev* 33:213–251.

Guyton A, Jones C, Coleman T (1973): *Circulatory Physiology: Cardiac Output and Its Regulation*. Philadelphia: WB Saunders.

Hokfeld B, Bydgeman S (1961): Increased adrenaline production following administration of 2-deoxy-d-glucose in the rat. *Proc Soc Exper Biol Med* 106:537–539.

Holzbauer M, Vogt M (1954): The concentration of adrenaline in the peripheral blood during insulin hypoglycemia. *Br J Pharmacol* 9:249–252.

Iadecola C, Lacombe P, Underwood M, Sved A, Reis DJ (1986): Adrenal catecholamines participate in the cerebrovascular vasodilation elicited by electrical stimulation of the dorsal medullary reticular formation in rat. *Acta Physiol Scand* 127(suppl 552): 74–77.

Iriuchijima J, Teranishi J (1982): Cardiac output in conscious and almost unrestrained spontaneously hypertensive rats. *Hiroshima J Med Sci* 31:259–266.

Johnson M, Smith P, Mills E, Schanberg S (1983): Paradoxical elevation of sympathetic activity during catecholamine infusion in rats. *J Pharmacol Exp Ther* 227:254–259.

Kahan T, Danlof C, Hjemdahl P (1987): Facilitation of nerve stimulation evoked noradrenaline overflow by isoprenaline but not by circulating adrenaline in the dog in vivo. *Life Sci* 40:1811–1818.

Katafuchi T, Oomura Y, Niijima A, Yoshimatsu H (1985): Effects of intracerebroventricular 2-DG infusion and subsequent hypothalamic lesion on adrenal nerve activity in the rat. *J Auton Nerv Syst* 13:81–84.

Kvetnansky R, McCarty R, Thoa N, Lake C, Kopin I (1979): Sympatho-adrenal responses of spontaneously hypertensive rats to immobilization stress. *Am J Physiol* 236:H457–H462.

Majewski H, Rand M (1986): A possible role of epinephrine in the development of hypertension. *Medicinal Res Rev* 6:467–486.

Majewski H, Tung L, Rand M (1981a): Adrenaline-induced hypertension in rats. *J Cardiovasc Pharmacol* 3:179–185.

Majewski H, Tung L, Rand M (1981b): Hypertension through adrenaline activation of prejunctional beta-adrenoceptors. *Clin Exp Pharmacol Phys* 8:463–468.

Majewski H, Rand M, Tung L (1981c): Activation of prejunctional beta-adrenoceptors in rat atria by adrenaline applied exogenously or released as a co-transmitter. *Br J Pharmacol* 3:669–679.

Majewski H, Tung L, Rand M (1982): Adrenaline activation of prejunctional beta-adrenoceptors and hypertension. *J Cardiovasc Pharmacol* 4:99–106.

McDougal D, Ferrendelli J, Yip V, Pusateri M, Carter J, Chi M, Norris B, Manchester J, Lowry O (1990): Use of nonradioactive 2-deoxyglucose to study compartmentation of brain glucose metabolism and rapid regional changes in rate. *Proc Natl Acad Sci USA* 87:1357–1361.

Medvedev O, Delle M, Thoren P (1988a): 2-deoxy-D-glucose–induced central glycopenia differentially influences renal and adrenal nerve activity in awake SHR rats. *Clin Exp Hypertens* A10 (suppl 1):375–381.

Medvedev O, Esler M, Angus J, Cox H, Eisenhofer G (1990): Simultaneous determination of plasma noradrenaline ana adrenaline kinetics: Responses to nitroprusside-induced hypotension and 2-deoxyglucose-induced glucopenia in the rabbit. *Naunyn-Schmiedeberg's Arch Pharmacol* 341:192–199.

Medvedev O, Hoque A (1986): Differential regional haemodynamic effects of centrally administered angiotensin II (ANG-II) in conscious rats. *J Hypertens* 4(suppl 6):S428–S430.

Medvedev O, Kuzmin A, Khulup G, Anosova O (1988b): 2-deoxyglucose as a tool for analysis of humoral component of the cardiovascular response to stress. *Bull Exper Biol Med* 95:143–145 (in Russian).

Medvedev O, Kuzmin A, Oranovskaja E, Khulup G, Hoque A, Matsievsky D (1989): Cardiovascular correlates of metabolic stress elicited by 2-deoxy-D-glucose. In: *Stress: Neurochemical and Humoral Mechanisms*, Van Loon G, Kvetnansky R, McCarty R, Axelrod J, eds. New York: Gordon and Breach Science.

Medvedev O, Murashev A, Meertsuk F (1986): Hemodynamic correlates of immobilization stress in rats. *Sechenov Physiol J USSR* 72:363–367.

Niijima A (1975): The effect of 2-deoxy-D-glucose and D-glucose on the efferent discharge rate of sympathetic nerves. *J Physiol* 251:231–243.

Okajima T, Ikuyama S, Kato K and Ibayashi H (1984): Naloxone inhibits the plasma epinephrine response to ACTH but not to 2-deoxy-d-glucose in rats. *Life Sci* 35:2177–2181.

Racz K, Kuchel O, Bun N (1985): In vivo release of adrenal catecholamines in rats by fusaric acid. *Eur J Pharmacol* 109:1–7.

Ricksten S, Thoren P (1980): Reflex inhibition of sympathetic activity during volume load in awake normotensive and spontaneously hypertensive rats. *Acta Physiol Scand* 110:77–82.

Sato A, Sato Y, Shimamura K, Suzuki H (1986): An increase in the sympathoadrenal medullary function in stroke-prone spontaneously hypertensive rats under anesthetized and resting conditions. *Neurosci Lett* 72:309–314.

Schwartz D, Eikenburg D (1986): Cardiovascular responsiveness to sympathetic activation and chronic epinephrine administration. *J Pharmacol Exp Therap* 238:148–154.

Smithe G, Grunstein H, Bradshaw J, Nicholson M, Compton P (1984): Relationships between brain noradrenergic activity and blood glucose. *Nature* 308:65–67.

Stjarne L, Brundin J (1975): Dual adrenoceptor-mediated control of noradrenaline secretion from human vasoconstrictor nerves: Facilitation by beta-receptors and inhibition by alpha receptors. *Acta Physiol Scand* 94:139–141.

Sun C, Thoa N, Kopin I (1979): Comparison of the effects of 2-deoxyglucose and immobilization on plasma levels of catecholamines and corticosterone in awake rats. *Endocrinology* 105:306–311.

Thompson D, Campbell R, Lilavivat U, Welle S, Robertson G (1981): Increased thirst and plasma arginin vasopressin levels during 2-deoxy-D-glucose–induced glucoprivation in humans. *J Clin Invest* 67:1083–1093.

Trippodo N, Yamamoto J, Frohlich E (1981): Whole-body venouse capacity and effective total tissue compliance in SHR. *Hypertension* 3:104–112.

Yamamoto J, Trippodo N, Ishise S, Frohlich E (1980): Total vascular pressure-volume relationship in the conscious rat. *Am J Physiol* 238:H823–H828.

Zabludowski J, Clark S, Ball S, Brown A, Inglis G, Lever A, Murray G (1984): Pressor effects of brief and prolonged infusions of epinephrine in the conscious rat. *Am J Physiol* 246:H683–H689.

# 18
# High-Renin Renal Hypertension Depresses the Baroreflex Control of Heart Rate and Sympathetic Activity

Maria C. Irigoyen, Robinson D. Moreira, Edson D. Moreira, and Eduardo M. Krieger

Centrally acting angiotensin II (Ang II) is well known to participate in several mechanisms leading to hypertension, as demonstrated by anatomical and functional studies (Ganten et aL, 1975; Weyhenmeyer and Phillips, 1982). Ang II may cause a centrally induced augmentation in sympathetic nerve activity (Ferrario et al., 1976) while decreasing the parasympathetic action on the heart (Potter and Reid. 1985) and influencing the activity of the peripheral sympathetic nervous system (Zimmerman, 1981). Its actions comprise the facilitation of adrenergic function through enhancing the release (Hyghes and Roth, 1971) and restraining the reuptake (Campbell and Jackson, 1979) of norepinephrine from sympathetic nerve terminals. Ang II stimulates the release of catecholamines from the adrenal medulla (Feuerstein et al, 1977) and increases vascular responsiveness to norepinephrine (Struthers et al.,1987). Finally, the inhibition of the baroreceptor reflexes may be an important component of the central effect of Ang II. Impairment of baroreflex bradycardia by Ang II has been demostrated in sheep (Lee et al., 1980), dogs (Fukiama, 1973), monkeys (Wasserstrum and Herd, 1977), rabbits (Guo and Abboud, 1984, a) and rats (Moreira et al., 1988). On the other hand, the pattern of pressure changes during natural sleep in rats, which is a sensitive index of the functional integrity of the baroreceptor reflex, is altered after intracerebral Ang Il infusion (Moreira and Krieger, 1988) or during hypertension accompanied by overactivity of the renin angiotensin system (RAS) (Moreira and Krieger, 1984), thus resembling the changes caused by sino-aortic denervation (SAD). After SAD the pattern of blood pressure during sleep varies from unchanged to a rise in synchronized sleep (SS) and from slight increase to a marked drop in desynchronized sleep (DS). In rats with hypertension accompanied by overactivity of RAS the pattern of MAP changes during sleep was similar to SAD rats. Overactivity of RAS rather than the severity of hypertension "per se" seems to be responsible for the alterations, since DOCA-salt rats with severe hypertension showed a normal pattern. The MAP drop during DS in rats with RAS overactivity more than compensates for the increase in MAP in SS, partially reducing the degree of hypertension in the conscious state. This fact may indicate that high-renin renal hypertension is partially dependent on elevated sympathetic drive, as has been known to other investigators using different methodological approaches (Krieger et al., 1988). The hypothesis that the RAS overactivity impairs baroreceptor function and thus changes the blood pressure pattern in high-renin hypertensive rats was tested by intracerebroventricular infusion of Ang II in normotensive rats. The alterations of the blood pressure pattern were similar to those observed in high-renin hypertensive rats during natural sleep (Moreira and Krieger, 1984).

In a previous study we demonstrated that the baroreflex control of heart rate is impaired in rats with high-renin renal hypertension of short and long duration, regardless of the severity of the hypertension (Moreira et al., 1988). Both the reflex bradycardia and tachycardia, elicited by phenylephrine and nitroglycerine, respectively, were depressed. In rats with one-kidney, one-clip hypertension, the reflex bradycardia and tachycardia were attenuated by 81% and 77%, respectively. In rats with mild or severe hypertension induced by aortic ligation there was a similar marked inhibition of the reflex bradycardia (90%) and tachycardia (62%). Normalization of RAS activity in rats with mild hypertension coincided with normalization of the bradycardic responses while the alteration persisted in those rats with severe hypertension in which hyperactivity of RAS also persisted. The reduced sensitivity of the baroreceptor control of heart rate (HR) may not always reflect a similar change in the peripheral circulation, because of the asymmetry of the system (Mancia et al., 1986). The possibility that the reflex regulation of vascular resistance is also abnormal in rats with high-renin hypertension deserves closer scrutiny. The purpose of the present study has been to determine the baroreflex control of HR and renal sympathetic nerve activity (RSNA) during increases and decreases in arterial pressure in rats with high-renin hypertension.


## Methodology

Male Wistar rats weighing 250–300g were used. Aortic ligation between the renal arteries (Chatelain et al., 1980) was performed under ether anesthesia. The rats were studied 12 days after surgery. One day prior to the experiment, the animals were instrumented under ether anesthesia with arterial (carotid) and venous (jugular) catheters. On the day of the experiment the animals were anesthetized with alpha-chloralose and implanted with a bipolar platinum electrode insulated with silicone rubber (Wacker SIL GEL 604) around a branch of the right renal nerve. The arterial cannula was connected to a strain-gauge transducer (P23-Db, Gould-Statham, Oxnard, California). RSNA was pre-amplified (high input impedance differential amplifier), filtered (100 Hz-2 KHz) and stored on a tape recorder (model 7754A, Hewlett-Packard, San Diego, CA, USA) simultaneously with the arterial pressure signals. The recorded signal was rectified, integrated and processed via an analog-to-digital converter using a data acquisition system to quantify nerve discharges and associated changes in arterial pressure and HR (Irigoyen et al., 1988). Increasing doses of phenylephrine (0.25–8 $\mu$g/ml) and sodium nitroprusside (2.5–80 $\mu$g/ml) were given (0.1 ml) as bolus injections to produce at least four pressure responses ranging from 5 to 40 mm Hg. Peak increases or decreases in MAP after phenylephrine or nitroprusside injections and the corresponding peak reflex changes in HR and RSNA were recorded for each dose of the drug (Figure 18.1). Baroreflex sensitivity was expressed by the measured values as well as by values derived by fitting a regression line through points relating the changes in RSNA or HR to the changes in MAP. The slope (sensitivity) for baroreceptor control of HR and RSNA was determined for each

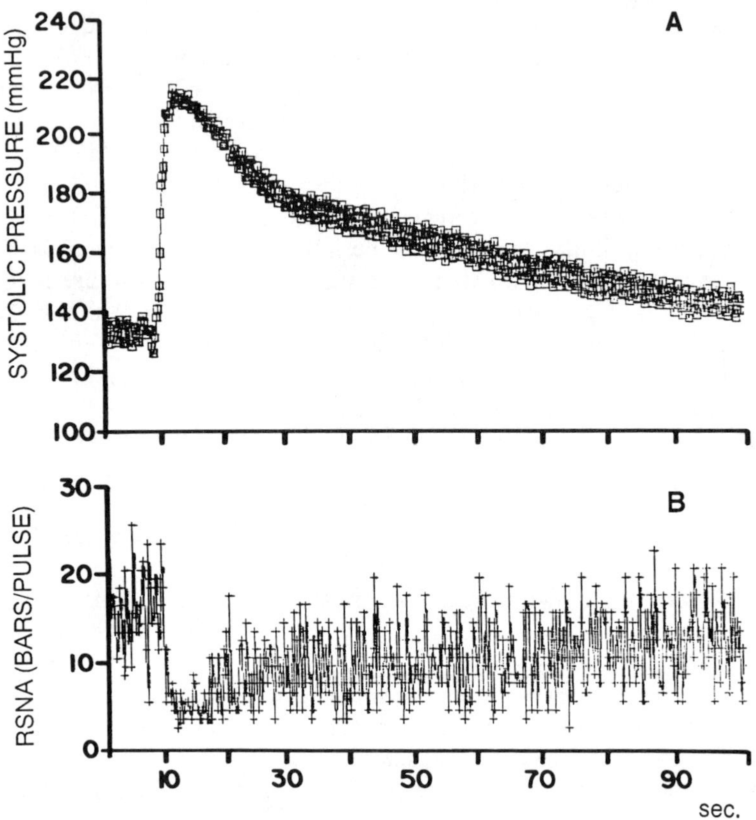

FIGURE 18.1. Peak increase in systolic pressure after phenylephrine injection. **A**: Arterial systolic pressure change during injection of vasoactive drug in normotensive rat. **B**: Associated change in rental sympathetic nerve activity (RSNA) during the same vasoactive drug injection. Beat-to-beat analysis.

rat. From slopes of individual rats the group means were calculated. The basal nerve activity was obtained by averaging the activity of RSNA in the first 40 cycles immediately before the drug injection.

Plasma renin activity (PRA) was measured by radio-immunoassay. In 4 hypertensive subjects the renin-angiotensin system activity was assessed indirectly by the depressor responses produced by administration of the converting enzyme inhibitor, captopril (10 mg/kg i.v.).

Data were expressed as mean ± SEM and the unpaired T test was used to compare slopes of the relations between control and hypertensive animals. To compare absolute actual values we normalized the pressure responses and associated changes in HR and RSNA. A statistical significance was assumed when $p < 0.05$.

## Results

Twelve days after aortic ligation MAP was $169 \pm 3$ vs $110 \pm 2$ mm Hg in control rats, and the HR was $420 \pm 20$ vs $375 \pm 17$ beat/min. Compared with normotensives, hypertensive rats exhibited a decreased baroreflex control of HR during changes in MAP (Figure 18.2). When MAP was raised, the slope of the relation between delta-MAP and delta-HR for hypertensives $(-0.18 \pm 0.04, r = 0.7 \pm 0.14)$ was significantly smaller than that for controls $(-0.98 \pm 0.09, r = 0.98 \pm 0)$. When MAP was lowered, the slope for

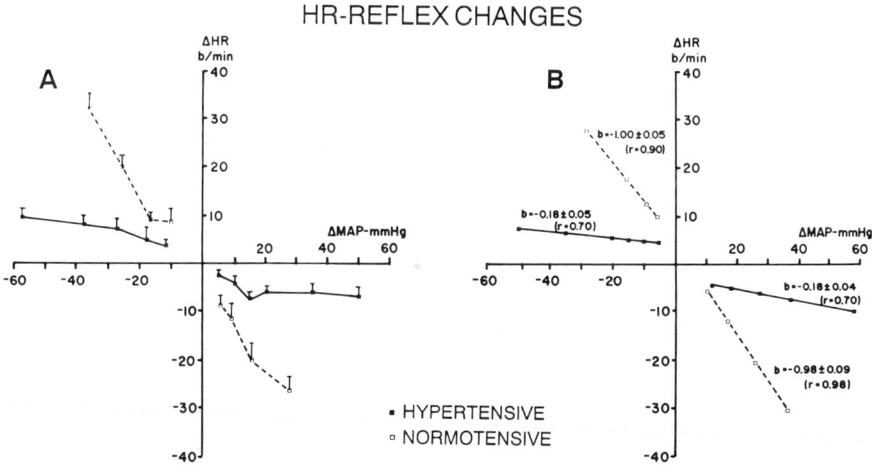



FIGURE 18.2. Effects of high-renin hypertension on the bradycardic and tachycardic responses to pressor changes induced by increasing doses of phenylephrine and sodium nitroprusside, respectively. **A**: Actual values of reflex bradycardia (lower right) and reflex tachycardia (upper left). **B**: Regression lines. Solid straight lines: hypertensive rats. Dashed lines: normotensive rats.

hypertensives $(-0.18 \pm 0.05, r = 0.7 \pm 0.18)$ was again smaller than that for controls $(-1.0 \pm 0.05, r = 0.90 \pm 0.03)$. High-renin hypertensive rats also had an impaired sensitivity for baroreflex control of RSNA, when compared with normotensive rats (Figure 18.3). When blood pressure was increased, the slopes of the relation between delta-MAP and delta-RSNA for hypertensives and normotensives were $-0.2 \pm 0.07, r = 0.98 \pm 0.01$, and $-0.9 \pm 0.01, r = 0.90 \pm 0.02$, respectively. When blood pressure was decreased, the slopes for renal hypertensive and control rats were $-0.1 \pm 0.05, r = 0.8 \pm 0.08$ and $-0.9 \pm 0.08, r = 0.90 \pm 0.02$, respectively. All differences between hypertensives and normotensives were statistically significant $p < 0.05$.

When the baroreflex was assessed through the actual measured parameters, the hypertensive rats exhibited marked inhibition of the bradycardic and tachycardic responses to bolus injection of phenylephrine and sodium nitroprusside by 75% $(-0.3 \pm 0.03$ vs $-1.2 \pm 0.16$ beat/mmHg) and 73% $(-0.25 \pm 0.07$ vs $-0.9 \pm 0.08$ beats, mmHg), respectively. The decreases were slightly smaller than the corresponding decreases in the slope of the regression line (82% for both increases and decreases of MAP).

The evaluation of baroreflex control of RSNA by the actual measured parameters during rises and falls in MAP showed an impairment of 73% $(-0.3 \pm 0.03$ vs $-1.1 \pm 0.1$ bars/mmHg) and 79% $(-0.2 \pm 0.03$ vs $-0.94 \pm 0.12$ bars/mmHg),respectively. The impairment evaluated by slope was greater (78 and 81% respectively).

The decrease in pressure produced by captopril was significantly greater

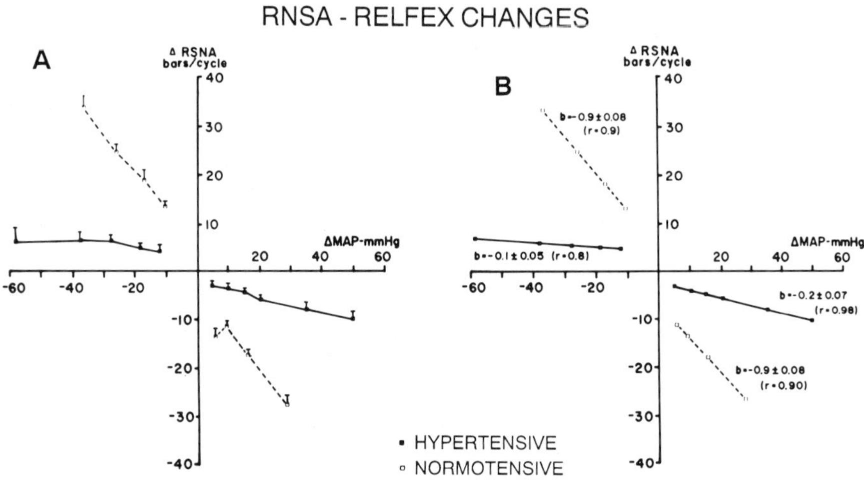


FIGURE 18.3. Effects of high-renin hypertension on the baroreflex control of renal sympathetic activity. Same as in Figure 18.2.

in the hypertensive rats 12 days after aortic ligation than in normotensive rats, (40 ± 4 vs 9 ± 5 mmHg). PRA values were increased in the hypertensives (40 ± 5 vs 2 ± 1 ng AngI/ml per h).

Another interesting finding is that hypertensive rats showed increased sympathetic activity during the control period (1000 cardiac cycles) and in each cardiac cycle (23.8 ± 2.8 vs 17.6 ± 2.7 bars/sec/cycle).

## Discussion

The major finding of the present experiments is that high-renin renal hypertensive rats not only have impaired reflex control of HR during increases and decreases in arterial pressure, but their reflex responses of RSNA to loading and unloading of the baroreceptors are also attenuated. These deficits were quite substantial (70–80%) and were similar for both the bradycardic and tachycardic responses as well as for the changes in renal sympathetic activity. Overactivity of RAS was demonstrated by the increase in plasma renin activity and by the increased depressor responses to injected captopril. Impaired reflex bradycardia during peripheral administration of Ang II, probably due to a central effect, has been demonstrated in sheep (Lee et al., 1980), dogs (Fukiyama 1973) and rabbits (Guo and Abboud. 1984a). We have also shown in a previous study that baroreflex attenuation of HR responses in high-renin hypertension in rats is probably caused by a central mechanism (Moreira et. al, 1988). Regarding the sites where the central pathways of the baroreflex are altered in high-renin renal hypertension, the ability of Ang II to impair the baroreceptor reflex directly at the nucleus tractus solitarius was demonstrated in rats (Castro and Phillips, 1986; Michelini and Bonagamba, 1990). It was also shown that an Ang II antagonist facilitated the baroreflex when injected into the nucleus tractus solitarius of rats (Campagnole-Santos et al., 1987). In dogs, rabbits and humans the central pressor response to i.v. administration of Ang II appears to be mediated by the area postrema, which has extensive interconnections with the nucleus tractus solitarius (Ferrario, 1983; Ferrario et al., 1985). In the rat, the area postrema also participates in the cardiovascular effects of Ang II (Skoog and Mangiapane, 1985), but the circumventricular organs, organum vasculosum of the lamina terminalis and subfornical organ, represent another important site of action for i.v. Ang II (Lappe and Brody,1984; Fink et al., 1986). It is also possible that impairment of the baroreflex is partially due to Ang II formed locally within the brain by the so-called intrinsic brain renin-angiotensin system (Ganten et al., 1981; Phillips et al., 1977). Central chronic captopril administration reversed the decrease in baroreflex sensitivity in spontaneously hypertensive rats (Berecek et al., 1983), which also showed overactivity of the cerebral RAS (Phillips et al., 1977).

The reduced sensitivity of the baroreceptor control of HR in experimental hypertension has been thought to reflect overall impairment of the cardiovascular influence exerted by arterial baroreceptors. However, recent studies have demonstrated that baroreceptor control on HR may not always reflect the influence of baroreceptors on the peripheral circulation (Ludbrook et al., 1980). Chloralose anesthesia in rats depresses both the reflex tachycardia and the pressor responses to carotid occlusion unchanged (Bedran-de-Castro et al., 1990). Regarding the reflex control of vascular resistance, the pressor effect produced by carotid occlusion in dogs was not affected by Ang II while the depressor responses mediated by the baroreflex were altered (Marker et al., 1980). The decrease in lumbar sympathetic nerve activity in the rabbit was inhibited by Ang II but not the increased discharges observed during hypotension (Guo and Abboud, 1984a). It seems that the acute administration of Ang II effectively blocks the inhibition exerted by the baroreceptors on the sympathetic outflow, thus exaggerating the pressor response, but leaving the reflex increase in sympathetic activity elicited by hypotension relatively unaltered. Ang II antagonists injected directly into the nucleus tractus solitarius selectively enhanced the reflex bradycardia but not the reflex tachycardia (Campagnole-Santos et al., 1987). Similarly, nitroprusside induced tachycardia was not altered by saralasin or Ang II microinjection into NTS in conscious rats (Michelini and Bonagamba, 1990).

However, different results were obtained when the baroreflex was studied in rabbits with renal hypertension. From 1 to 40 days after induction of hypertension, loss of baroreflex bradycardia was observed (Alexander and DeCuir, 1966). After 6 weeks of hypertension, baroreflex control of HR in response to increases and decreases in pressure was impaired, but reflex regulation of lumbar sympathetic nerve activity remained unaltered (Guo and Thames, 1983). With 4 months of renal hypertension bradycardic responses worsened and tachycardic responses, which had been severely depressed, did not progress, but the lumbar sympathetic nerve response also became attenuated (Guo and Abboud, 1984b). When the renal nerve, instead of the lumbar sympathetic nerve traffic, was analyzed, an abnormality of the baroreflex control of the sympathetic outflow was already detected after 6 weeks of hypertension (Thames et al., 1984).

Our data showed clearly that chronic overactivity of RAS in high-renin hypertension produced a general impairment of the baroreflex control of the circulation. Not only the bradycardia and tachycardia responses are similarly attenuated but the reflex sympathetic activity is also impaired, both when the baroreceptors are loaded or unloaded.

Recently it was demonstrated that captopril attenuated the pressor responses to bilateral carotid occlusion in conscious rabbits (Isaacson and Reid, 1990). The inhibitory effect was attributed mainly to the removal of the postsynaptic action of Ang II to facilitate sympathetic transmission rather than to alteration in the baroreflex per se. We obtained similar results, showing that captopril attenuated the neurogenic hypertension produced by sinoaortic denervation in rats (Longo et al., 1989). However, lifetime oral captopril treatment enhances baroreflex control of HR and lumbar sympathetic activity in SHR (Cheng et al., 1989), and intra-cerebroventricularly infused enalapril in normotensive rats augments the reflex bradycardia and sympathetic nerve inhibition in response to phenyl-ephrine, but not the opposite reflex response produced by sodium nitro-prusside (Bunag et al., 1990). Therefore, when endogenous Ang II levels are lowered by chronic converting enzyme inhibition, the enhancement of the central reflex during the unloading of the baroreceptors may be counteracted by the removal of the facilitation exerted by Ang II on the sympathetic system. In the present experiment the rats with increased endogenous Ang II exhibited an overall impairment of the baroreflex con-trol of circulation (HR and RSNA) accompanied by increased sympa-thetic activity (RSNA).

Another aspect to be discussed in connection with the general impair-ment of the baroreflex control of circulation in high-renin renal hyperten-sive rats is that in this model of hypertension hypertrophic heart is pro-duced (Rojo-Ortega and Genest, 1968), because of hypertension as well as the action of Ang II on the myocardium (Hirakata et al., 1990). The re-duced RSNA responses to changes in MAP may be the result of an en-hanced inhibitory influence of cardiac afferents of the hypertrophic heart on the arterial baroreflex regulation of RSNA, as shown in endurance-trained rabbits (DiCarlo and Bishop, 1990). In SHR, Rickstein and Thoren (1979) also showed a "hyperreactive" volume receptor mechanism, in which a decreased distensibility of the low-pressure capacitance would offset the receptor resetting. The exaggerated natriuretic response to saline load in hypertensives (DiBona, 1977), favors the possible participation of cardiac afferents in reflex RSNA inhibition.

In summary our data clearly show that chronic overactivity of the renin–angiotensin system in high-renin hypertension produces a general im-pairment of the baroreflex. This involves a blunting of both the reflex bradycardic and tachycardic responses as well as an impairment of reflex sympathetic activity, either when the baroreceptors are loaded or when they are unloaded.

*Acknowledgments.* This project is supported by FINEP, Fundacao EJ. Zerbini and CAPES.

# References

Alexander N, DeCuir M (1966): Loss of baroreflex bradycardia in renal hyperten-sive rabbits. *Circ Res* 19:7–13.

Bedran-De Castro MT, Farah VMA and Krieger EM (1990): Influence of general anesthetics on baroreflex control of circulation. *Braz J Biol Res* 23:1185–1193.

Berecek KH, Okuno T, Nagahama S and Oparil S (1983) Altered vascular reactivity and baroreflex sensitivity induced by chronic central administration of captopril in the spontaneously hypertensive rat. *Hypertension* 5:689–700.

Bunag RD Eriksson L and Tanabe S (1990): Baroreceptor reflex enhancement by enalapril in normotensive rats. *Hypertension* 15:284–290.

Campagnole-Santos MJ, Diz DI and Ferrario CM (1987): Facilitation of the baroreflex by bilateral injections of an angiotensin II antagonist into the nucleus tractus solitaii. *Hypertension* 9:534.

Campbell WB and Jackson EK (1979): Modulation of adrenergic transmission by angiotensin in the perfused rat mesenting. *Am J Physiol* 236:H-211–H-217.

Castro R and Phyllips MI (1986): Angiotensin II attenuates baroreflexes at nucleus tractus solitarius of rats. *Am J Physiol* 250:R-193–R-198.

Chatelain RE, Dibello PM and Ferrario CM (1980): Experimental benign and malignant hypertension with malignant nephrosclerosis. *Br J Exp Path* 61:401–410.

Cheng SWT, Swords BH, Kirk KA and Berecek KH (1989): Baroreflex function in lifetime captopril-treated spontaneously hypertensive rats. *Hypertension* 13:63–69.

DiBona GF (1977): Neurogenic regulation of renal tubular sodium reabsorption. *Am J Physiol* 233:F-73–F-81.

DiCarlo SE and Bishop VS (1990): Exercise training enhances cardiac afferent inhibition of baroreflex function. *Am J Physiol* 258: H-212–H-220.

Ferrario CM (1983): Neurogenic actions of angiotensin II. *Hypertension* 5 (suppl V): V-73–V-79.

Ferrario CM, McCubbin JW and Berti G (1976): Centrally mediated hemodynamic effects of angiotensin. In: *Regulation of blood pressure by the central nervous system*. Onesti G, Fernandes M, Kim KE eds. New York, Grune and Stratton, Inc, pp. 175–182.

Ferrario CM, Mikami H, Michelini LC, Kawamo Y and Brosnihan KB (1985): Interaction of vasopressin with central neurogenic mechanisms of blood pressure regulation. In: *Vasopressin*, Schrier RW ed. New York: Raven Press, pp. 47–57.

Feuerstein G, Boonyaviroj P and Gutman Y (1977): Renin-angiotensin mediation of adrenal cathecholamine secretion induced by hemorrhage. *Eur Phyarmacol* 44:131–112.

Fink GD, Bruner CA and Mangiapane ML (1986): Median preoptic nucleus ablation does not affect angiotensin II induced hypertension. *Am J Physiol* 252:H-148–H-152.

Fukiyama K (1973): Central modulation of baroreceptor reflex by angiotensin. *Jpn Heart J* 14:135–139.

Ganten D, Hutchinson JS and Schelling P (1975): The intrinsic brain isorenin-angiotensin system inthe rat: Its possible role in central mechanisms of blood pressure regulation. *Clin Sci Mol Med* 48:265s–268s.

Ganten D, Unger T, Scholkens B, Rascher W, Speck G and Stock G (1981): Role of neuropeptides in regulation of blood pressure. In: Disturbances in neurogenic control of the circulation. Bethesda. *Am Physiol Soc* pp. 139–151.

Guo GB and Abboud FM (1984a): Angiotensin II attenuates baroreflex control of heart rate and sympathetic activity. *Am J Physiol* 246:H-80–H-89.

Guo GB and Abboud FM (1984b): Impaired central mediation of the arterial baroreflex in chronic renal hypertension. *Am J Physiol* 246:H-720–H-727.

Guo GB and Thames MD (1983): Abnormal baroreflex control in renal hypertension is due to abnormal baroreceptors. *Am J Physiol* 246:H-420–H-428.

Hirakata H, Fouad-Tarazi FM, Bumpus FM, Khosla M, Healy B, Husain A, Urata H and Kumagai H (1990): Angiotensin and the failing Heart. *Circ Res* 66:891–899.

Hughes J and Roth RH (1971): Evidence that angiotensin enhances transmitter release during sympathetic nerve stimulation. *Br J Pharmacol* 41:239–255.

Irigoyen MC, Cestari IA, Moreira ED. Oshiro MS and Krieger EM (1988): Measurements of renal sympathetic nerve activity in conscious sinoaortic denervated rats. *Braz J Med Biol Res* 21:869–872.

Isaacson JS and Reid LA (1990): Importance of endogenous angiotensin II in the cardiovascular responses to sympathetic stimulation in conscious rabbits. *Circ Res* 66:662–671.

Krieger EM, Moreira RD and Padilha JU (1988): Central angiotensin alters blood pressure regulation during natural sleep. *Clin and Exper. Theory and Practice* A10 (suppl 1):123–129.

Lappe RW and Brody MJ (1984) Mechanisms of the central pressor action of angiotensin II in conscious rat. *Am J Physiol* 246:R-56–R-62.

Lee WB, Ismay MJ and Lumbers ER (1980): Mechanisms by which angiotensin II affects the heart of conscious sheep. *Circ Res* 47:286–292.

Longo VL, Farah VMM, Gutierrez MA and Krieger EM (1989): Attenuation of neurogenic hypertension by chronic converting enzyme inhibition. *J Hypertens* (suppl 6):S-44–S-45.

Ludbrook J Mancia G and Zanchetti A (1980): Does the baroreceptor-heart rate reflex indicate the capacity of the arterial baroreceptors to control blood pressure? *Clin Exp Pharmacol* 7:499.

Mancia G, Ferrari AU, Zanchetti A (1986): A reflex control of the circulation in experimental and human hypertension. In: *Handbook of Hypertension–Regulatory Mechanisms*, Zanchetti A, Tarazi RC, eds. Amsterdam: Elsevier Science Publishers. New York: Oxford University Press, pp. 47–68.

Marker JD, Miles TS and Scrop GC (1980) Modulation of the baroreceptor reflex by angiotensin II and other vasoactive drugs in anesthetized greyhounds. *Clin Sci* 58:7–13.

Michelini LC and Bonagamba LGH (1990): Angiotensin II as a modulator of baroreceptor reflexes in the brainstem of conscious rats. *Hypertension* 15 (suppl I): I-45–I-50.

Moreira ED, Oliveira M and Krieger EM (1988): Impaired baroreflex control of heart rate in high-renin renal hypertension. *J Hypertens* 6:619–625.

Moreira RD and Krieger EM (1984): Alterations of the pattern of pressure changes during sleep of rats with overactivity of the renin-angiotensin system. *Clin Exp Hypertens* (A) 6:2123–2126.

Moreira RD and Krieger EM (1988): Abnormal blood pressure behaviour produced by intracerebral angiotensin during natural sleep. *J Hypertens* 6 (suppl 4):s452–s454.

Phillips Ml, Felix D, Hoffman WE and Ganten D (1977): Angiotensin-sensitive sites in the brain ventricular system In: *Society for Neuroscience Symposia*, Cowan E.W.M., Ferrendeli J.A.E. eds. Bethesde: Society of Neuroscience, vol II, pp 139–151.

Potter EK and Reid IA (1985): Intravertebral angiotensin II inhibitis cardiac vagal efferent activity in dogs. *Neuroendocrinology* 40:493–196.

Ricksten SE and Thoren P (1979): Reflex inhibition of sympathetic activity during volume load in awake normotensive and spontaneously rats. *Acta Physiol Scand* 110:77–82.

Rojo-Ortega JM and Genest J (1968): A method for production of experimental hypertension in rats. *Can J Physiol Pharmacol* 46:883–885.

Skoog KM and Mangiapane ML (1985): Transient hypotension following area postrema lesions in the rat. *Neurosci Abstr* 11:190.

Struthers AD, Pai S. Seidelin PH, Contre WJR and Morton JJ (1987): Evidence in humans for a postsynaptic interaction between noradrenaline and angiotensin II with regard to systolic but not diastolic blood pressure. *J Hypertens* 5:671–676.

Thames MD, Gupta BN and Ballon BJ (1984): Central abnormality in baroreflex control of renal nerves in hypertension. *Am J Physiol* 246:H-843–H-850.

Wasserstrum N and Herd JA (1977): Heart rate and oxygen uptake response to angiotensin in the squirrel monkey at 10 C. *Am J Physiol* 233:H-10–H-14.

Weyhenmeyer JA and Phillips MK (1982): Angiotensin-like immunoreactivity in the brain of the spontaneously hypertensive rat. *Hypertension* 4:514–523.

Zimmerman BG (1981): Adrenergic facilitation by angiotensin: Does it serve a physiological function? *Clin Sci* 60:343–345.

# 19
# Opioidergic-Dopaminergic Interaction in Hypertension

CSABA FARSANG AND ALEXANDER ALFÖLDI

## Dopaminergic System and Blood Pressure Regulation

Dopamine has important physiological functions in the central nervous system, peripheral nervous system, and cardiovascular system (Snider and Kuchel, 1983), where specific dopaminergic receptors have been identified (Stoof and Kebabian, 1984). The neurotropic dopaminergic receptors are located in various regions of the peripheral sympathetic nervous system as well as in different parts of the central nervous system. These include the presynaptic membranes of the postganglionic sympathetic nerve terminals, the sympathetic ganglia, and the centers of cardiovascular control. Activation of neurotropic dopamine receptors results in an inhibition of central sympathetic outflow and a subsequent lowering of blood pressure and heart rate (Cavero et al., 1982).

The existence of two dopaminergic receptor subtypes (D-1 and D-2, or, DA-1 and DA-2, postsynaptic and neurotropic, respectively) has been supported by the identification of selective agonists and antagonists. The selective D-1 and DA-1 agonists stimulate the vascular and renal DA-1 receptors, some of them are currently undergoing clinical trials as antihypertensive drugs (Casagrande et al., 1989). The relatively selective D-2 and DA-2 agonists, bromocriptine, pergolide mesylate, and quinpirole, inhibit prolactin secretion (Stoof and Kebabian, 1983). SCH 23390 and R-sulpiride are selective antagonists of the D-1 and DA-1 receptors, whereas domperidone, S-sulpiride, and metoclopramide block the D-2 and DA-2 receptors, but not the D-1 and DA-1 receptors (MacLeod and Lehmeyer, 1974).

Data are also available for the regulatory role of dopamine in patients with essential hypertension. These patients are more sensitive to the depressor effect of dopamine and dopaminergic agonists (Kikuchi et al., 1982). A decrease in central dopaminergic tone is believed to contribute to the increase in blood pressure in essential hypertension (Kolloch et al., 1980). Furthermore, a decrease in the secretion of renal dopamine may cause fluid and water retention, which also increases blood pressure (Worth et al., 1985, Kuchel et al., 1979). However, the failure of dopaminergic antagonists to influence arterial blood pressure either in normotensive or in hypertensive patients (Thorburn and Sowton, 1973) does not support the role of endogenous dopaminergic "tone" in the control of arterial blood pressure.

## Interaction Between the Dopaminergic and Opioidergic Systems

The opioidergic system may contribute to the control of arterial blood pressure by the stimulation of different opiate receptors in the central nervous system as well as at the periphery. Beta-endorphin and dynorphin, the endogenous ligands with affinity for mu and kappa receptors, respectively, are considered to have a blood pressure lowering effect that, in certain conditions, is associated with bradycardia (Laubie et al., 1977). On the other hand, the enkephalins, which have a higher affinity for delta receptors, appear to increase blood pressure and heart rate after central administration (Simon et al., 1978; Yukimura et al., 1981). Opioid peptides can presynaptically inhibit the release of noradrenaline from the sympathetic nerve terminals (Gaddis and Dixon, 1982). The opiate antagonist naloxone, in a dose that selectively blocks mu opiate receptors, has no effect on blood pressure and heart rate either in rats (Pickar et al, 1982) or in patients with essential hypertension (Farsang et al., 1982). However, naloxone has been reported to alter the pressor response to hand-grip and bicycle exercise (Lam et al., 1986; Staessen et al., 1985), and can cause a pressor effect in a subset of clonidine-treated patients with essential hypertension (Farsang et al., 1984).

Opiate and dopamine receptors are colocalized in several brain regions intimately involved in blood pressure regulation (Morel and Pelletier, 1986). It is well known that both opioids and dopamine can modulate the secretion of different hormones, such as prolactin, adrenocorticotropic hormone (ACTH), cortisol, beta-endorphin, and aldosterone.

The pituitary secretion of ACTH and beta-endorphin is inhibited by dopaminergic mechanisms in rats (Przewloczki et al., 1979). The dopaminergic antagonist, metoclopramide, increases the plasma level of beta-endorphin and the content of this opioid in the hypothalamus of rats (Höllt and Bergman, 1982). In contrast, we are unaware of any data in humans on a possible opioidergic-dopaminergic interaction in the regulation of plasma beta-endorphin.

Aldosterone secretion from the adrenal cortex is probably also under dopaminergic control because metoclopramide increases the plasma aldosterone response to various stimuli, such as angiotensin II (ANG II) or physical exercise (Aguilera et al., 1984; Gilchrist et al., 1984). The possible involvement of opioids in this dopaminergic inhibition is supported by the finding that naloxone administered before hand-grip exercise potentiates the increase in plasma aldosterone concentration (Lam et al., 1986).

# Aim of the Study

As no effect of naloxone or metoclopramide was noted on the blood pressure or heart rate of patients in steady-state resting condition, we hypothesized that the endogenous dopaminergic and opioidergic systems may be activated during stress situations, resulting in a blunted pressor response. Therefore, we investigated the possible interaction between these two systems not only in the regulation of basal blood pressure, but also in the baroreflex control of heart rate. We further hypothesized that the interaction between the opioidergic and dopaminergic systems could be reflected by changes in the plasma levels of beta-endorphin, ACTH, renin activity, cortisol, and aldosterone.

# Patients and Methods

Male and female patients with uncomplicated borderline essential hypertension, aged 18 to 49 years, were selected for this study. Informed consent was obtained from all patients participating in the study, which was approved by our institutional Ethics Committee. The patients were off all medications for at least 7 days prior to their being tested.

## *Hemodynamic Study*

A randomized, double-blind, placebo-controlled, cross-over study was performed on nine patients with borderline essential hypertension (four women and five men, mean age $38 \pm 9$ years, range 18 to 45 years). Thirty min after the intravenous (i.v.) injection of 10 mg metoclopramide (Cerucal, VEB GDR) or physiological saline (placebo) a submaximal (85%) bicycle exercise was performed in the sitting position. The test was repeated at the same time on a different day, after the administration of the alternative drug (placebo or metoclopramide). Immediately before and at every minute during the exercise arterial blood pressure was measured by sphygmomanometry and the heart rate was also determined.

## *Hormonal Study*

A randomized, double-blind, placebo-controlled, cross-over study was performed on 13 patients with borderline essential hypertension (six women and seven men, mean age $35 \pm 8$ years, range 19 to 48 years). A cannula was inserted into the antecubital vein for i.v. injections and for taking blood samples. Sixty min after the i.v. injection of 10 mg metoclopramide or physiological saline, 0.4 mg naloxone (Narcan, DuPont) or placebo was given i.v. Ten min after the administration of naloxone or the second dose of placebo a submaximal (85%) bicycle ergometry test was performed for 9 to 12 min. Immediately before and 30 and 60 min after the administration of metoclopramide, and also immediately before and 30

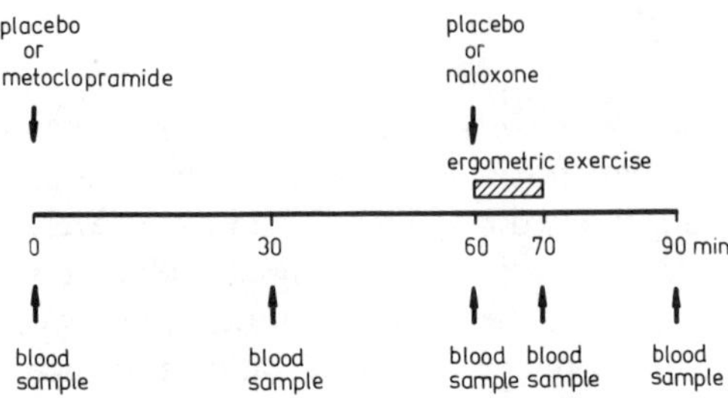


FIGURE 19.1.  Study protocol.

min after the bicycle ergometry test, blood samples were taken for the determination of plasma ACTH, beta-endorphin, cortisol, and aldosterone levels and of plasma renin activity (Fig. 19.1). At baseline and 60 min after the injection of metoclopramide the plasma level of prolactin was determined by radioimmunoassay.

Hormone concentrations were measured by commercially available radioimmunoassay kits [Beta-endorphin: Immuno-Nuclear Co., USA; ACTH: Oris, France; cortisol, prolactin: Frederic Joliot-Curie National Research Institute for Radiation Biology, Hungary; aldosterone: Serono, Italy; renin activity (angiotensin I): Pharmacia, Sweden].

Comparisons were made using student's paired $t$ test (with the Bonferroni modification) and the multiple linear regression analysis. Values are presented as means ± SEM.

# Results

## Hemodynamic Study

Neither placebo nor metoclopramide nor naloxone affected the resting arterial blood pressure and heart rate of our patients. The exercise-induced increase in systolic blood pressure was also unaffected. The exercise-induced tachycardia was significantly potentiated by metoclopramide between the third and sixth min of exercise (Table 19.1).

TABLE 19.1. The effect of metoclopramide on exercise-induced tachycardia in patients with essential hypertension.

| | Baseline | 1 | 2 | 3 | 4 | 5 | 6 min |
|---|---|---|---|---|---|---|---|
| Placebo | 85 ± 4 | 107 ± 5 | 112 ± 5 | 112 ± 6 | 130 ± 8 | 130 ± 7 | 127 ± 6 |
| Metoclopramide | 85 ± 5 | 109 ± 4 | 118 ± 5[a] | 118 ± 7[a] | 138 ± 7[a] | 136 ± 6[a] | 132 ± 6[a] |

Values represent ± SEM for heart rate (beats/min).
[a] Indicates significant difference from corresponding placebo value.

TABLE 19.2. Regression analysis of systolic blood pressure/heart rate relationship measured before and at every minute during exercise.

| y | $=a \pm s_a$ | $+bx \pm s_b$ |
|---|---|---|
| Placebo | $-35.0 \pm 26.8$ | $+0.98 \pm 0.09$ x |
| Naloxone | $-31.2 \pm 18.2$ | $+0.97 \pm 0.14$ x |
| Metoclopramide | $-50.3 \pm 8.9$ | $+1.20 \pm 0.14$ x[a,b] |
| Metoclopramide plus naloxone | $-69.8 \pm 41.4$ | $+1.21 \pm 0.19$ x |

Intercepts (a) and slopes (b) are given with their standard errors (s). Significant difference ($p < 0.05$) from placebo ([a]) or from naloxone ([b]).

Heart rate values corresponding to the same systolic blood pressure were higher after metoclopramide than after placebo. When systolic blood pressure values were plotted against the corresponding heart rate values and a linear regression calculated, the slope of the regression was significantly increased by metoclopramide (Table 19.2), indicating decreased baroreflex sensitivity. Naloxone did not influence the pressor response to submaximal bicycle exercise or the slope of the blood pressure/heart rate regression line (Table 19.2).

## Hormonal Study

The plasma beta-endorphin concentration was not affected by placebo, metoclopramide, naloxone, or metoclopramide plus naloxone administration, but it was moderately increased by physical exercise. Naloxone potentiated the plasma beta-endorphin response to ergometry, and this potentiation was blocked when metoclopramide was given prior to naloxone (Fig. 19.2).

An essentially similar picture emerges when plasma ACTH and cortisol levels are analyzed. The plasma concentrations of both hormones increased slightly by exercise, and these increases were markedly potentiated by naloxone. Metoclopramide had no effect of its own but blocked the potentiation caused by naloxone (Fig. 19.2).

A significant positive linear correlation was found between the postexercise plasma ACTH and beta-endorphin levels both in the absence of naloxone ($r = 0.7638$, $p<0.01$) and in its presence ($r = 0.8063$, $p<0.01$). Furthermore, there was a significant positive linear correlation between the naloxone-induced changes in postexercise plasma ACTH and plasma cortisol levels ($r = 0.7042$, $p<0.01$).

Plasma prolactin levels showed a marked, more than 20-fold increase (from $3.9 \pm 0.8$ to $86.3 \pm 13.9$ nM, $p<0.001$) 60 min after metoclopramide, indicating tonic inhibitory dopaminergic control of prolactin secretion.

Plasma renin activity increased significantly after ergometry; this in-

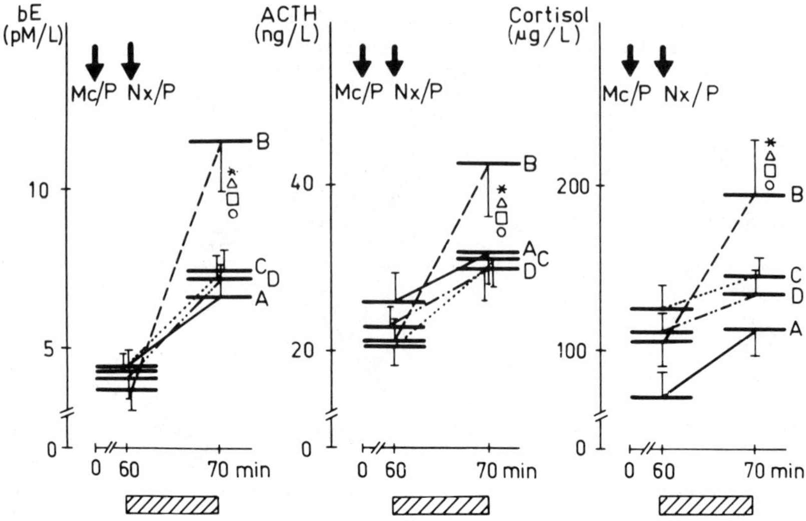

FIGURE 19.2. Changes in plasma levels of beta-endorphin (bE), ACTH, and cortisol after submaximal bicycle ergometry and/or **A**: placebo, **B**: naloxone, **C**: metoclopramide, **D**: naloxone plus metoclopramide. The dashed bar indicates the time of the exercise. Significant difference ($p<0.05$) from placebo (*) metoclopramide ($\triangle$), naloxone plus metoclopramide ($\square$) or baseline ($\bigcirc$).

crease was not affected by naloxone, metoclopramide, or their combination (Fig. 19.3). Plasma aldosterone levels were also significantly increased by ergometry. Metoclopramide significantly increased both basal aldosterone levels and the exercise-induced increase, whereas naloxone did not affect either parameter or the metoclopramide-induced changes in plasma aldosterone (Fig. 19.3). The effects of metoclopramide on plasma aldosterone levels were similar to earlier findings by others (Aguilera et al., 1984; Gilchrist et al., 1984).

## Discussion

### Circulatory Changes

The results presented confirm earlier observations (Thorburn and Sowton, 1973) that resting arterial blood pressure or heart rate are not under tonic dopaminergic control. On the other hand, metoclopramide significantly increased the heart rate response to physical exercise and increased the slope of the systolic blood pressure/heart rate relationship, suggesting decreased baroreflex sensitivity. On the basis of these data we propose that endogenous dopamine may tonically facilitate the baroreflex in patients with essential hypertension, as also suggested by Snider and Kuchel (1983), and

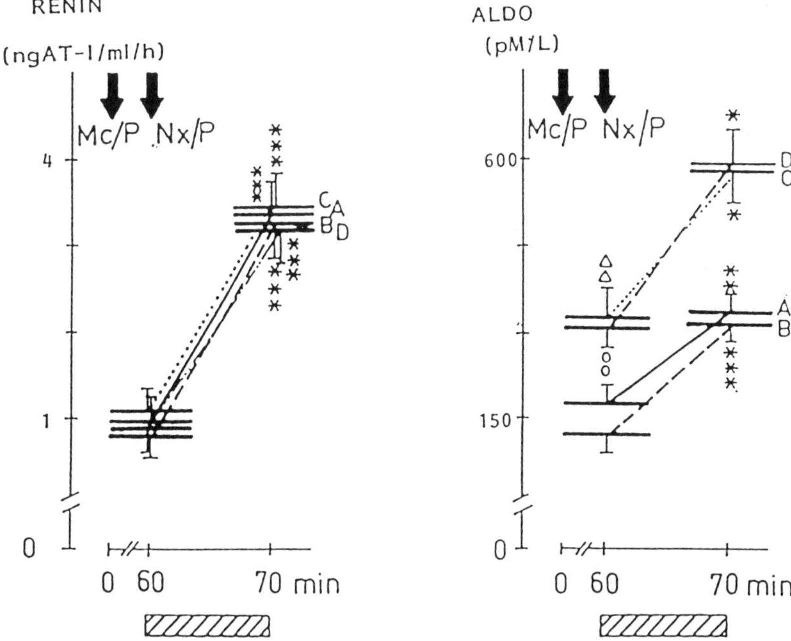


FIGURE 19.3. Changes in plasma renin activity (RENIN) and plasma aldosterone levels (ALDO) after submaximal bicycle ergometry and/or A: placebo, B: naloxone, C: metoclopramide, D: naloxone plus metoclopramide. The dashed bar indicates the time of the exercise. Significant difference ($p<0.05$) from baseline (*) or from value obtained after metoclopramide treatment. Significant difference ($p<0.01$) from baseline obtained after metoclopramide ($\triangle$) or metoclopramide plus naloxone ($\bigcirc$) treatment.

that this effect is amplified by physical exercise. Another process under tonic dopaminergic control is the secretion of prolactin, where tonic inhibition is indicated by the marked increase of plasma prolactin levels after metoclopramide treatment.

At the low dose used in the present study, naloxone selectively inhibits the $\mu$ subtype of opiate receptors (Egan and North, 1981). The observed lack of cardiovascular effects of naloxone indicates the absence of tonic control of blood pressure and heart rate by endogenous opioids acting at $\mu$ receptors in patients with essential hypertension. Naloxone also failed to influence the pressor response to submaximal bicycle exercise, in agreement with the results of a previous study in normotensive volunteers (Lam et al., 1986).

## Hormonal Changes

Our results reinforced earlier observations in normotensive volunteers (Carey et al., 1979) and indicated that in patients with essential hypertension there is no evidence for tonic dopaminergic control of resting plasma levels of beta-endorphin, ACTH, or cortisol. In rats (Höllt et al., 1982) and in some studies in men (Genazzani et al., 1988) the dopaminergic antagonist, metoclopramide, increased the beta-endorphin content of the hypothalamus and the plasma level of this endogenous opioid. In humans exogenous opioids can inhibit ACTH and cortisol secretion, and this action is antagonized by naloxone (Delitala et al., 1983). Furthermore, naloxone was found to increase basal as well as stress-stimulated ACTH and corticosterone levels in some (Volavka et al., 1979) but not in other studies (Staessen et al., 1985). To our knowledge, there are no published data concerning the possible interaction of endogenous opioids and dopamine in the regulation of plasma beta-endorphin, ACTH, cortisol, and aldosterone levels in humans.

During the activation of the sympathoadrenal system by physical exercise we observed a significant facilitatory effect on pituitary hormone secretion by the opiate antagonist, naloxone. Similar observations have been reported in normotensive individuals (Hargreaves et al., 1986). This supports the existence of a tonic opioidergic inhibitory mechanism in the regulation of plasma beta-endorphin, ACTH, and cortisol levels in both normotensive individuals and patients with mild essential hypertension. It is possible that naloxone blocks the effect of an endogenous opioid peptide that inhibits pituitary beta-endorphin and ACTH release either directly or through modulation of the secretion or effect of corticotropin-releasing factor (CRF). There is some evidence that morphine can blunt the ACTH response to exogenous CRF in vivo, although morphine was without effect on CRF-induced ACTH release from dispersed rat pituitary cells (Rittmaster et al., 1985). Alternatively, naloxone's effect may be due to its interaction with a beta-endorphin autoreceptor in the hypothalamopituitary axis (Weihe et al., 1988). An action of naloxone at the level of the pituitary is supported by the significant correlation between the plasma beta-endorphin and ACTH responses to ergometric exercise observed after naloxone pretreatment in the present study. The additional correlation with plasma cortisol levels probably reflects stimulation of cortisol secretion by the increased levels of circulating ACTH.

Our results indicate that metoclopramide blocks the ability of naloxone to potentiate the exercise-induced increase in plasma beta-endorphin. As the dose of naloxone used only blocks the $\mu$ and $\varepsilon$ opiate receptors (Egan and North, 1981) for which the preferred endogenous ligand is beta-endorphin, these findings suggest an interaction between stimulatory dopaminergic and inhibitory beta-endorphinergic mechanisms in the regulation of beta-endorphin, ACTH, and cortisol secretion. Our finding that this interaction became more prominent during physical exercise may be related to the fact that exercise appears to activate both systems: during exercise there is an increase in the plasma levels of beta-endorphin (our findings) as well as an increase in both circulating dopamine (Snider and

Kuchel, 1983) and dopamine release in the central nervous system (Bortz et al., 1981).

A high intravenous dose of naloxone has been reported to potentiate the exercise-induced increases in plasma aldosterone and plasma renin activity (Grossmann et al., 1984). In contrast, at the low dose used in the present study naloxone failed to influence the same parameters. Therefore, it seems unlikely that endogenous beta-endorphin acting at $\mu$ or $\varepsilon$ receptors would tonically inhibit aldosterone, renin, and prolactin secretion, at least in patients with mild essential hypertension.

Our finding of a marked increase in plasma prolactin after metoclopramide treatment has been interpreted in terms of removal of a tonic dopaminergic inhibition of prolactin secretion. Metoclopramide is primarily a dopamine antagonist, and the dose used is sufficient for blocking the effects of endogenous dopamine at dopamine receptors (MacLeod, 1976). However, metoclopramide can also inhibit the actions of serotonin (Fozard and Mobarok, 1978). As serotonergic antagonists can block the stimulatory effect of CRF on the pituitary release of proopiomelanocortin-derived peptides in the rat (Saland et al., 1988), metoclopramide may also owe some of its effects to blockade of serotonin receptors. Further studies are required to clarify this issue.

# References

Aguilera G, Mendelsohn AO, Catt KJ (1984): Dopaminergic regulation of aldosterone secretion. In: *Frontiers in Neuroendocrinology*, Martini L, Ganong WF, eds. New York: Raven Press, pp. 265–655.

Bortz WM, Angwin P, Mefford IN, Boarder MR, Noyce N, Barchas JD (1981): Catecholamines, dopamine and endorphin levels during extreme exercise. N *Engl J Med* 305:466 (letter).

Carey RM, Thorner MD, Ortt EM (1979): Effects of metoclopramide and bromocryptine on the renin-angiotensin-aldosterone system in man: dopaminergic control of aldosterone. *J Clin Invest* 63:727–735.

Casagrande C, Merlo L, Ferrini R, Miragoli G, Semeraro C (1989): Cardiovascular and renal action of dopaminergic prodrugs. *J Cardiovasc Pharmacol* 14(suppl 8):S40–S59.

Cavero I, Massingham R, Lefevre-Borg F (1982): Peripheral dopamine receptors, potential targets for a new class of antihypertensive agents *Life Sci* 35:1243–1273.

Delitala G, Grossman A, Besser M (1983): Differential effects of opiate peptides and alkaloids on anterior pituitary secretion. *Neuroendocrinology* 37:275–279.

Egan TM, North RA (1981): Both u and d opiate receptors exist on the same neuron. *Science* 214:923–924.

Farsang C, Kapocsi J, Juhász I, Kunos G (1982): Possible involvement of an endogenous opioid in the antihypertensive effect of clonidine in patients with essential hypertension. *Circulation* 66:1268–1272.

Farsang C, Kapocsi J, Vajda L, et al. (1984): Reversal by naloxone of the antihypertensive effect of clonidine: Involvement of the sympathetic nervous system.

274     C. Farsang and A. Alföldi

*Circulation* 69:461–467.

Fozard JR, Mobarok ATM (1978): Blockade of neural tryptamine receptors by metoclopramide. *Eur J Pharmacol* 49:109–112.

Gaddis RR, Dixon WR (1982): Modulation of peripheral adrenergic neurotransmission by methionin-enkephalin. *J Pharmacol Exp Ther* 221:285–288.

Genazzani AR, Petraglia F, Facchinetti F, et al. (1988): Evidence for a dopamine-regulated peripheral source of circulating beta-endorphin. *J Clin Endocrinol Metab* 66:279–282.

Gilchrist NL, Espiner EA, Nicholls MG, Donald RA (1984): Effect of metoclopramide on aldosterone and regulatory factors in man. *Clin Endocrinol* 21:1–7.

Grossman A, Boloux P, Price P, et al. (1984): The role of opioid peptides in the hormonal responses to acute exercise in man. *Clin Sci* 67:483–491.

Hargreaves KH, Dionne RA, Mueller GP, Goldstein DS, Dubner R (1986): Naloxone, fentanyl and diazepam modify plasma beta-endorphin levels during surgery. *Clin Pharmacol Ther* 40:165–172.

Höllt V, Bergmann M (1982): Effects of acute and chronic haloperidol treatment on the concentrations of immunoreactive beta-endorphin in plasma, pituitary and brain of rats. *Neuropharmacology* 21:147–154.

Kikuchi K, Miyama A, Nakao T (1982): Hemodynamic and natriuretic responses to intravenous infusion of dopamine in patients with essential hypertension. *Jpn Circulat J* 46:486–493.

Kolloch R, Kobayashi K, DeQuattro W (1980): Dopaminergic control of sympathetic tone and blood pressure: evidence in primary hypertension. *Hypertension* 2:380–397.

Kuchel O, Buu NT, Unger T, Lis M, Genest J (1979): Free and conjugated plasma and urinary dopamine in human hypertension. *J Clin Endocrinol Metab* 48:425–429.

Lam KSL, Grossmann A, Bouloux P, Drury PL, Besser GM (1986): Effect of an opiate antagonist on the responses of circulating catecholamines and the renin-aldosterone system to acute sympathetic stimulation by hand-grip in man. *Acta Endocrinol* 111:252–257.

Laubie M, Schmitt H, Falq E (1977): Dopamine receptors in the femoral vascular bed of the dog as mediators of a vasodilator and sympathoinhibitory effect. *Eur J Pharmacol* 16:67–71.

MacLeod RM (1976): Regulation of prolactin secretion. In: *Frontiers in Neuroendocrinology*, Martini L, Ganong WF, eds. New York: Raven Press, pp 4:169–194.

MacLeod RM, Lehmeyer JE (1974): Studies on the mechanism of the dopamine-mediated inhibition of prolactin secretion. *Endocrinology* 94:1077–1084.

Morel G, Pelletier G (1986): Endorphinergic neurons are contracting the tubero-infundibular dopaminergic neurone in the rat brain. *Peptides* 7:1197–1202.

Pickar D, Cohen MR, Naber D, Cohen RM (1982): Clinical studies of the endogenous opioid system. *Biol Psychiat* 17:1243–1276.

Przewloczki H, Höllt V, Voigt KH, Herz A (1979): Modulation of in vitro release of beta-endorphin from the separate lobes of the rat pituitary. *Life Sci* 24:1601–1608.

Rittmaster RS, Cutler GB, Sobel DO Jr, Goldstein DS, Koppelmann MCS (1985): Morphine inhibits the pituitary-adrenal response to ovine corticotropine-releasing hormone in normal subjects. *J Clin Endocrinol Metab* 60:891–895.

Saland LC, Guttierez L, Kraner J, Samora A (1988): Corticotropin-releasing factor (CRF) and neurotransmitters modulate melanotropic peptide release from rat neurointermediate pituitary in vitro. *Neuropeptides* 12:59–66.

Simon W, Schaz K, Ganten U, Stock G, Schlor KH, Ganten D (1978): Effects of enkephalins on arterial blood pressure are reduced by propranolol. *Clin Sci Mol Med* 55:237s–241s.

Snider SR, Kuchel O (1983): Dopamine: an important neurohormone of the sympathoadrenal system. Significance of increased peripheral dopamine release for the human stress response and hypertension. *Endocrine Rev* 4:291–309.

Staessen J, Fiocchi R, Bouillon R, Fagard R, Amery A (1985): The nature of opioid involvement in the hemodynamic respiratory and humoral responses to exercise. *Circulation* 72:982–990.

Stoof JC, Kebabian JW (1984): Two dopamine receptors: biochemistry, physiology and pharmacology (minireview). *Life Sci* 35:2281–2296.

Thorburn CW, Sowton E (1973): The hemodynamic effect of metoclopramide. *Postgrad Med J* 49(suppl):22–24.

Yukimura T, Unger T, Rascher W, Lang RE, Ganten D (1981): Central peptidergic stimulation in blood pressure control, role of enkephalins in rats. *Clin Sci* 61:347s–350s.

Volavka J, Cho D, Mallaya A, Bauman J (1979): Naloxone increases ACTH and cortisol levels in man. *N Engl J Med* 300:1056–1057.

Weihe E, Nohr D, Millan MJ, et al. (1988): Peptide neuroanatomy of adjuvant-induced arthritic inflammation in rat. *Agents Actions* 25:255–260.

Worth DP, Harvey JN, Brown MJ, Lee MR (1985): Gludopa (g-l-glutamyl-l-DOPA) is a dopamine prodrug, relatively specific for the kidney in normal subjects. *Clin Sci* 69:207–214.

# Index